# Anxiety Disorders - The New Achievements

*Edited by Vladimir V. Kalinin,*
*Cicek Hocaoglu and Shafizan Mohamed*

Published in London, United Kingdom

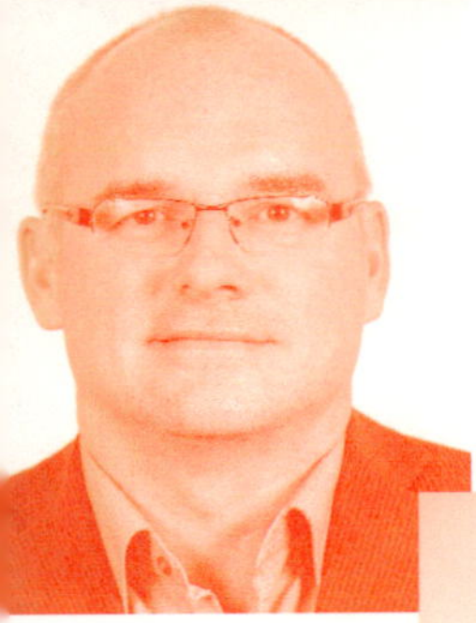
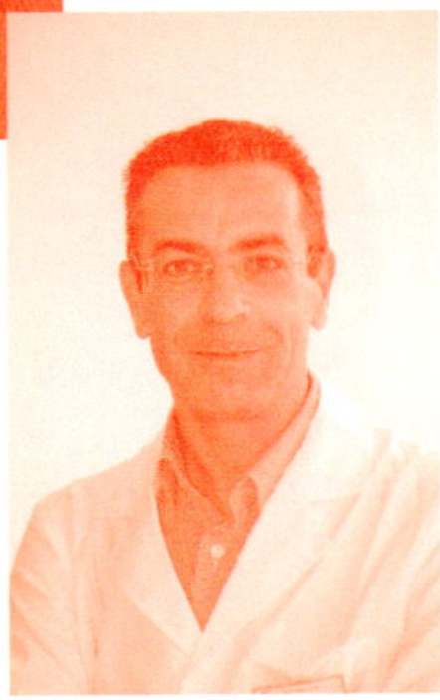
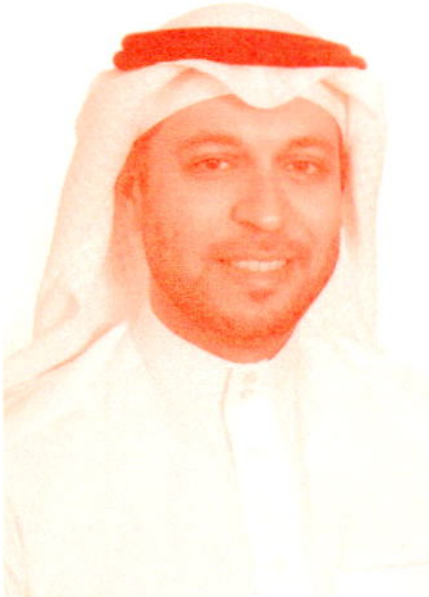
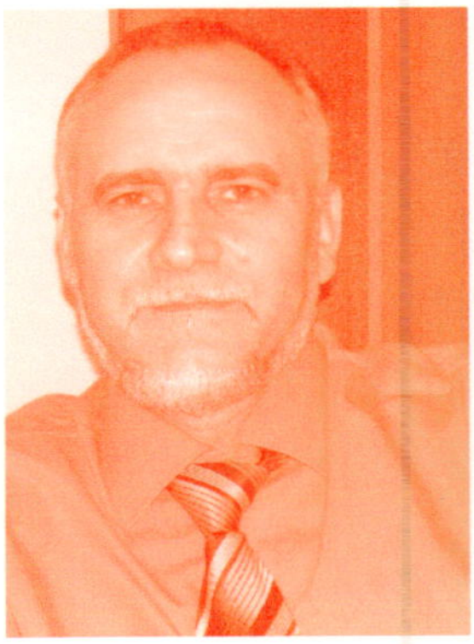
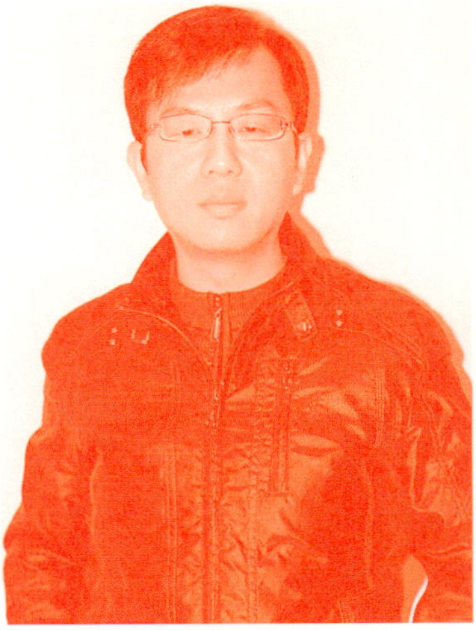
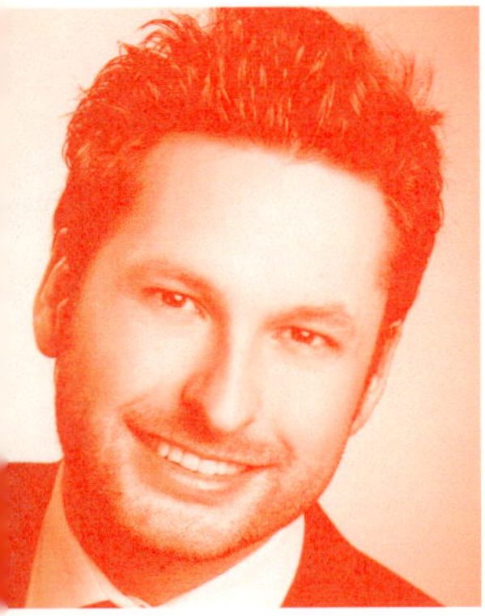
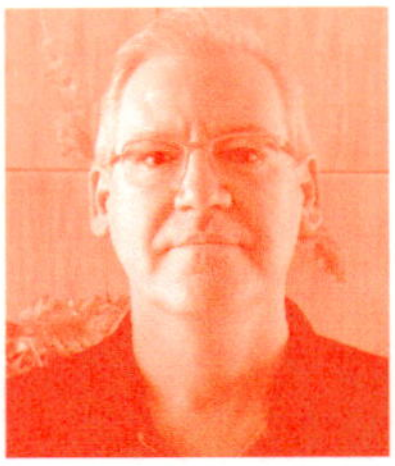

IntechOpen

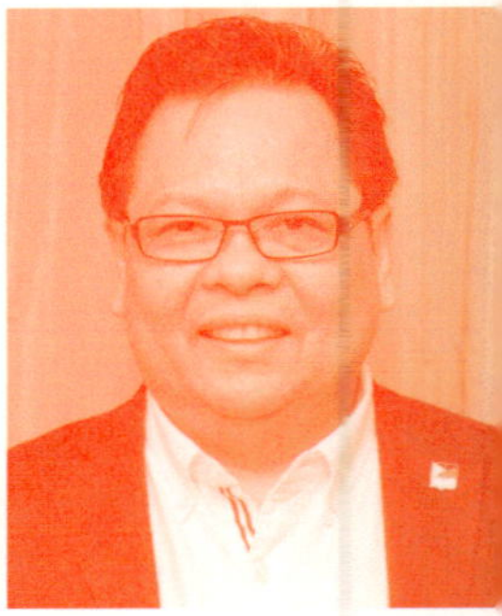
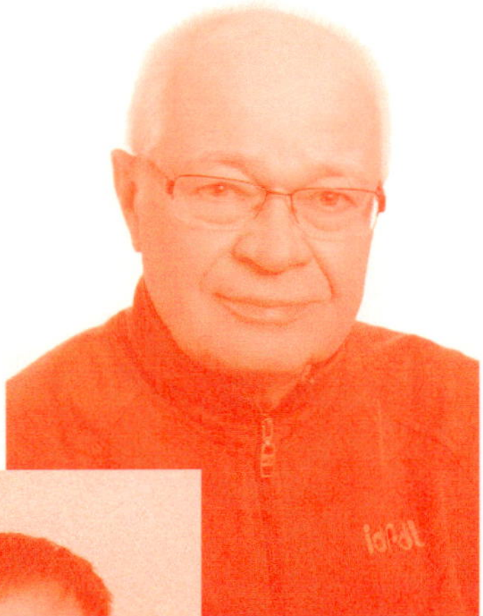
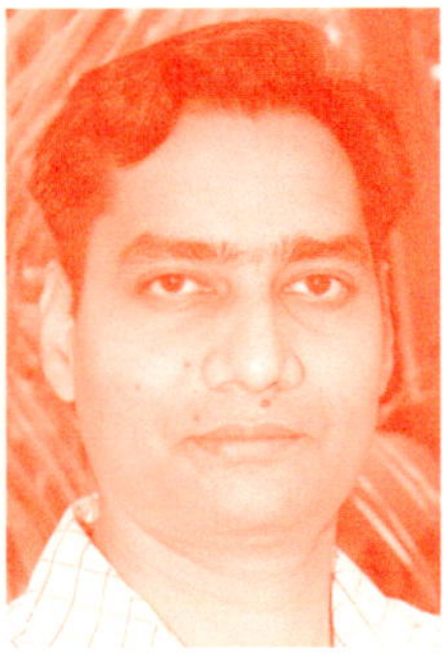
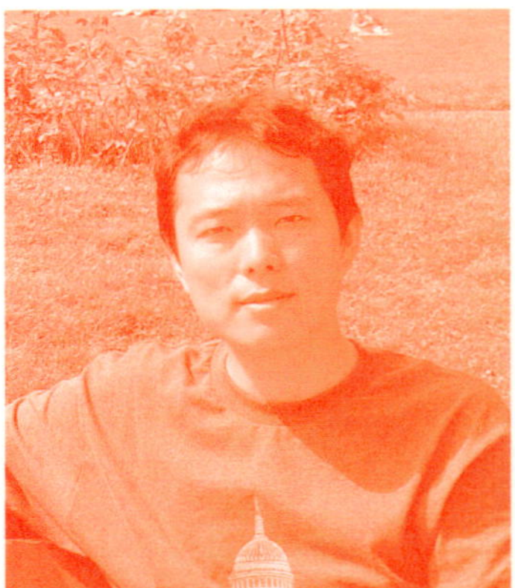
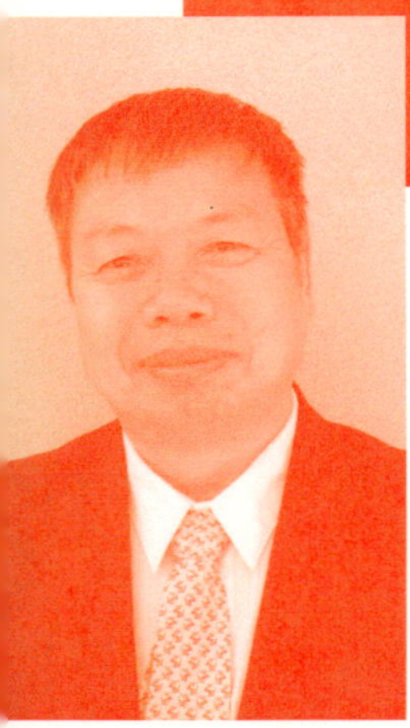
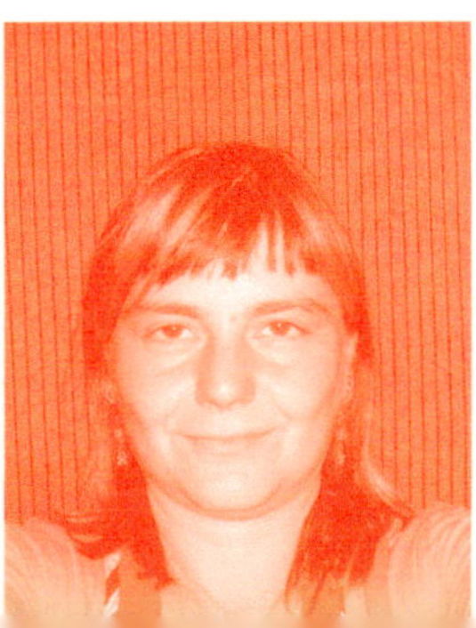

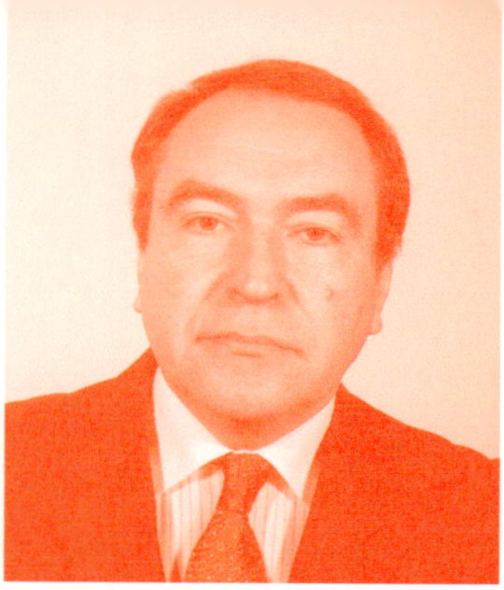
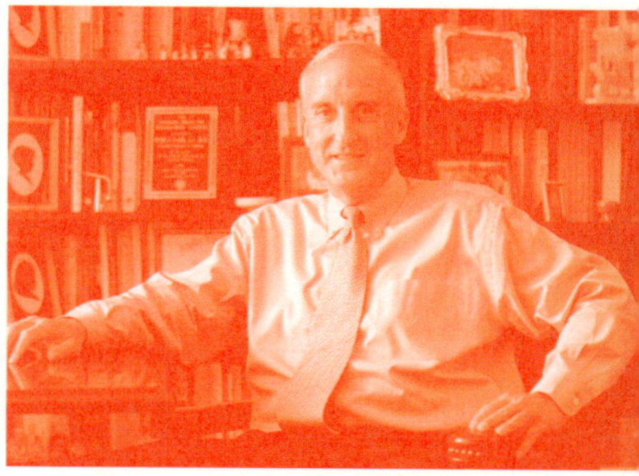
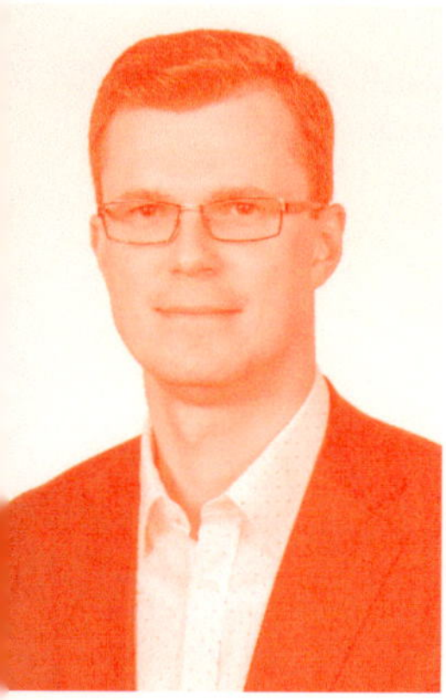
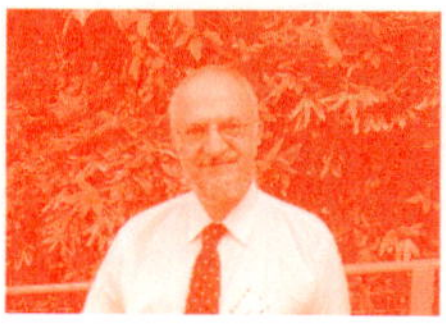
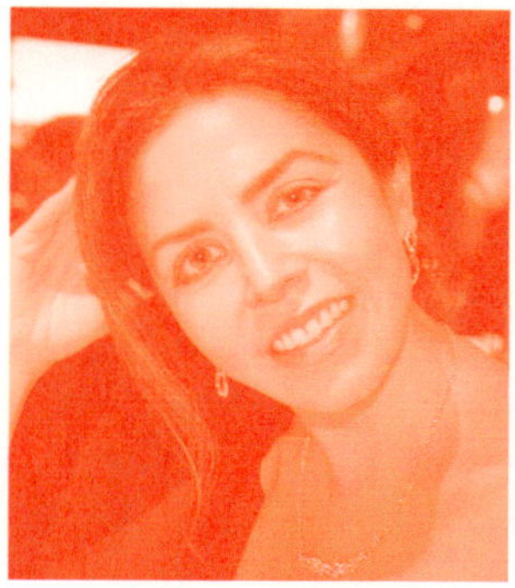

*Supporting open minds since 2005*

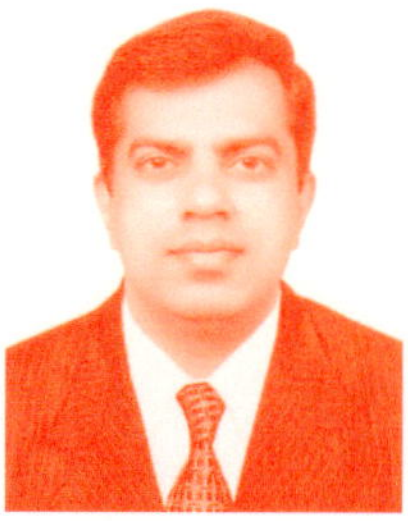
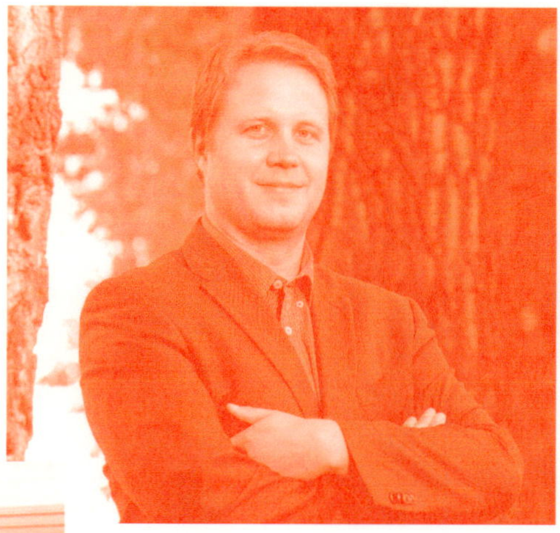
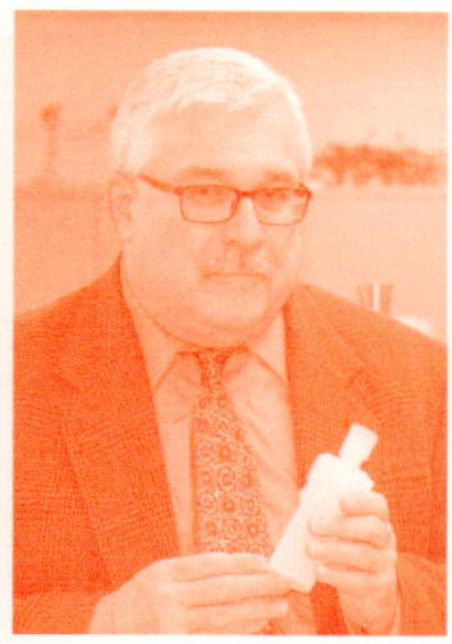
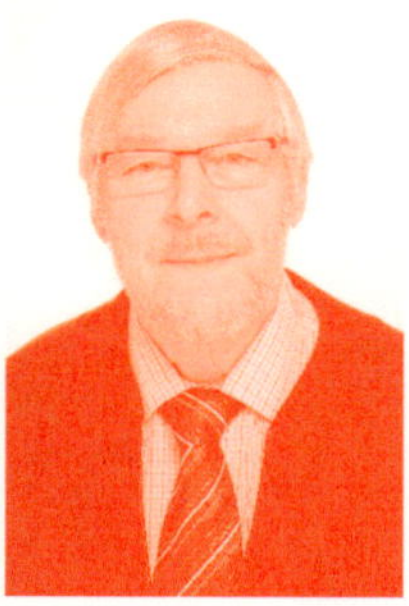
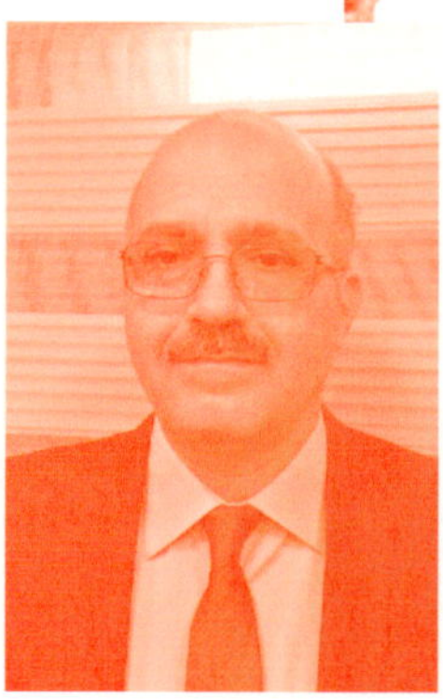
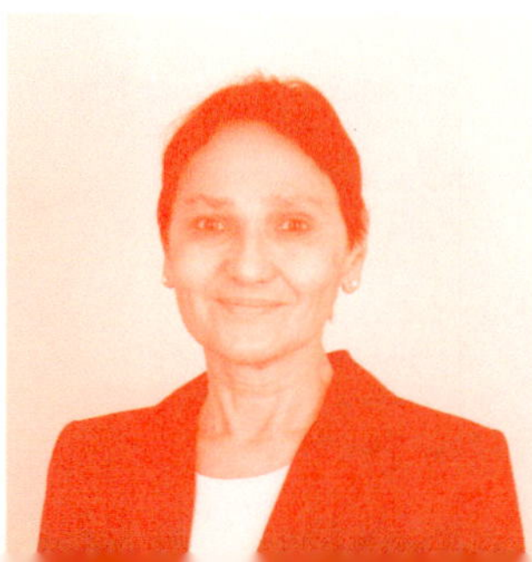
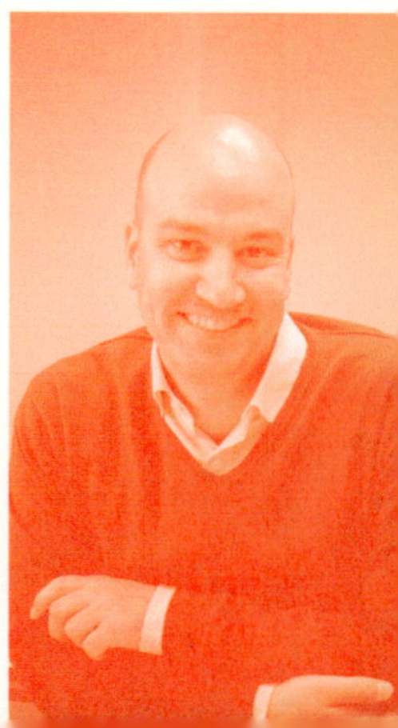

Anxiety Disorders - The New Achievements
http://dx.doi.org/10.5772/intechopen.87325
Edited by Vladimir V. Kalinin, Cicek Hocaoglu and Shafizan Mohamed

Contributors
Timothy Oblad, Olawunmi Olagundoye, Olalekan Popoola, Morenike Alugo, Tulika Ghosh, Minkesh Chowdwary, Cicek Hocaoglu, Aslı Enzel Koc, Sergio De Figueiredo Rocha, Nabila Y. AlKandari, Rubaba Azim, Victoria Fateeva, Kristina Konstantinovna Khacheva, Alexey Glazunov, Khakimova Gulnara Rinatovna, Hülya Kök Eren, Elena Gromova, Valery Gafarov, Igor V. Gagulin, Almira V. Gafarova, Vladimir N. Maksimov, Kumiko Muramatsu, Hitoshi Miyaoka, Kunitoshi Kamijima, Yoshiyuki Muramatsu, Katuya Fuse, Fumitoshi Yoshimine, Ichiro Mashima, Yutaka Tanaka, Michio Hosaka, Kikuchi Toshiaki, Natsue Shimizu, Baba Shigeji, Vladimir V. Kalinin, Kirill Y. Subbotin, Natalia G. Yermakova, Anna A. Zemlyanaya, Lyudmila V. Sokolova



First published in London, United Kingdom, 2021 by IntechOpen
IntechOpen is the global imprint of INTECHOPEN LIMITED, registered in England and Wales, registration number: 11086078, 5 Princes Gate Court, London, SW7 2QJ, United Kingdom
Printed in Croatia

British Library Cataloguing-in-Publication Data
A catalogue record for this book is available from the British Library

Additional hard and PDF copies can be obtained from orders@intechopen.com

Anxiety Disorders - The New Achievements
Edited by Vladimir V. Kalinin, Cicek Hocaoglu and Shafizan Mohamed
p. cm.
Print ISBN 978-1-83968-428-9
Online ISBN 978-1-83968-429-6
eBook (PDF) ISBN 978-1-83968-430-2

For EU product safety concerns:
IN TECH d.o.o., Prolaz Marije Krucifikse Kozulić 3, 51000 Rijeka, Croatia, info@intechopen.com or visit our website at intechopen.com.

# Meet the editors

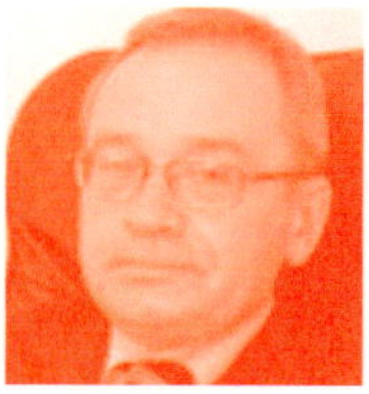

Vladimir V. Kalinin was born in1952 into a family of physicians in Orenburg (Russian Federation). He obtained an MD from Moscow State Medical Stomatological University in 1976. In 1976-1977 he completed an internship in Psychiatry. In 1978 he became a scientific researcher at Moscow Research Institute of Psychiatry of Ministry of Health and Social Development where he is currently the department head. His scientific interests concern a broad range of psychiatry problems. The topic of his doctoral thesis in 1996 was the psychopathology and therapy of anxiety disorders with an emphasis on panic disorder. Prof. Kalinin has authored 222 publications, including research articles in professional journals (in Russian and English), three monographs in Russian, and three monographs in English.

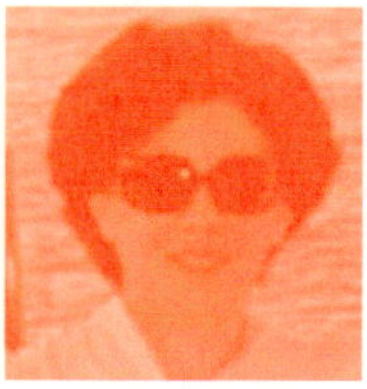

Cicek Hocaoglu obtained her medical degree from Uludag University Faculty of Medicine, Bursa, Turkey. She received postgraduate training in psychiatry at the Medical School of Karadeniz Technical University, Trabzon, Turkey. She is currently Professor and Head of the Department of Psychiatry at the Recep Tayyip Erdogan University Medical School, Rize, Turkey. She has many published national/international scientific articles, book chapters, and papers presented in congresses. Her interests include consultation-liaison psychiatry, suicide, schizophrenia, anxiety disorders, bipolar disorder, and psychopharmacology.

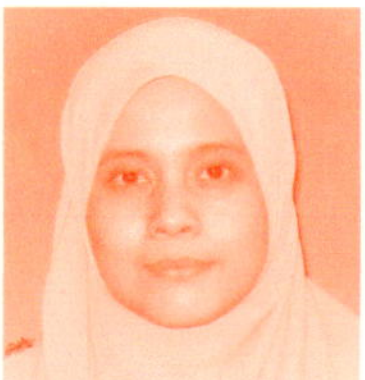

Shafizan Mohamed is an assistant professor in the Communications Department, International Islamic University of Malaysia. She holds a Ph.D. in Media Studies from Monash University, Australia. She is the author, co-author, and editor of several books, journal articles, monographs, and newspaper articles on media and communication. Her research covers the fields of new media theory, political communication, health communication, and digital media literacy. Her two recent research projects examined the digital media skills of underprivileged children and the communication of vaccination in mainstream and social media. Both studies are based on the experience of Malaysia. Aside from teaching and research, Dr. Mohamed loves food, music, and interior design.

# Contents

# Preface

Anxiety seems to be a widespread and universal phenomenon. It includes protective properties against possible future threats and additionally may cause severe psychopathological experiences disturbing an individual's everyday life.

All anxiety symptoms are divided into the subjective and the objective. The first group includes psychologically unpleasant experiences such as fear, emotional worries, feelings of threat, fear of dying, and other similar symptoms. The second group represents somatic complaints, including heart palpitations, dizziness, vertigo, tremor, hyperventilation, breathlessness, and headache. All these symptoms should be considered when treating anxiety and may require different therapeutic approaches.

At present, several so-called independent anxiety disorders exist, and each one is thought to have its own psychopathological structure and pathogenesis. Nevertheless, the level of our knowledge is not sufficient to explain the mechanisms of anxiety's origin in each concrete case. This book is an attempt at clarification.

This book is organized into three sections containing chapters related to multifarious problems of anxiety. In the first section, chapters are related to various social aspects of anxiety. The second section includes data on clinical aspects of anxiety and some other psychopathological syndromes in which anxiety may be evident. It also presents the psychopathology of Capgras syndrome and de Clerambault's syndrome. The third section includes chapters related to neurobiological data and the pathogenesis of anxiety disorders. The section also presents results of immunological and neurochemical studies of some anxiety states.

This book is intended for neurologists, psychiatrists. and physicians interested in anxiety.

**Vladimir V. Kalinin MD, Ph.D.**
Professor,
Department of Brain Organic Disorders and Epilepsy,
Moscow Research Institute of Psychiatry—The Branch of Serbsky's National Center of Psychiatry and Narcology of Ministry of Health of Russian Federation,
Russia

**Cicek Hocaoglu**
Recep Tayyip Erdoğan University,
Turkey

**Shafizan Mohamed**
International Islamic University Malaysia,
Malaysia

## Section 1

# The Social Aspects of Anxiety

Chapter 1

# Social Media and Suicide

*Olalekan Popoola, Olawunmi Olagundoye and Morenike Alugo*

## Abstract

Today, online social media are as ubiquitous as they are inextricable, especially as they have become critical to every aspect of our everyday lives. In the face of this upsurge in social media use, particularly in the adolescent age-group, rates of suicide, attempted suicide, and deliberate self-harm have spiked. This chapter aims to elucidate on current-day definitions of these terminologies as well as their epidemiology regionally and globally. Furthermore, it explores any established causality as well as possible associations and contributory factors such as cyberbullying and substance abuse. The chapter also explores how trending issues such as celebrity suicide and suicide reporting have impacted on the prevalence of suicide and examines its comorbidities. Novel concepts such as the Werther and Papageno effect are highlighted. It explicates on present-day recommendations to curb this menace while also examining the possibilities and merits of using social media as a prohibitive and rehabilitative tool against suicidal behavior.

**Keywords:** social media, suicide, mental health, suicidal ideation, suicide prevention, suicidal behavior

## 1. Introduction

Over the past decade, suicide has gained prominence across all social groups as the world experienced a significant change in lifestyle with the rise in technological advancement. There is a significant change in the way humans connect and the way information is being shared. The advent of social media has sparked the popularization of certain terms and it serves as a go-to place for firsthand information on happenings all over the world. These come with a need for equilibrium in other to avert the dire consequences it poses on mental health and wellbeing. Unfortunately, social media usage has popularized the act of suicide both directly and indirectly, from its means of information sharing to the influence and consequences it has on emotional health. Social media have indeed resulted in an upsurge of suicide risk factors and suicide-related behaviors.

This chapter elucidates the existing affiliation between social media use and suicide. It also showcases the connection between social media and suicide on one hand and the potential of social media as a positive tool for wellbeing on the other hand.

### 1.1 Social media, its use and popularity today

In a world where there is a constant need to enhance communication and connect with people, it is only inevitable for humans to find means of easing the process. The fact that man is a social being who does not exist in isolation spells out the importance of Communication to human survival. With the dawn of the information age, the internet era birthed a resolution to this dire human need of communication. The twentieth century experienced a surge in technological advancement, and this heralded the more sophisticated means of information sharing via social media. Social media are a platform or are platforms that make it possible to connect with other people all over the world by enabling communication through the sharing of content and information via a computer, a website or an application. The different platforms can be categorized base on the type of content being shared and the mode of sharing. There are now social networking sites like Facebook, Instagram, Twitter, Myspace, Snapchat, WhatsApp which provides an avenue for people all over the world to connect, communicate and share various contents in forms of pictures, videos, voice recordings, events, podcasts, web links and more. With this, people can share their day to day activities with family and friends. Although there is now a wide range of online activities that help ease work and day to day living, social media top the list as being the most popular online activity. From estimated statistics, the year 2018 revealed 2.65 billion constantly using social media worldwide. This statistic is also projected to increase to an estimate of 3.2 billion people constantly using social media in the year 2021 [1]. In Nigeria alone, 2018 statistics revealed an estimate of 29.3 million social network users which is projected to increase to an estimate of 36.8 million users in the year 2023 [1].

Social networking platforms now facilitates the ability to detect the happenings in the life of others even without reaching out, people are able to project the type of lives they so desire to be displayed for others to see even when it is dissimilar to reality. There is now the possibility of having a social media life where people's decisions are constantly being influenced by the activities of others. With these possibilities, come various gains as well as losses. Social media platforms are also a great source of news, information, entertainment, products, as well as tools for learning. Blogging websites, business directory, E-commerce website, informational websites, online communities and more are such veritable avenues for learning and obtaining information that people no longer have to physically present themselves in an educational setting in other to acquire skills. With the advent of such a video site as YouTube, there is now growing confidence in the opinion that anything can be learnt online. The advent of the internet and social media has indeed made life fluid. E-learning, E-commerce, E-banking, E-governance has changed the face of the world as it becomes more sophisticated and advanced. Social media have impacted the lifestyle of many from the way we develop social skills, relate to our loved ones, discover self and choose a career to the way we do business. There has been a significant shift and especially for the younger generation who are found to be the most avid users of social media.

A crucial point to note is the pitfalls which accompany the use of social media, it comes with experiences such as loss in concentration/motivation, comparison, lower grades, poor effects on physical and mental health, reduced social skills in real human contact, time wastage, wrong influences, quick access to vulgar information, internet Freud, cyberbullying and many more negativities. There is a prevailing irony with social media usage; could it be that the same medium which was created to ease social behavior might be the one destroying it? These evident factors demand that we get a full understanding of all precipitating and perpetuating factors of behavioral change due to social media usage, to find ways that balance can be attained. Indeed, social media are here to stay, hence; it is only important that humans establish means to unravel and unhinge its downsides.

## 2. Suicide and suicide-related behavior

Suicide is a calamitous act that calls to take antecedence as a major global health concern. It is simply the act of an individual ending his/her own life intentionally. According to other definitions, Suicide is defined as a death caused by one engaging in injurious behaviors toward self to die as a result of the behavior [2]. It can also be defined as purposeful behavior carried out either to manage or eradicate unbearable levels of pain in one's present life circumstances [2].

### 2.1 The burden of suicide

Suicide is a leading cause of death, particularly among young people. Suicide occurs all over the world in all regions, across cultures, economic and social status and indeed all age groups. Although suicidal behaviors might differ across age groups, sex and geographic regions, no human is immune to it.

Suicide accounts for high rates of deaths in all regions of the world today. According to the WHO [3], statistics reveal close to 800,000 who take their own life every year and this estimated amount differentiates from those who attempt that act alone which sometimes can be more. Suicide is also known to occur throughout the life span with the highest occurrence happening during adolescence. Suicide is the third leading cause of death among 15-19-year-olds. In America, suicide is one of the 10 leading causes of death overall and in persons within the age group of 10–64 years [4]. Every suicide is both an individual tragedy and a part of a public health crisis that imposes a great burden on society [5]. The burden of suicide reaches beyond the deaths themselves, extending to family, friends, and colleagues of the individuals who have died by suicide [6]. According to the Centers for Disease Control and Prevention [7] it is estimated that between six and 32 survivors (e.g. close family and friends) are personally affected by suicide mortality in terms of increased mental health risk, and this may include increased risk of suicide for the bereaved. Concomitantly, suicide results in financial burdens, costing society approximately US$44.6 billion per year in combined medical and work loss costs [7]. Thus, the prevention of suicide has become a matter of paramount public health importance globally.

### 2.2 Risk factors

Suicide is preventable as it comes with lots of warning signs that, if detected early enough, can be cured. The more common cause of suicide known to many is depression. Although this majorly leads to suicide, many other factors come to play in explaining the cause of suicide. A combination of social, psychological, environmental, biological, medical and genetic factors could result in suicide. Various studies have been carried out in assessing the risk factors for suicide. Some risk factors associated with suicide are family history of suicide and child maltreatment, family history of alcohol/substance abuse and mental illnesses particularly depression, previous attempts at suicide, impulsive and aggressive behavioral tendencies, feelings of hopelessness, isolation, loss of loved ones, job or financial difficulties, physical illness, lack of access to mental health care, abuse, local epidemics of suicide, stigma and other factors that hinders one from seeking help [8].

In a study [9] on suicide trajectories, it was revealed that although mental illnesses as depression and anxiety result in Suicidal Behaviors across the lifespan, past and present studies have revealed that other factors as impulsive aggression, conduct disorder, interpersonal conflict, antisocial behavior, and alcohol and substance abuse more prominently result in suicidal behaviors among adolescents and young adults.

### 2.3 Suicide related behavior

The suicide-related behaviors to always look out for are:

- Feelings of worthlessness and hopelessness
- Neglect of personal welfare
- Lack of interest in usual fun activities
- Irregular sleeping and eating habits
- Social withdrawal and isolation
- Overwhelmed feelings of pain
- Anxiety and irritability
- Suicidal ideation in which the individual engages with thoughts on how to end one's life
- Suicidal plan in which the individual makes plans and preparations toward ending his/her own life
- Suicidal attempt in which the individual attempts self-injurious behavior with an intent to die

Although suicide is commonplace globally, there is still an existing stigma associated with this act and with any form of mental illness in some parts of the world today. This often prevents those who are at risk from speaking up and from seeking help. A study [10] revealed that although there has been a reduction in the stigmatization of mental illnesses, suicide remains as stigmatized as ever. Many developing countries of the world today, including Nigeria, do not have meaningful statistical records of suicide and suicide-related behaviors. Because there is no proper record of deaths and their causes in most developing countries, it can be said that suicide rates are grossly underreported globally.

## 3. Social media and mental health

The relationship between social media and mental health is extant as social media are being linked to mental health problems like stress, psychological distress, anxiety and depression. In recent times, there is a rising research interest on this topic as research works carried out have established a link between mental health, lifestyle and social media. Social media have been linked to high rates of depression, anxiety and poor sleep, and research has revealed a 70% increase in depression and anxiety resulting from social media use in the past 25 years [11]. Other literatures have also described social media as being more addictive than substances like alcohol and cigarette [11]. There are now such terms as 'Facebook depression' which occurs as a result of spending so much time on Facebook and being exposed to the intensity of online activities of others that one starts to exhibit depressive symptoms. FOMO—Fear of Missing Out is another issue of mental health concern that results from the constant use of social media. It is a form of anxiety aroused by the fear that others might be having exciting and rewarding experiences from which one is missing out on. It results in the constant desire to be everywhere events are taking place, the constant need to check one's phone for the latest updates, the obsessive desire to always stay connected with what others are doing [12]. FOMO often affects both mental and physical health, and it results in the feeling of inferiority, life dissatisfaction, mood swings, low self-esteem, loneliness, increased negative feelings and depression [12].

Social media also encourage attitudes that are unhealthy to mental health such as unhealthy comparisons, jealousy, emulations, and counterfeit appearances. Most people put up only the best version of their lives on social media and with this might torture others who follow them and aspire to be like them. It has encouraged the living of fake lives just for social media presence.

The change in lifestyle that results from social media use has become an issue of concern globally due to the rising rate of mental health disorders. It has become important for people to learn proper ways of using social media to their benefit and not otherwise.

### 3.1 Social media exposure: risks and safety

Social media and its effect on suicide related behavior have now become a topic of growing concern and debate [13]. The question that results is if social media help in suicide prevention or helps in increasing suicidal behaviors. Social media and the internet, in general, have helped in the advancement of communication, social connections, and businesses, which have helped make man's life better. This being the case, in promoting suicide prevention, social media come in handy as a powerful tool, as this same platform is now evidently being associated with enhancing suicidal behaviors especially among teenagers. The risk of social media usage today is now more associated with adolescents simply because they are the more vulnerable population who are likely to be influenced. The adolescent stage is a stage of significant developmental changes where there is an increased risk of experimentation and peer emulation, teens at this stage are trying to form an identity that leads them to be more susceptible to peer pressures. With adolescence comes the tendency to engage in risky behaviors which also explains why there is a high rate of social media misuse among adolescents.

There is no doubt that adolescents have a lot to benefit from the use of social media both socially, academically and personally. It helps in enhancing communication skills and connecting with others. They can experiment with self-expression, share ideas and learn from others. It also helps in developing new interests and skills as there are basic social and technical skills important to everyday functioning that are learnt through social media use [14]. Most adolescents utilize social media as an extension of activities and relationships that take place at school; with social media, they can build on their social skills and enrich their friendships [14]. With this, it can be said that teen deprivation of social media could take its toll on their social skills and learning experiences.

Social media also serve as a useful tool to reach people in crises by providing information, guidance, and support. In present times, the internet has been employed as a tool of intervention for those facing several types of mental difficulties. With social media, online resources/information, counseling/therapy, and support groups can be easily accessed. On the downside, there is the risk of accessing vulgar, distressing and negative information that affects more vulnerable people. There are now series of contents that not only encourage risky behaviors like substance abuse, casual sex, sexting, pornography, inappropriate sexual behaviors, and suicide but also go out to attack or bully others into these behaviors.

## 4. Suicide risk factors associated with social media usage

### 4.1 Cyberbullying

This is also referred to as cyber-harassment or online bullying. It is a form of bullying or harassment that takes place online using electronic devices like mobile phones and computers and social media are the main platform often used in carrying out this act. In cyberbullying, the perpetrator harasses the victim by putting out negative, harmful and false posts, comments and contents about the victim [15]. It could also involve the perpetrator sending out private information about the victim to embarrass or humiliate the other party [15]. An eminent example is an act of cyberbullying that led to the death of a college student in 2010 called Tyler Clementi who committed suicide after a fellow student posted her private sexual encounter with another male student on social media [16]. Cyberbullicide is suicide which results from cyberbullying. Cyberbullying has led to suicide and suicidal behaviors among adolescents. Victims of cyberbullying are at a higher risk of experiencing self-harm and suicidal behaviors than those who are not [17]. Teenagers who experience any form of bullying including cyberbullying are at a higher risk of anxiety, sleep deprivation, poor academic performance, dropping out of school and depression [18]. It has been recorded that Seven in ten young people have experienced cyberbullying, with 37% of them saying they experience cyberbullying on a high-frequency basis [11]. Research [19] also revealed that students who experience any form of bullying and cyberbullying are twice more likely to attempt suicide. In a study [20], 33.8% of students reported that they have been cyberbullied in their lifetime while 11.5% admitted to having cyberbullied others.

### 4.2 Body image dissatisfaction

This can be defined as the feelings and negative attitudes a person has about their body and is usually influenced by certain factors such as the cultural norms relating to an ideal body, personal perceptions toward weight gain, and body appearance [21]. In a study [22] social media were revealed to influence the attitude of young women and adolescent girls causing them to engage in social comparisons which often leads to the feeling of inadequacy and body dissatisfaction. Concerns with body image lead people to depression and suicidal thoughts. Body image dissatisfaction occurs in both male and female although it tends to be more common in females, both genders are exposed to images online which they tend to fix as their perfect and ideal body. The activities and images portrayed by celebrities and social media influencers play a huge role in shaping standards for young people as they strive to emulate their admirers online.

Body image dissatisfaction often results in feelings of low self-esteem, depression, low body confidence, eating disorders. Results from a study revealed a link between suicide ideation and how both male and female adolescents perceive their body image [23].

### 4.3 Substance abuse

The link between social media use and substance abuse cannot be overlooked as social media are not only capable of pressuring one to use substances but also provide a platform that eases the process of accessing hard drugs. Drug dealers now use social media to connect with their buyers all over the world which makes it easy to purchase hard drugs online. Adolescents through social media are being constantly exposed to the popularity of drug use, it has become commonplace to see celebrities display their use of hard drugs online [24]. The behavior of celebrities and social media influencers who glamorize and normalize the abuse of substances on social media goes a long way in influencing the attitude of adolescents who follow them [24]. Most adolescent engages in comparison with such social media influencers and by these, they begin to lose their values as they seek to emulate the popular behaviors they perceive online. Such social comparison could lead to depressive symptoms and other mental health difficulties which could in turn fuel the abuse of substances. The view that friends and fans on social media are having fun with their lifestyle can tempt adolescents into risky behaviors just to fit in. All these experiences are detrimental to mental health and can increase suicide risk.

### 4.4 Suicide contagion

This is a possible increase in suicide or suicide-related behaviors that results from exposure to information on suicide-related behaviors and actual suicide occurrences within one's immediate group. This form of information is often passed across through social media and can become popular within a very short time. The term 'Werther effect' explains a case of suicide that occurs as a result of a person copying cases of suicidal behaviors seen or heard of from various online platforms. Werther effect also referred to as copycat suicide and it explains the process of suicide contagion [16]. A person who has prior suicidal thoughts but is unable to carry out the act for several contingent issues of concern can suddenly become motivated to carry out the act after learning of another's case of suicide on media. The term 'Werther' was derived from a book written by Johann Wolfgang von Goethe titled 'The Sorrows of Young Werther', in which the principal character in the book named Werther, ends his own life by shooting himself at his desk [25]. After the book was published, several suicide cases were recorded with similar methods to the suicide case described in the book. This made it evident that the suicide cases that followed were influenced by that of Werther's character in the novel. Reporting of suicide cases especially celebrity suicide has popularized the incidence of suicide among the general public and it has now become very crucial that guidelines be adhered to, to reduce the popularity of suicide through Werther Effect.

## 5. Suicide prevention via social media usage

As has been reiterated severally, and with good reason, Social media have changed the world as we have come to know it, and this includes the mental health of the populace. The potential detrimental, stressor and suicidal capacity of social media use has been largely investigated and somewhat accepted. Dissimilarly, however, the potential use of online social media in suicide prevention is only in its infancy as it is only recently started accruing mainstream attention.

Logically, preventing any menace will center majorly on efforts to handicap its perpetrating factors, and in the same vein, involve an in-depth understanding of its underlying mechanism and attempting to impede it at any and several stages in its evolution.

Almost all cases of successful and failed suicidal attempts have a Diagnostic and Statistical Manual of Mental Disorders, Fourth Edition (DSM-IV) psychiatric illness. Mood disorders, principally major depressive disorder and bipolar disorder are associated with about 60% of suicides [26–28].

Consequently, any efforts at using social media to avert suicide must cater for mental health broadly; increasing its awareness, diagnosis and treatment alongside providing a means to access appropriate help.

Nowadays, in the age of the internet, young people can effortlessly access and share content across the globe in the snap of a finger using varying platforms including but not exclusive to collaborative projects (e.g. Wikipedia and social bookmarking), blogs and microblogs (e.g. Twitter), content communities (e.g. YouTube), social networking sites (e.g. Facebook, WhatsApp), virtual game and social worlds [29]. These avenues can and have been used by youth to find out about suicide and varying means of perpetrating it as well as making suicide pacts with other distressed individuals. Alas, fortunately, this provides an opportunity to find and intervene early if someone expresses suicidal intent as well as an avenue for people who have felt suicidal in the past to help persons currently feeling so.

In a small-scale internet survey administered by Robinson et al. they noted that respondents had identified social media as an avenue to provide support and equally receive help as relating to suicide, with the respondents acknowledging increased feelings of well-being by being able to help and support suicidal persons; the latter further accentuating previous reports that social media users found the ability to help therapeutic in and of itself. This beneficial reversibility of roles provided by social media is not applicable in one-on-one therapy. Another immense advantage of social media also highlighted by respondents was the potential to intervene swiftly if and when persons expressed suicidal intent online. Two previous studies cited this as a unique benefit of social media [30, 31]. One of these reports [31] described a successful intervention in a suicide attempt following the posting of a suicide note on Twitter.

A more representative and personal experience is shared by Reidenberg, the Executive director of the United States-based prevention organization Suicide Awareness Voices of Education (SAVE) [32].

Daniel Reidenberg was scanning Facebook for his suicide-prevention organization on a Friday evening in the spring of 2014 when he noticed the post of a clearly suicidal young widow who had declared the intent to take her life and that of her baby. As he had a wealth of experience working with Facebook and other digital companies on the prevention of suicide, he knew exactly what to do: he contacted Facebook's safety center. Although, there was no indication in the post of the woman's location, he knew Facebook would still be able to find her, and that they did in very few minutes. Facebook employees determined the woman had posted her message from an Internet café in a small village in South America. They contacted the local police. Holding a picture from the woman's Facebook page, police officers walked through the village. Within ten minutes of leaving the café, the police found were able to find her and get her into a hospital and get her childcare [32].

With 2 billion people using social media and 500 million people posting on Facebook alone, there is "a lot of opportunity for intervention and prevention," says Reidenberg. "It's critical that everyone starts looking at this new era with technology being involved in the field of suicide prevention. It isn't just going to a doctor's office any longer—it is that 'plus.'"

"In a few short years since some of the big social media companies began meeting periodically at Facebook's California head office in 2011 to brainstorm about what to do, the world's largest social network has rolled out a direct intervention. In 25 of the 50 American states, when a user posts a message on Facebook containing a phrase that its algorithms flag as indicating suicidal thoughts or intentions, a banner pops up on the user's page. Friends viewing the post can also click on an icon that reports the message, sending it to the Facebook safety centre to review" [32].

The automatic banner asks whether the user needs help and provides the number of the National Suicide Prevention Lifeline. Facebook then contacts the user and offers to connect him or her to the distress line. The message includes tips and links to support videos aligned with best prevention practices. Facebook may also freeze the user's page until the person in distress has interacted with the support applications. The program is billed to be expanded to the entire country and is even said to piloted in some undisclosed countries [32].

A psychiatrist has said that Facebook's program raises a 'thorny' issue as users can post content they don't intend to act on. Reidenberg acknowledged that companies are wrestling with the privacy issue, but he reminded the audience at the International Association for Suicide Prevention's annual conference in Montréal, Quebec, that once someone posts anything on a social media site—even if it's personal health information—it is no longer private [32].

## 6. Novel approaches to suicide prevention

Current efforts at suicide prevention center largely on reducing suicidal desire among individuals hospitalized for suicidality or being treated for related psychopathology. Such efforts have yielded evidence-based treatments, and yet the national suicide rate has continued to climb [33]. The contrast between the robust evidence base for several treatments and the continually increasing suicide rate points toward a vital disconnect between the primary problem and the tools we are using to address it [33].

Rightly so, new frontiers and novel approaches to suicide prevention are emerging by the day. One such compelling proposal was made by Michael et al. [33], who propose that this disconnect is heavily influenced by an unmet need to consider population-level interventions aimed at reducing the capability for suicide.

HIV death rates peaked in 1965, necessitating the need for national-level intervention strategies. However, one that was noted to have been quite effective was the needle exchange program whose aim was to reduce needle sharing, which at the time was the main means of contracting the disease. It also provided an avenue for counseling and health education on safe sex and intravenous drug use. A similar approach was employed to drastically reduce the incidence and prevalence of lung cancer by aggressive public education, increased taxation of cigarette companies, policies limiting places where smokers could publicly smoke as well as the introduction of cigarette filters. By the same token, vehicular accidents were massively reduced by laws imposing the use of seatbelts, child passenger safety and bans on alcohol consumption whilst driving.

Drawing from these largely successful interventions that quelled major public health concerns, Michael et al. resolved that a similar population-level means restriction approach be undertaken. They postulate that achieving a position of strength as regards suicide prevention will stem from a more adept understanding of the mechanism underpinning various aspects of suicide risk. A recent meta-analysis by Franklin et al has shown no increased predictive value of the past few decades of research examining traditional risk factors of suicide. Besides, research has shown that lots of people who think about taking their own lives, never do and the great majority who do try do not die by suicide. The failure of these traditional methods has led to a new approach in suicidology, "ideation to action framework", which has heralded the various psychological theories of suicide. Foremost and oldest amongst these theories is the interpersonal theory of suicide.

The interpersonal theory of suicide (ITS) [34] posits that individuals are at greatest risk of suicide ideation when they feel a sense of burdensomeness to others, lack a sense of belonging, and feel hopeless that these states will change. Although, the ability to make a suicidal attempt is acquired through exposure to painful and provocative events, such as experiences that heighten individuals' pain tolerance and fearlessness about death. Examples of such painful and provocative events include starvation [35], risky illegal behaviors [36], and combat [37]. Additionally, research has indicated that genetic factors may influence individuals' capability for suicide [38]. Conclusively, both suicidal ideation and suicidal capacity must be present for suicidal behavior to ensue [33]. O'Connor's Integrated Motivational–Volitional Model of Suicidal Behavior (IMV) [39] is another suicidal theory influenced by the ITS. Both the IMV and ITS have been empirically tested and supported [40]. Klonsky and May [41] have proposed and empirically tested the most recent of theory within the ideation to action framework, the Three-Step Theory (3ST).

All three theories posit that suicidal intent and suicidal capacity must be present for suicide to ensue. Although defined somewhat differently across each theory, they posit that for a suicidal or lethal attempt to occur, suicidal capacity must be in play. It is important to note that capacity is not in and of itself pathological, in actual fact it is beneficial and can be adaptive in the right circumstances. For instance, increased comfort with blood would prove beneficial to emergency doctors and nurses, likewise, an increased fearlessness of death would enable soldiers to complete a dangerous mission. However, in conditions where persons with an elevated capacity for suicide also experience danger and an increased suicidal desire, the odds for a fatal suicidal attempt increase substantially. Consequently, this offers a promising opportunity for the development of broader-scale national level preventive interventions that target suicidal capacity, even in individuals who deny suicidal thoughts. The most prominent example of such approaches currently in practice, albeit sporadically, is means safety [33]. Novel as this may seem, it's actually an age long, veritably tested and acknowledged measure as evinced by the significant reduction in suicide rates following reduced packaging and access to drugs known to be lethal in high doses, restriction of access to suicide hotspots (bridge barriers), detoxification of gas, ban on popular insecticides frequently used to execute suicide. This effect was witnessed in 2006 in Israel as the Israeli defense Force prevented soldiers from taking their firearms home over the weekend having noted that firearm suicide was high over weekends. As much as a 40% reduction was noted in suicide rates amongst soldiers aged 18–21 following the intervention. Literature, scientific and historical, is fraught with successful campaigns of means restriction/safety. Decreased access to and safe use/storage of lethal means might represent an opportunity to address an important aspect of the capability for suicide without diminishing the ability of individuals to succeed in their chosen professions and environments [33].

A reasonable concern among individuals first hearing about means safety is the possibility that limiting access to one specific method for suicide will simply result in individuals dying by another method. Importantly, this argument has been largely refuted by available research [33]. In his review of means restriction and means substitution research, Daigle [42] found little evidence in favor of means substitution, Similarly, Sarchiapone et al. [43] also examined the effect of broad-scale means safety efforts and found that means substitution was uncommon across a variety of methods.

The overwhelming evidence for means restriction and safety, as a means of suicide prevention, lends credence to the recommendation that it be promulgated into law. Whilst a few countries have passed laws and regulations encouraging means restriction, most are yet to. Social media advocacy can be a veritable tool to ensure legislation of means restriction and safety globally, public education on the importance of the subject matter and ultimately shift public perception and cultural views on means safety.

Another budding and promising endeavor for the cause of suicide prevention, presented by recent advancements in science and technology, is 'big data'. Generally, big data is high-volume, high-velocity and high-variety data usually in its raw inedited format and coming from diverse sources. This large data set potentially offers scientists and researchers alike, the access to an unprecedented sample size to experiment and test hypothesis and published data. More so, analytics of text, images, videos, audio and social media information can be used to extract information, patterns, relationships and diversities which can in turn be used to predict suicide risk in varying demographics the world over. Additionally, this may also impel the development of online and app-based interventions to extend even to persons who are unawares of their suicidal capacity. One such app is Therapeutic Evaluative Conditioning, TEC, which aims to alter an individual's association with suicidal behavior. Although, caution has been advised with its use, it exemplifies the burgeoning opportunities the use of big-data will afford the world in preventing suicide.

## 7. The way forward-striking a balance between the risks associated with social media use and its capacity and potential use in suicide prevention

The media are a something of a double-edged sword as concerning its effect on mental health and suicide, making its use in suicide prevention fraught with a lot of danger; hence, caution must be exercised in this undertaking. Albeit, this chapter is replete with means by which the internet can be used to prevent suicide, it can also exacerbate suicide risk by glamorizing suicide or promoting it as a solution to life's problems. As elucidated by Pirkis and Blood [44, 45] and Gould [46], the latter could encourage distressed and suicidal individuals to actually attempt suicide or be drawn to suicide hot spots portrayed in various media. The Internet is of increasing concern, particularly the effects of suicide chat rooms, the provision of instruction in methods for suicide, and the active solicitation of suicide-pact partners [47]. Media blackouts on reporting suicide have coincided with decreases in suicide rates [48]. A 1987 campaign [49] to decrease media coverage of subway suicides in Austria cut subway suicides by 80%. This only goes to show how vital the education of journalists and reporters is, as well as the regulation of suicide reporting. The American Foundation for Suicide Prevention [50] and Annenberg Public Policy Center, and The Centers for Disease Control and Prevention [51] in the United States have produced guidelines for the responsible reporting of suicide; however, no published studies have evaluated their impact [47].

Additionally, in an online survey by Robinson et al. [29], most organizations that facilitated user-user interaction via their social media sites had trained moderators in situ; however, few had clear safety protocols or a code of ethics underpinning their work. The need for clear protocols and ethical standards for suicide prevention activities using social media platforms has been emphasized before [52]. The subsequent implementation of these guidelines will be an important step toward enhancing the safe delivery of suicide prevention initiatives using the internet [29].

Robinson et al. [29] identified the need for more interventional studies for persons at risk of suicide, and bereaved due to suicide; they also noted the need for additional research investigating the safety and ethics of delivering interventions via social media.

The unstructured, formless and anonymous nature of social media has constituted not only systematic but also ethical challenges for researchers and other stake holders looking to use social media to curb suicide. It has therefore become something of a necessity that if this endeavor were to be successful, the development of methodologies that can be rigorously and aptly applied to researches that utilize social media as a platform has become imperative. In the same vein, service-related guidelines that will ensure the acceptability, utility, efficacy, and ethical standards of social media-based suicide prevention services must be formulated. In doing this, researchers must work more closely with agencies and organizations involved in using social media for suicide prevention to ensure the practical applicability of these guidelines as well as their implementation.

### 7.1 Media reporting and guidelines

Locally and internationally, researchers have shown that detailed and sensationalized reporting of suicide is associated with suicidal behavior especially in persons in the same sex-age demographics as the deceased even after accounting for reporting and methodological and reporting bias.

Following the release of JW Von Goethe's novel 'The Sorrows of Jung Werther', imitative suicides of young men across European countries were identified leading to the coining of the term 'The Werther effect'. Similarly, there was an increase of about 12% in suicide rates after the suicidal death of famous American model and actress, Marilyn Monroe. Numerous studies have shown that the copycat and imitation effects of media reporting are primarily found for vulnerable people, such as people with depression and those who have engaged in self-harm [53].

The provision and compliance with media reporting guidelines have heralded applaudable impact with reduction in suicide rates and use of lethal weapons. However, Bohanna and Wang report that media guidelines can be effective only when 'accompanied by media endorsement, active dissemination strategies and ongoing training and monitoring' [54].

## 8. Conclusion

The internet has heralded an age of global interconnection via social media and this wave of modernization has become ingrained in almost all human endeavors leaving an indelible mark of positives as well as negatives on the very fabric of society. In this time, suicide and suicidal behavior have snowballed especially amongst young people, the most avid social media users.

This chapter is replete with empirical evidence to disprove any coincidentally in this simultaneous pattern of events as well as establish that social media usage is associated with mental health problems such as anxiety, depression, etc. Phenomena such as cyber-bullying, body image dissatisfaction, substance abuse, suicide contagion and celebrity suicide that are caused or promoted by social media are contributory to self-harming and suicidal behavior.

We have examined the existing channels of suicide prevention via social media as well as the potential and novel avenues it presents for the prevention of suicide and suicidal behavior. Emphasis was placed on the use of 'big data' and appropriate reporting of suicide following laid down guidelines. A major talking point was the adoption of a new approach to exploring the mechanism of suicide and reducing the capacity for it.

Future priorities identified included more inquiry and research into the safety and ethics of delivering suicide prevention interventions online whilst developing and enforcing service-related guidelines. Additionally, legislative enforcement and media endorsement of suicide reporting guidelines should be acidly pursued.

**Author details**

Olalekan Popoola[1], Olawunmi Olagundoye[2]* and Morenike Alugo[3]

1 National Primary Healthcare Development Agency, Abuja, Nigeria

2 Lagos State Health Service Commission, General Hospital Lagos, Nigeria

3 Psychology Department, University of Lagos, Nigeria

*Address all correspondence to: olabima@yahoo.com

## References


[1] Clement J. Statista. Number of social network users worldwide from 2010 to 2021. 2019. Available from: https://www.statista.com/statistics/278414/number-of-worldwide-social-network-users/

[2] Nero RL. The link between social media and suicide. In: Hope and Healing Center Seminar Series. 2015. Available from: https://hopeandhealingcenter.org/wp-content/uploads/2015/10/The-Link-between-Social-Media-and-Suicide1.pdf

[3] World Health Organization (WHO). Suicide. 2019. Available from: https://www.who.int/news-room/fact-sheets/detail/suicide

[4] Centers for Disease Control and Prevention. Increase in suicide in the United States, 1999-2014. 2016. Available from: http://www.cdc.gov/nchs/products/databriefs/db241.htm#ref4

[5] World Health Organization. Suicide: Factsheet. 2014. Available from: http://www.who.int/mediacentre/factsheets/fs398/en/ [Accessed: 8 June 2015]

[6] National Action Alliance for Suicide Prevention. A prioritized research agenda for suicide prevention: An action plan to save lives. 2014. Available from: http://actionallianceforsuicideprevention.org/sites/actionallianceforsuicideprevention.org/files/Agenda

[7] Centers for Disease Control and Prevention. Suicide: Consequences. 2015. Available from: http://www.cdc.gov/violenceprevention/suicide/consequences.html [Accessed: 2 June 2015]

[8] National Center for Injury Prevention and Control, Division of Violence Prevention. Risk and protective factors. 2019. Available from: https://www.cdc.gov/violenceprevention/suicide/riskprotectivefactors.html

[9] Seguin M, Beauchamp G, Robert M, DiMambro M, Turecki G. Developmental model of suicide trajectories. The British Journal of Psychiatry. 2014;**205**(2):120-126

[10] Sudak H, Maxim K, Carpenter M. Suicide and stigma: A review of the literature and personal reflections. Academic Psychiatry. 2008;**32**:136

[11] Royal Society for Public Health (RSPH). Status of Mind, Social Media and Young People's Mental Health and Wellbeing. London: Royal Society for Public Health; 2017

[12] Berla N. How FOMO is affecting your mental health and needs to be addressed. The Economic Times. 2018. Available from: https://economictimes.indiatimes.com/magazines/panache/between-the-lines/fomo/articleshow/62550811.cms

[13] Fiedorowicz JG, Chigurupati RB. The internet in suicide prevention and promotion. In: Sher L, Valens A, editors. Internet, and Suicide. New York: Nova Science Publishers; 2009. pp. 1-12

[14] Mir E, Novas C. Social Media and Adolescents' and Young Adults' Mental Health. Washington, DC: National Center for Health Research; 2020. Available from: http://www.center4research.org/social-media-affects-mental-health/

[15] Stopbullying.Gov. What is Cyberbullying? Washington, DC: Stopbullying.Gov; 2019. Available from: https://www.stopbullying.gov/cyberbullying/what-is-it

[16] Ortiz P. The werther effect: Suicide contagion and the media. Washington Psychiatirst. 2017;**6**(3):5-7. Available

from: https://cdn.coverstand.com/26559/440251/91d8b446e304b90e028b75c863a116871c0efe7b.2.pdf

[17] John A, Glendenning AC, Marchant A, Montgomery P, Stewart A, Wood S, et al. Self-Harm, suicidal behaviours, and cyberbullying in children and young people: Systematic review. Journal of Medical Internet Research. 2018;**20**(4):e129

[18] Centers for Disease Control and Prevention. Youth risk behavior surveillance—United States, 2017. Morbidity and Mortality Weekly Report—Surveillance Summaries. 2018;**67**(SS08). Available from: https://www.cdc.gov/healthyyouth/data/yrbs/pdf/2017/ss6708.pdf

[19] Hinduja S, Patchin J. Connecting adolescent suicide to the severity of bullying and cyberbullying. Journal of School Violence. 2018;**18**:1-14. DOI: 10.1080/15388220.2018.1492417

[20] Hinduja S, Patchin JW. Cyberbullying fact sheet: Identification, prevention, and response. Cyberbullying Research Center. 2019. Available from: https://cyberbullying.org/Cyberbullying-Identification-Prevention-Response-2019.pdf

[21] Phillips N, De Man AF. Weight status and body image satisfaction in adult men and women. North American Journal of Psychology. 2010;**12**(1):171-183

[22] Alperstein N. Social comparison of idealized female images and the curation of self on Pinterest. The Journal of Social Media in Society. 2015;**4**:5-27

[23] Kim DS. Body image dissatisfaction as an important contributor to suicidal ideation in Korean adolescents: Gender differences and mediation of parent and peer relationships. The Journal of Psychosomatic Research. 2009;**66**(4):297-303. DOI: 10.1016/j.jpsychores.2008.08.005

[24] Hilliard J. The influence of social media on teen drug use. In: Addiction Centre. 2019. Available from: https://www.addictioncenter.com/community/social-media-teen-drug-use/

[25] Moody A. The two effects: Werther vs Papageno. PleaseLive.org. 2015. Available from: https://www.pleaselive.org/blog/2015/06/

[26] Barraclough B, Bunch J, Nelson B, Sainsbury P. One hundred cases of suicide: Clinical aspects. The British Journal of Psychiatry. 1974;**125**:355-373

[27] Bertolote JM, Fleischmann A, DeLeo D, Wasserman D. Suicide and mental disorders: Do we know enough? The British Journal of Psychiatry. 2003;**183**:382-383

[28] Isometsä E, Henriksson M, Marttunen M, et al. Mental disorders in young and middle-aged men who commit suicide. British Medical Journal. 1995;**310**:1366-1367

[29] Robinson J, Rodrigues M, Fisher S, Bailey B, Herrman H. Suicide and suicide prevention. Shanghai Archives of Psychiatry. 2015;**27**(1):27-35

[30] Greidanus E, Everall R. Helper therapy in an online suicide prevention community. British Journal of Guidance & Counselling. 2010;**38**(2):191-204 [CrossRef] [Google Scholar]

[31] Ogburn KM, Messias E, Buckley PF. New-age patient communications through social networks. General Hospital Psychiatry. 2011;**33**(2):200.e1-200.e3 [PubMed] [CrossRef] [Google Scholar]

[32] Eggertson L. Social media embraces suicide prevention. Canadian Medical Association Journal. 2015;**187**(11):E333

[33] Michael D, Anestis P, Keyne C, Law MA, Jin H, Claire BA, et al. Treating the capability for suicide: A vital and understudied Frontier in suicide prevention. Suicide and Life-Threatening Behavior. 2016;**47**(5):523-537

[34] Van Orden KA, Witte TK, Cukrowicz KC, Braithwaite SR, Selby EA, Joiner TE. The interpersonal theory of suicide. Psychological Review. 2010;**117**:575-600

[35] Selby EA, Smith AR, Bulik CM, Olmsted MP, Thornton L, Cfarlane M, et al. Habitual starvation and provocative behaviors: Two potential routes to extreme suicidal behavior in anorexia nervosa. Behavior Research and Therapy. 2010;**48**:634-645

[36] Mitchell SM, Jahn DR, Cukrowicz KC. The relation between illegal risk behaviors and the acquired capability for suicide. Crisis. 2014;**35**:368-377

[37] Bryan CJ, Cukrowicz KC, West CL, Morrow CE. Combat experience and the acquired capability for suicide. Journal of Clinical Psychology. 2010;**66**:1044-1056

[38] Smith AR, Ribeiro JD, Mikolajewski A, Taylor J, Joiner TE, IACONO WG. An examination of environmental and genetic contributions to the determinants of suicidal behavior among male twins. Psychiatry Research. 2012;**197**:60-65

[39] O'connor RC. The integrated motivational-volitional model of suicidal behavior. Crisis. 2011;**32**:295-298

[40] O'connor RC, Smyth R, Ferguson E, Ryan C, Williams JMG. Psychological processes and repeat suicidal behavior: A four-year prospective study. Journal of Consulting and Clinical Psychology. 2013;**81**:1137-1143

[41] Klonsky ED, May AM. The three-step theory (3ST): A new theory of suicide rooted in the 'ideation-to-action' framework. International Journal of Cognitive Therapy. 2015;**8**:114-129

[42] Daigle MS. Suicide prevention through means restriction: Assessing the risk of substitution. Accident Analysis and Prevention. 2005;**37**:625-632

[43] Sarchiapone M, Mandelli L, Iosue M, Andrisano C, Roy A. Controlling access to suicide means. International Journal of Environmental Research and Public Health. 2011;**8**:4550-4562

[44] Pirkis J, Blood RW. Suicide and the media, I: Reportage in nonfictional media. Crisis. 2001;**22**:146-154

[45] Pirkis J, Blood RW. Suicide and the media, II: Portrayal in fictional media. Crisis. 2001;**22**:155-162

[46] Gould MS. Suicide and the media. Annals of the New York Academy of Sciences. 2001;**932**:200-221

[47] Mann J, Apter A, Bertolote J, Beautrais A, Currier D, Haas A, et al. Suicide prevention strategies a systematic review. Journal of the American Medical Association. 2005;**294**:2064-2074

[48] Motto JA. Newspaper influence on suicide: A controlled study. Archives of General Psychiatry. 1970;**23**:143-148

[49] Etzersdorfer E, Sonneck G. Preventing suicide by influencing mass-media reporting: The Viennese experience 1980-1996. Archives of Suicide Research. 1998;**4**:67-74

[50] American Foundation for Suicide Prevention. Reporting on suicide: Recommendations for the media. 2002. Available from: http://www.afsp.org/index-1.html

[51] O'Carroll PW, Potter LB. Suicide contagion and the reporting of suicide:

Recommendations from a national workshop. MMWR Recommendations and Reports. 1994;**43**(RR-6):9-17

[52] Birbal R, Maharajh HD, Birbal R, Clapperton M, Jarvis J, Ragoonath A, et al. Cybersuicide and the adolescent population: challenges of the future. International Journal of Adolescent Medical Health. 2009;**21**(2):151-159

[53] Sisask M, Värnik A. Media roles in suicide prevention: A systematic review. International Journal of Environmental Research and Public Health. 2012;**9**(1):123-138

[54] Bohanna I, Wang X. Media guidelines for the responsible reporting of suicide: A review of effectiveness. Crisis. 2012;**33**:190-198

Chapter 2

# Mental Distress among Medical Students

*Syeda Rubaba Azim*

## Abstract

Depression, anxiety, and stress affect the mental health of an individual. Previous studies have shown high rates of depression, anxiety, and stress among medical students throughout the world. Medical students are future doctors, but mental distress among them has negative effects on their output, which ultimately affects patient care and quality of life. This chapter will discuss various reasons of mental distress among medical students and proposed solutions for the well-being of medical undergraduates like providing proper student support service and more opportunities for extracurricular activities.

**Keywords:** mental distress, medical students

## 1. Introduction

The World Health Organization defines health as: "A state of complete physical, mental and social well-being and not merely the absence of disease" [1]. Many of us perceive health merely as being physical fitness and neglect the importance of mental health. Depression, anxiety, and stress levels are considered as significant pointers for the psychological well-being of the population. It is predicted that by the year 2020, depression will become the second most common reason of disability globally [2]. Failure to identify and cure of these mental disorders might have unwanted bearings on the lives of individuals [3].

Mental distress has been well identified in undergraduate medical students and is a matter of concern in both developed and developing countries [4]. The young students are the most susceptible group of the population to stressful life events, especially those who are pursuing a higher professional education in a competitive setting [5]. It is noted that medical undergraduates have higher levels of mental distress than the general population and their fellow peers [6]. Medical education encompasses challenging curriculum and clinical training [7]. The duration of the medical course is different across countries; some have 4-year graduate programs, and others have 5- or 6-year undergraduate programs [8]. The medical curriculum is usually divided into basic or preclinical (1st and 2nd years), clinical (3rd, 4th, and 5th years), and clinical house job (6th year) periods. The curriculum of preclinical phase focuses on basic medical science subjects, i.e., anatomy, physiology, and biochemistry, whereas the clinical phase emphasizes on clinical subjects, i.e., surgery, general medicine, pediatrics, community medicine, forensic medicine, and gynecology. In the clinical internship period, medical graduates have to rotate in different wards in the hospital and emergency units for 1 year under direct supervision.

Medical students learn specialized knowledge, skills, and attitudes which prepare them to become a competent physician; this highly demanding medical curriculum may have undesirable effects on the learner's physical and mental health [9, 10].

A high prevalence of stress, anxiety, and depression among medical students has been identified globally [11–14]. Medical education can cause a considerable amount of psychological stress on undergraduates [7]. Various psychological morbidities have been reported among medical students, ranging from stress, anxiety, social problems, depression, burnout, and suicidal ideation [15]. Due to the heavy educational workload in undergraduate medicine, medical students are more prone to psychiatric complaints such as depression, anxiety, and stress than their nonmedical peers [16]. Depression and anxiety in medical undergraduates can also continue during internship and residency periods and later in the medical professional life [9].

One of the major aims of medical education is to produce knowledgeable, skilled, and proficient doctors. The medical profession is considered as one of the prestigious professions in society. Students enter in the medical field for various reasons, including fulfilling their own passions, parental pressure, financial and job security, to secure a respected place in society, etc. [17].

Studies suggest that medical education may have an unintended harmful effect on students' mental health, resulting in high prevalence of depression, anxiety, and stress among medical students [10, 17–19]. It has been hypothesized that various factors are responsible for the decline in mental health of medical students, including academic pressure [20], increased workload [13], financial issues [20], sleep deprivation, and exposure to patients' suffering and deaths [7]. Mental distress adversely affects the learning and cognitive abilities of students [21] which might have an influence on their academic performance [10]. A study in the UK showed a high dropout rate in psychologically ill students [9]. It is crucial to recognize students' mental distress and their causes so that it can help the medical educationist to develop necessary amendments in the curriculum to ensure production of graduates who are emotionally fit for their difficult training to deal with various aspects of life like human suffering and death [17].

## 2. Prevalence of depression, anxiety, and stress among medical students

A widely distributed body of literature indicates that the prevalence of mental distress is increasing among students studying medicine [16, 20, 22]. It is evident that mental health problems are prevalent in the whole society, but university students are significantly more affected than the general population [14, 23]. This might be due to numerous challenges that university students have to face such as competition to succeed, high academic demands, teacher and parent's expectations, increased workload, financial problems, and apprehension about the future [24]. And among all university students, medical students exhibit higher mental distress than both the general population and their age-matched peers [20]. Worldwide medical undergraduates have been found at risk of mental distress and reduced life satisfaction [7, 24, 25]. Medical training involves many risk factors for mental illness, including academic burden, lack of sleep, minimal physical activities, and decreased time for social activities. A large study conducted in the USA, including six medical schools (582 students), concluded that when medical students enrolled in a medical institute, they had better or similar mental health than the general population. It shows that higher rates of distress reported in medical students are the result of the over-competitive training process of medical education that can have an unfavorable effect on the mental health of students [26].

## 3. Prevalence of mental distress among medical students in western countries vs. non-western medical students

Dyrbye found the significantly higher frequency of mental distress among US and Canadian medical students than the general population [20]. Dahlin et al. [10] reported that 13% of Swedish medical students were depressed as compared to 7.8% in an age-matched control sample and, of further concern, one-third of the students reporting suicidal thoughts during the course of training. Another research study conducted in Australia involved 1811 medical students and concluded that one in five students reported suicidal thoughts over the past 1 year [27].

Studies from non-western countries also reported a high prevalence of mental distress [5, 7, 9, 13, 28–30]. There is a small but growing body of research that has recently emerged that attempts to determine the prevalence and the causes of mental distress among medical students of Pakistan. Pakistani study findings are not different from rest of the globe, and they also found high mental distress among medical students [17, 19, 31–33].

It is clearly obvious from the above discussion that the prevalence of mental distress is higher in non-western countries than western ones. This might be due to low knowledge and awareness about mental health in developing countries [34]. But there is evidence that western institutes did introduce curricular changes, better assessment, and innovation to cope with stress [20].

## 4. Potential causes of depression, anxiety, and stress in medical students

This section will explore the sources of psychological distress among medical students. Various potential sources of mental distress found in literature among medical students are discussed below.

### 4.1 Academic demands

#### *4.1.1 Vast syllabus*

The medical curriculum had long been identified as one of the important risk factors for distress among students. Several studies recognized assessments and academic-associated elements as the most substantial stressors [7, 22, 25, 32]. A longitudinal study in the UK concluded that the enormous academic load is the most significant reason of mental distress among medical students [35]. Studies have shown that the mental health of many students deteriorates after their enrollment in medical school and remains low throughout their training [9, 17, 22].
The poor mental health of medical undergraduate affects not only their physical well-being but also their educational achievements during their training period [9]. Some degree of stress facilitates learning and performance, but intense pressure and huge demands of the medical curriculum may have undesirable effects on vulnerable students' behavior which reduces their learning abilities [36]. There is evidence that prolonged stress exposure may affect the prefrontal area of the brain, which is responsible for higher cognitive functions and learning [37]. Stress and anxiety not only cause underachievement but also result in low-level self-esteem and reduced motivation and effort to complete educational tasks [6]. Poor and unsatisfactory academic achievement may further increase the mental distress among students [15] which may have serious consequences, e.g., dropout from medical course or suicide in extreme cases [38].

#### *4.1.2 Frequent exams*

Frequent examinations are found to be another main reason for mental stress. A study revealed that the amount of stress almost doubled during or near the examination [25]. Moreover, due to frequent examination and assessments throughout the academic year, it becomes difficult for students to prepare for the exams properly; as a result, they get an average or poor grade [39]. Adults are motivated to learn mostly by internal factors, but external sources such as assessments also contribute strongly to motivate the learner to learn [40]. Too many examinations do not let students study deep, and they failed to produce intended outcome or good grades, hence becoming demotivated and distressed [41].

#### *4.1.3 Inadequate feedback*

Dahlin et al. [10] mention that insufficient feedback is also related to increased distress of students. It is very crucial to give effective feedback to students because it enables the learner to analyze their actions and helps them plan for the future; learners can be confused if left unsupervised [42]. Effective feedback practice from teachers permits students to develop positive insights about the task, and corrective feedback is essential for effective learning; without it the level of performance attained is lower [40].

#### *4.1.4 Lack of time*

In a semi-structured interview-based study, students revealed that huge academic tasks render them to have limited or no time for sleep and recreational activities; this lack of sleep might reduce the emotional well-being of students [43]. Due to high academic demands of medical education, most of the medical students fail to take time out for physical activities like exercise and other healthy activities [39]. People who have minimal physical activity are at higher risk of mood disorders like depression, anxiety, and stress [44]. Medical students get fewer opportunities for extracurricular activity, and that might have a negative effect on their mental health. Due to lack of time and the heavy burden of study, students could not find enough time for self-care; they are not able to take proper sleep and time for leisure activities which have a further bad effect on their well-being [45].

### 4.2 Transition

The literature offers evidence of the association between transitions and students' mental distress [5, 7, 10, 16, 31]. Transition is a dynamic process in which students experience cultural, social, and cognitive challenges while passing from a familiar to a less familiar environment. The medical curriculum is interrupted by two major transitions, first from the high school to the first year of medicine and another from preclinical to clinical, i.e., third year. Dahlin et al. [10] explored the distress among different years of students and found higher mental distress among first-year and third-year students than senior level year students.

#### *4.2.1 Transition from high school to the first year of medicine*

Students of the first year are overburdened with huge subjective curriculum, the pace of study is too fast, and they have little time to cover the syllabus. However, Dyrbye et al. [20] argued that many junior students might face the challenges of being displaced from friends and family and experience difficulty in adjusting to a new environment along with heavy academic toll. So this high mental distress might be a part of the adjustment process to the new educational setting. According to the U-curve theory, this stage of adjustment is known as "culture shock" in which a medical student faces isolation, stress, anxiety, and emptiness [46, 47]. The successful adjustment at this stage depends on the self-confidence of students in their ability to cope with the stressors [48, 49]. In this stage, a student must face numerous challenges to adapt in a new environment as well as meet academic demands [48, 49]. So, in this context, self-efficacy seems to be the most suitable principle to deal with stress [50]. Bandura [21] concludes that cooperative learning strategies, in which learners work together and help one another, tend to improve both self-efficacy and academic achievement. Furthermore, constructive feedback is also important in developing self-efficacy in students [21].

#### *4.2.2 Transition to clinical phase*

A study done in a Thai school revealed a higher mental stress among third-year medical students [5]. Students are susceptible to become depressed during their initial clinical years of study when they rotate through the hospitals, because at that time students often detach from their friends and peer group and must work with constantly changing groups of residents and attending physicians at different hospitals [43]. Furthermore, clinical rotations anticipate a number of stress-provoking tasks, such as interactions with senior doctors and staff during ward rounds; dealing with patients, diseases, and death may also contribute to the poor mental health of medical students during their initial clinical years [15], because at this stage, students are not able to contribute enough to the patient care which makes them feel insecure about not having enough knowledge and skills [43]. Students, when entering into the clinical stage, are not confident enough to communicate effectively with clinical staff and are hesitant to participate in teamwork. It is evident that stress has been associated with poor communication, reduced quality of patient care, and medical errors [51].

#### *4.2.3 Lack of communication skills*

Students find it difficult to deal with newly added tasks and interacting with critically ill patients. Undergraduate curriculum mostly does not contain any information about communication skills. Effective communication builds a strong relationship between students, clinical staff, and patient which ultimately reduces the distress of students and enhances learning [52], and this will ultimately affect the quality of care delivered to the patient and quality of life [53]. These transitions might have negative effects on the learning process due to the lack of social interaction. Students who are distressed may face isolation and stigma which further affect their learning. Social constructivism theory describes that the adult learner learns through interaction and collaboration with other people in their natural setting [54]. Students learn better when they interact with their friends and peers regularly [55].

These large changes during the period of transitions need coping strategies in order to function effectively in the new environment. Critical reflection is the most desirable quality for a smooth transition [56, 57]. Experience is converted into learning by reflection, and this process can be improved by the cooperation of a facilitator or teacher [58]. Encouraging reflection in learners will lead to the development of reflective practice which is a significant element of professionalism [59]. Learners should be involved in assessing their own learning process. Critical reflection on experience promotes deep and self-directed learning among students [40]. Mann [53] argues that introduction of activities like reflective portfolios, feedback, and peer review helps students cope with the stress during the transition and avail opportunity of learning during the transition phase. It is also noted that early introduction of clinical medicine also aids to stimulate smooth transitions [60].

### 4.3 Miscellaneous causes of mental distress

In addition to the aforementioned reasons, some other causes are also mentioned in the literature, e.g., personal life events, the death of family members, marriage, the birth of a child, family history of depression, etc. These reasons are also recognized to contribute to depression, anxiety, and stress in medical students, the same as the general population [61]. Financial problems are another factor mentioned in various studies, as a cause of increased stress levels in medical students [25]. A study discovered that the poorer the background, the more stress is experienced by students [25]. Medical education is considered a costly course which is also associated with other demands such as expensive textbooks, suitable clothing, and medical equipment. Some medical students suffer financial problems. Long academic hours do not allow students for part-time jobs to fulfill their financial needs [15]. Finances would be one of the main factors of the distress among students. As a medical educationist, we cannot do much about this issue, but we can suggest stakeholders create more scholarship opportunities for students.

### 4.4 Educational interventions that contribute to student well-being

Literature is largely focused on the efforts to improve student mental health through improving access to mental health provider and decreasing the stigma to mental health treatment and implementing of wellness programs. But there are only a few studies focused on innovative models that build to address the root causes of stress, i.e., academic related. The few most frequent curricular-related recommendations to improve the well-being of students are as follows.

#### *4.4.1 Grading system*

Implementation of the pass/fail grading is the most common curricular innovation mentioned in the literature. Reed et al. [60] found in a multi-institutional study that levels of mental distress are higher in students of the medical institute that used grading system with three or more levels than the students of the medical institute that used pass/fail grading [62]. Students always do a competition for getting better grades, and that consistently caused distress. Implementation of the pass/fail grading system, especially during the initial 2 years of medical school, helps students not to over-occupy themselves with competition for the high grade [15].

#### *4.4.2 Clear learning objectives*

Evans and Brown [61] proposed that students can be helped to reduce academic burden by offering them a clear learning objective so that students will know what they have to learn. It reduces the distress and thus fosters the well-being of students [63]. A predetermined clear learning objective not only lets students focus on them but also motivates them to achieve those [64].

#### *4.4.3 Teaching strategies*

Offering a variety of teaching strategies for delivering of course material such as small group activities, team-based learning, and flipped class is also known to reduce mental distress [65]. Small group learning is a more effective tool in gaining student-teacher bonding than didactic traditional lectures and thus helps the transfer of knowledge efficiently [66]. Furthermore, a small group setup provides a secure state in which students can argue and discuss their perceptions and assumptions. This problem solving and peer interaction can result in deep understanding; group discussion complements the situational learning of professionalism [66] which is known to enhance the well-being of students [57].

#### *4.4.4 Self-efficacy and critical reflection*

The practice of self-efficacy and reflection also mentioned reducing stress among medical students. The introduction of the reflective practice for students causes them to become the self-directed learner, and they become responsible for their own learning, which greatly alleviates mental distress [67]. The most frequently used tools for reflection are reflective journals, reflective dialogical exercises, and portfolios [68]. A learner should be involved in reflective practices because it provides them a chance to assess their own learning style. Reflection allows students' knowledge to be actively integrated and thus encourages self-directed, deep, and continued learning [55]. Problem-based learning (PBL) is known to promote self-efficacy and self-directed learning and hence endorse easy transitions during medical education [67].

#### *4.4.5 Vertical curriculum*

Vertical curriculum, which is defined as the assimilation between the basic science and clinical segments of the curriculum [64], is known to reduce mental distress because in that there is the early introduction of clinical medicine and students can relate theory to practice [69]. Early exposure of students to clinical medicines gives them instantaneous opportunities to apply the basic science knowledge to the clinical setting and help them in smooth transition through their educational journey [64].

#### *4.4.6 Longitudinal electives*

Longitudinal electives (e.g., communication skills or coping with stress) and other community-based activities seem promising in reducing stress among students [69]. Stress reduction teaching modules or electives intended to raise self-awareness and self-reflection and hence engage in self-care [26].

#### *4.4.7 Promoting professionalism*

Professionalism in medicine can be described as the collection of values, attitudes, and behavior that a health professional show when they deal with a patient, colleagues, and society [70]. Brazeau et al. [26] observed a positive relationship between medical mental well-being and professionalism [71]. Professionalism is mostly considered as a part of the hidden and informal curriculum [72]. The inclusion of professionalism in the formal curriculum is relatively a newer concept, but it becomes today's requirement [73]. Every medical institute should develop their own institutional specific curriculum for professionalism with faculty and students' help along with a structured teaching and learning methods and assessments [18].

## 5. Conclusion

Medical students experience a substantial amount of distress during their training, which has been shown to contribute to substandard academic performance, dishonesty, pessimism, and substance abuse [20]. A good physician requires the sound mental health to nurture and increase compassion, professionalism, and tolerance [20]. The main stresses identified during literature search are academic related. An undue amount of stress during medical education had the negative effect on students, who might have experienced difficulties in social encounters and a lack of concentration which leads to increased frequency of blunders, carelessness, and negligence [45]. Poor psychological health not only upsets students' lives but also has undesirable effects on patients' care in the long run [39]. Increased frequency of depression and anxiety within medical professionals may put the future of health care in danger; it may cause reduced productivity, low quality of life, and learning difficulties which will ultimately have a negative effect on the quality of patient care [20]. Depression, anxiety, and stress can have profound negative effects on the learning abilities of students [24], and this will ultimately affect the quality of care delivered to the patient and quality of life [53]. Evaluation of the literature shows that students and doctors who are suffering from mental distress are more likely to have poor professionalism, ranging from cheating, plagiarism, and providing substandard patient care [45]. So as a medical educator, this is a real state of urgency to introduce innovation in the curriculum to improve mental health, for this effort existing literature on curricular factors may serve as a model.

## 6. Recommendation for practice

The recommendations to reduce mental distress among medical students are discussed as follows:

- Provide an engaging curriculum which offers different styles, e.g., small group tutorials, team-based learning, and flipped classes.

- Exams should be prescheduled with proper gaps between different subjects. Proper time off should be given to students between their clinical rotations so that they can relax.

- Promote reflective activities, e.g., reflective diaries and portfolios throughout the curriculum, and timely and constructive feedback should be provided to students.

- Early introduction of clinical medicine, so that students can easily relate theory to practice.

- Longitudinal workshops or module on communication skills and stress management should be part of the curriculum for the medical undergraduate to become self-aware of their own well-being during their course of training. Special presentations by the faculty should be given to students about challenges in work-life balance.

- Provide opportunities for extracurricular activities to students, and encourage students to promote their well-being with regular physical exercise and sufficient sleep. Give students in the campus opportunity for sporting and cultural activities to lessen their distress.

- Include elements of professionalism in the core curriculum.

It is needed to convince stakeholders of medical institute, i.e., head of medical education and principal, that we need to establish a strong support system for students for counseling, with whom they can discuss their problems, whether it is related to their psychological health or academics. Merely identifying the mental distress of a student does not seem to contribute to reducing the psychological morbidity; it is crucial to provide personalized support to the stressed students once they are recognized [15]. Students are reluctant to take available support because of the stigma related to the mental illness; they are not comfortable enough in taking consultations from their own institution. Such students should be given a chance to have an off-campus psychological support or online help with full confidentiality. These support systems increase the awareness and practice of positive coping approaches. These distress management programs should advise students about the negative effects of mental distress on human functioning and enlighten students on how to recognize the sources of mental distress and how to manage it. These groups provide an opportunity to students to express themselves and to share their feelings fearlessly, and thus it decreases the possibility of burnout. Such support groups help students to realize that they are not the only ones who are suffering but many others are also in the same situation. It also gives them a chance to realize how their colleagues solve such issues. Students should be given the chance to express their vision on the curriculum, so that they can give their unique insights to curriculum committees. Regular feedback from students on teaching and training can play a vital role in reducing the stress among students [15, 74–77].

## 7. Recommendation for future research

The potential for mental health to improve medical undergraduates and graduates' professionalism is also mostly unexplored. Large-scale, prospective, multicenter, and hypothesis-based or phenomenological-based qualitative studies are much needed to provide effective and generalized evidence about this issue. Both quantitative and qualitative research should be done in the future to see the long-term outcomes of the curricular change project. Support and funding for such research program are also limited, which must be alleviated. Research studies to explore the causes and consequences of medical students' distress and to examine possible solutions are not only beneficial for the affected medical student but also useful for the patients to whom they deliver their services. Subsequently, the interventions to promote students' mental health will advantage the student, the physician, the patients, and the community as a whole.

## Acknowledgements

I dedicate this piece of writing to my loving father, Syed Azim-ur-Rahman (late), for his love and support throughout my life.

## Conflict of interest

None.

## Notes/thanks/other declarations

None.

## Author details

Syeda Rubaba Azim
Medical Education, Dow University of Health Sciences, Pakistan

*Address all correspondence to: rubaba.azim@duhs.edu.pk

## References

[1] Nutbeam D. Health promotion glossary. Health Promotion International. 1998;**13**(4):349-364

[2] World Health Organization. Mental Health: A Call for Action by World Health Ministers. Geneva: World Health Organization, Department of Mental Health and Substance Dependence; 2001

[3] Teh CK, Ngo CW, Binti Zulkifli RA, Vellasamy R, Suresh K. Depression, anxiety and stress among undergraduate students: A cross sectional study. Open Journal of Epidemiology. 2015;**5**(04):260

[4] Carson AJ, Dias S, Johnston A, McLoughlin MA, O'connor M, Robinson BL, et al. Mental health in medical students a case control study using the 60 item general health questionnaire. Scottish Medical Journal. 2000;**45**(4):115-116

[5] Saipanish R. Stress among medical students in a Thai medical school. Medical Teacher. 2003;**25**(5):502-506

[6] Saravanan C, Wilks R. Medical students' experience of and reaction to stress: The role of depression and anxiety. The Scientific World Journal. 2014;**2014**

[7] Melaku L, Mossie A, Negash A. Stress among medical students and its association with substance use and academic performance. Journal of Biomedical Education. 2015;**2015**

[8] Baldassin S, Alves TC, de Andrade AG, Martins LAN. The characteristics of depressive symptoms in medical students during medical education and training: A cross-sectional study. BMC Medical Education. 2008;**8**(1):60

[9] Abdulghani HM, AlKanhal AA, Mahmoud ES, Ponnamperuma GG, Alfaris EA. Stress and its effects on medical students: A cross-sectional study at a college of medicine in Saudi Arabia. Journal of Health, Population and Nutrition. 2011:516-522

[10] Dahlin M, Joneborg N, Runeson B. Stress and depression among medical students: A cross-sectional study. Medical Education. 2005;**39**(6):594-604

[11] Soh NLW, Norgren S, Lampe L, Hunt GE, Malhi GS, Walter G. Mental distress in Australian medical students and its association with housing and travel time. Journal of Contemporary Medical Education. 2013;**1**(3):163-169

[12] Moffat KJ, McConnachie A, Ross S, Morrison JM. First year medical student stress and coping in a problem-based learning medical curriculum. Medical Education. 2004;**38**(5):482-491

[13] Iqbal S, Gupta S, Venkatarao E. Stress, anxiety & depression among medical undergraduate students & their socio-demographic correlates. The Indian Journal of Medical Research. 2015;**141**(3):354

[14] Bayram N, Bilgel N. The prevalence and socio-demographic correlations of depression, anxiety and stress among a group of university students. Social Psychiatry and Psychiatric Epidemiology. 2008;**43**(8):667-672

[15] Dyrbye LN, Thomas MR, Shanafelt TD. Medical student distress: causes, consequences, and proposed solutions. Mayo Clinic Proceedings. 2005;**80**(12):1613-1622

[16] Inam SNB, Saqib A, Alam E. Prevalence of anxiety and depression among medical students of private university. Journal-Pakistan Medical Association. 2003;**53**(2):44-46

[17] Khan MS, Mahmood S, Badshah A, Ali SU, Jamal Y. Prevalence of depression,

anxiety and their associated factors among medical students in Karachi, Pakistan. Journal-Pakistan Medical Association. 2006;**56**(12):583

[18] Abdallah AR, Gabr HM. Depression, anxiety and stress among first year medical students in an Egyptian public university. International Research Journal of Medicine and Medical Sciences. 2014;**2**(1):11-19

[19] Hashmi AM, Aftab MA, Naqvi SH, Sajjad W, Mohsin M, Khawaja IS. Anxiety and depression in Pakistani medical students: A multicenter study. HealthMED. 2014;**8**(7):813-820

[20] Dyrbye LN, Thomas MR, Shanafelt TD. Systematic review of depression, anxiety, and other indicators of psychological distress among US and Canadian medical students. Academic Medicine. 2006;**81**(4):354-373

[21] Bandura A. Perceived self-efficacy in cognitive development and functioning. Educational Psychologist. 1993;**28**(2):117-148

[22] Kulsoom B, Afsar NA. Stress, anxiety, and depression among medical students in a multiethnic setting. Neuropsychiatric Disease and Treatment. 2015;**11**:1713

[23] Stallman HM. Psychological distress in university students: A comparison with general population data. Australian Psychologist. 2010;**45**(4):249-257

[24] Abdulghani HM. Stress and depression among medical students: A cross sectional study at a medical college in Saudi Arabia. Pakistan Journal of Medical Sciences. 2008;**24**(1):12

[25] Yusoff MSB, Liew YY, Ling HW, Tan CS, Loke HM, Lim XB, et al. A study on stress, stressors and coping strategies among Malaysian medical students. International Journal of Students' Research. 2011;**1**(2):45-50

[26] Brazeau CM, Schroeder R, Rovi S, Boyd L. Relationships between medical student burnout, empathy, and professionalism climate. Academic Medicine. 2010;**85**(10):S33-SS3

[27] Wu F, Ireland M, Hafekost K, Lawrence D. National mental health survey of doctors and medical students. 2013

[28] Oku AO, Owoaje ET, Oku OO, Ikpeme BM. Prevalence of stress, stressors and coping strategies among medical students in a Nigerian medical school. African Journal of Medical and Health Sciences. 2015;**14**(1):29

[29] Ahmed I, Banu H, Al-Fageer R, Al-Suwaidi R. Cognitive emotions: Depression and anxiety in medical students and staff. Journal of Critical Care. 2009;**24**(3):e1-e7

[30] Rab F, Mamdou R, Nasir S. Rates of depression and anxiety among female medical students in Pakistan. 2008

[31] Jadoon NA, Yaqoob R, Raza A, Shehzad MA, Zeshan SC. Anxiety and depression among medical students: A cross-sectional study. The Journal of the Pakistan Medical Association. 2010;**60**(8):699-702

[32] Rizvi F, Qureshi A, Rajput AM, Afzal M. Prevalence of depression, anxiety and stress (by DASS Scoring System) among medical students in Islamabad, Pakistan. British Journal of Medicine and Medical Research. 2015;**8**(1):69-75

[33] Shaikh BT, Kahloon A, Kazmi M, Khalid H, Nawaz K, Khan N, et al. Students, stress and coping strategies: A case of Pakistani medical school. Education For Health-Abingdon-Carfax Publishing Limited. 2004;**17**:346-353

[34] Sohail N. Stress and academic performance among medical students. Journal of College of Physicians and Surgeons of Pakistan. 2013;**23**(1):67-71

[35] Kaplan HI, Saddock BJ. Learning theory Synopsis of Psychiatry: Behavioural Sciences/Clinical Psychiatry. 8th ed. Philadelphia: Lippincott Williams & Wilkins; 2000. pp. 148-154

[36] Arnsten AF. Stress signalling pathways that impair prefrontal cortex structure and function. Nature Reviews Neuroscience. 2009;**10**(6):410-422

[37] Huberty TJ. Test and performance anxiety. Principal Leadership. 2009;**10**(1):12-16

[38] Rosenthal JM, Okie S. White coat, mood indigo—Depression in medical school. New England Journal of Medicine. 2005;**353**(11):1085-1088

[39] Kaufman DM, Mann KV. Teaching and learning in medical education: How theory can inform practice. Understanding Medical Education: Evidence, Theory and Practice. 2014;**2**:7-29

[40] Hutchinson L. Educational environment. British Medical Journal. 2003;**326**(7393):810

[41] Dennick R. Twelve tips for incorporating educational theory into teaching practices. Medical Teacher. 2012;**34**(8):618-624

[42] Radcliffe C, Lester H. Perceived stress during undergraduate medical training: A qualitative study. Medical Education. 2003;**37**(1)

[43] De Mello MT, de Aquino Lemos V, Antunes HKM, Bittencourt L, Santos-Silva R, Tufik S. Relationship between physical activity and depression and anxiety symptoms: A population study. Journal of Affective Disorders. 2013;**149**(1):241-246

[44] Wood DF. Mens sana in corpore sano: Student well-being and the development of resilience. Medical Education. 2016;**50**(1):20-23

[45] Perry C, Allard A. Making the connections: Transition experience for first-year education students. Journal of Educational Enquiry. 2003;**4**(2):74-89

[46] Denovan A, Macaskill A. An interpretative phenomenological analysis of stress. 2013

[47] Morton S, Mergler A, Boman P. Managing the transition: The role of optimism and self-efficacy for first-year Australian university students. Journal of Psychologists and Counsellors in Schools. 2014;**24**(1):90-108

[48] Smith HM, Betz NE. An examination of efficacy and esteem pathways to depression in young adulthood. Journal of Counseling Psychology. 2002;**49**(4):438

[49] Ibrahim MB, Abdelreheem MH. Prevalence of anxiety and depression among medical and pharmaceutical students in Alexandria University. Alexandria Journal of Medicine. 2015;**51**(2):167-173

[50] Teunissen PW, Westerman M. Opportunity or threat: The ambiguity of the consequences of transitions in medical education. Medical Education. 2011;**45**(1):51-59

[51] Jarwan BK. Depression among medical students of Faculty of Medicine, Umm Al-Qura University in Makkah, Saudi Arabia. International Journal of Public Health Research. 2015;**4**(2):184-191

[52] Kaufman DM. Applying educational theory in practice. BMJ. 2003;**326**(7382):213-216

[53] Mann KV. Theoretical perspectives in medical education: Past experience and future possibilities. Medical Education. 2011;**45**(1):60-68

[54] Booth A. Developing history students' skills in the transition

to university. Teaching in Higher Education. 2001;**6**(4):487-503

[55] Matheson D. An Introduction to the Study of Education. Routledge; 2014

[56] Schön DA. Educating the Reflective Practitioner: Toward a New Design for Teaching and Learning in the Professions. San Francisco; 1987

[57] Finlay L. Reflecting on 'Reflective practice' Practice-Based Professional Learning Centre. 2008. Retrieved January. 2015:13

[58] Wijnen-Meijer M, Ten Cate OTJ, Rademakers JJ, Van Der Schaaf M, Borleffs JC. The influence of a vertically integrated curriculum on the transition to postgraduate training. Medical Teacher. 2009;**31**(11):e528-e532

[59] Paykel ES. The evolution of life events, research in psychiatry. Journal of Affective Disorders. 2001;**62**(3):141-149

[60] Reed DA, Shanafelt TD, Satele DW, Power DV, Eacker A, Harper W, et al. Relationship of pass/fail grading and curriculum structure with well-being among preclinical medical students: A multi-institutional study. Academic Medicine. 2011;**86**(11):1367-1373

[61] Evans D, Brown J. Supporting students in difficulty. Learning and Teaching in Medicine. 2010;**78**

[62] Hassan S. Concepts of vertical and horizontal integration as an approach to integrated curriculum. Education in Medicine Journal. 2013;**5**(4)

[63] Slavin SJ, Schindler DL, Chibnall JT. Medical student mental health 3.0: Improving student wellness through curricular changes. Academic Medicine. 2014;**89**(4):573

[64] Thampy H, Gwynne C, Foulkes R, Codd R, Burling S. Teach professionalism. Education for Primary Care. 2012;**23**(4):297-299

[65] Altirkawi K. Teaching professionalism in medicine: What, why and how? Sudanese Journal of Paediatrics. 2014;**14**(1):31

[66] Cheng M. Quality Enhancement Themes: Transition Skills and Strategies, Critical Self-Reflection. 2015. Available from: http://www.enhancementthemes.ac.uk/docs/publications/transition-skills-and-strategies---critical-self-reflection.pdf?sfvrsn=12

[67] Shah SIA, Ahmed M. Medical students' anxiety on beginning clinical studies. Al Ameen Journal of Medical Sciences. 2013;**6**(3):195-201

[68] Saunders PA, Tractenberg RE, Chaterji R, Amri H, Harazduk N, Gordon JS, et al. Promoting self-awareness and reflection through an experiential mind-body skills course for first year medical students. Medical Teacher. 2007;**29**(8):778-784

[69] Working Party of the Royal College of Physicians. Doctors in Society. Medical professionalism in a changing world. Clinical Medicine (London, England). 2005;**5**(6 Suppl 1):S5

[70] Stern DT, Papadakis M. The developing physician—Becoming a professional. New England Journal of Medicine. 2006;**355**(17):1794-1799

[71] Cruess RL, Cruess SR. Teaching professionalism: General principles. Medical Teacher. 2006;**28**(3):205-208

[72] Porur RN. Perceptions of CRRIs on formal curriculum for professionalism. International Journal of Pure and Applied Bioscience. 2015;**3**(2):279-285

[73] Al-Faris EA, Irfan F, Van der Vleuten CPM, Naeem N, Alsalem A, Alamiri N, et al. The prevalence and correlates of depressive symptoms

from an Arabian setting: A wake up call. Medical Teacher. 2012;**34**(Suppl):S32-S36

[74] Johari AB, Hassim IN. Stress and coping strategies among medical students in national university of Malaysia, Malaysia University of Sabah and University Kuala Lumpur Royal College of Medicine Perak. Jurnal Kesihatan Masyarakat. 2009;**15**(2):106-115

[75] Mahmoud JSR, Staten RT, Hall LA, Lennie TA. The relationship among young adult college students' depression, anxiety, stress, demographics, life satisfaction, and coping styles. Issues in Mental Health Nursing. 2012;**33**(3):149-156

[76] Saravanan C, Wilks R. Medical students' experience of and reaction to stress:The role of depression and anxiety. The Scientific World Journal. 2014;**2014**

[77] Takeichi M, Sato T. Studies on the psychosomatic functioning of ill-health according to eastern and western medicine. 7. Psychoimmuno-endocrinological changes induced by Kampo medication and relaxation training. American Journal of Chinese Medicine. 2001;**29**(3-4):411-422

Chapter 3

# A Holistic Overview of Cyberbullying across the World: Review of Theories and Models

*Timothy Oblad*

## Abstract

This chapter reviews cyberbullying research from across the world. Not only it is important to be familiar with the range of impact and risks that commonly fall upon cyber victims, but much can be learned when reviewing a myriad of research focused on the bullies themselves. In addition to that, it provides some theoretical discussion for other researchers who wish to study cyberbullying through a specific lens that may help standardize the research and better understand what is truly happening behind the screens. This chapter also explores how those involved with cyber aggressive behaviors choose to cope, whether positively or negatively. In depth, this chapter explores cyberbullies in hopes of creating more awareness of signs for parents or educators that may be able to prevent perpetration or targeting.

**Keywords:** cyberbullying, cyber aggression, adolescents, emerging adults, depression, suicidal ideation

## 1. Introduction

The connection between mental illness and social media use has been well documented over the past decade [1, 2]. What has been most concerning, however, is the pervasive nature and impact of unwanted cyber aggression over the years. As social media has adapted and changed, there have been increased risks of suicidal ideation, suicide, sexual exploitation or solicitations and a myriad of other negative coping methods such as quitting school or losing self-control. Through a meta-analysis, a primary consequence of cyber victimization was found to be increased levels of depression, particularly among females [3]. Because of this phenomenon, it is important to address the impact cyberaggression has on various ages, primarily adolescent ages but also emerging adults and that have provided some insight into how they cope or manage cyberbullying. This chapter will also provide a review of theoretical frameworks that helps to explain motivation behind the screen and why some are more at risk than others. The secondary purpose of this chapter is to explore motivation of the bully or the harasser, connections between bullies and victim, self-harm, internalized and externalized coping.

### 1.1 Defining characteristics of cyberbullies and cyber victims

Prior to describing the impact from involvement in cyberaggressive activities, it is important to describe commonly found characteristics among individuals often identified as cyberbullies as well cyber victims, as well as the historical context from which cyberbullying ascended.

In the late 1990s and early 2000s, internet access within the home was becoming a normal available tool to have. Chatrooms had already existed for several years and social media was beginning to take off. By the year 2000, the term "cyberbullying" began to appear in anti-bullying laws but was not required until years later after cases of suicides and online bullying became the center of media attention and exposure [4].

Face-to-face bullying had already existed for decades but researchers began to notice online bullies were often not physically dominant over their victims. Olweus [5] claimed a bully had to have some physical dominance, or more power, thus a power imbalance over their victim(s). Unlike traditional bullies, today cyberbullies can be of any size or age and through anonymous accounts, can remove that necessary power-feature to be stronger or physically more dominant. Another characteristic found among cyberbullies are that they often report higher psychosocial challenges, depressive symptomatology and other problematic behaviors [6]. Sabella et al., [7] also found cyberbullies tend to be motivated by revenge-seeking behaviors (see [8]).

To understand key indications for cyber victimization, researchers had been exploring risks such as spending time online, little to no parental monitoring, peer-network connecting online, etc., These were each significantly associated with increases in cyber victimization [6]. However, little was still known about the psychosocial risks of involvement for online victims. To consider the cyber victims' perceptions and understanding, Campfield [9] explored psychosocial characteristics of both victims and bullies. Specifically among cyber victims, Campfield discovered that victims were significantly more likely to have low self-esteem, more feelings of loneliness and other emotional problems.

While researchers have found some differences among bullies and victims as described, it is important to note that the commonly shared element are elevated levels of psychosomatic disturbances (see [10]). As studies investigate these characteristics, unique differences, or similarities even, the research all suggest concerns for such individuals, especially those that behave as both bullies and victims [9, 11].

## 2. Impact cyberaggression leaves on targeted victims

Nearly the entire world is connected online in one form or another. Especially in the western world virtually everyone spends time on the internet connected to others socially [12]. Likewise, cyberbullying has quickly grown over the last decade, nearly parallel to the growth and interest in social media networking (SNS) [12]. While SNS are a wonderful tool that helps maintain relationships and allows for immediate connection to family and friends as well as potentially new and interesting people, cyber aggressive activities may constrain the benefits of using social networks. For example, a recent study of adolescent students reportedly found such online aggression led to elevated levels of fear and sadness among cyber victims [13]. Over the past decade, research has followed and uncovered coping methods including serious negative coping methods such as depression or suicide. This chapter describes cross-cultural research across the world to provide a more holistic lens of this phenomenon.

In the Czech Republic, [14] researchers explored the potential impact from being targeted. They were primarily interested in how cyber victims coped after receiving online abuse or attacks. Through open-ended responses, one of the immediate consequences was actually a primary prevention method: becoming more cautious and limiting trust in others, especially online. Some respondents reported as going as far as completely removing social network profiles, blocking individuals, or removing personal profile information (e.g., photos). Personal information became more restricted as a direct result of previous online attacks, which should be considered a positive coping response.

In terms of negative impact, Sleglova and Cerna [14] found some cyber victims had a negative psychological impact as well. While there were findings of resilience, some struggled with letting incidents (attacks) go, or moving on from them. As discussed, some reported loss of trust as well as feeling helpless, disillusioned, drop on self-confidence for some cyber victims. One of the participants shared incidence of recurring nightmares. In some other cases, some lost close friends or peer groups, traditional bullies started bullying as well. A major concern reported was that of self-harm. Respondents shared cutting became a method of coping, another had weight gain changes.

### 2.1 Victimization among emerging adults

Cyberbullying among emerging adults is also concern today. When considering emerging adults and all of their transitions and decisions they have to make, cyber victims within this age group may suffer from losing relationships due to online disagreements, harassment or targeting for their own worldviews or political opinions. Consistent targeting may also lead to unwanted attention that may obstruct their focus on academics as well as leading to decreased levels of self-esteem or increased levels of depression even [2]. However, its prevalence is somewhat uncertain according to one college study in the US [15].

Due to various approaches and new scales assessing cyber aggressive activity on each campus, research findings have projected a great range of results and experiences from victims. Research has shown some variability among findings concerning cyberbullying experiences among youth [16] as well, but majority of research in this field is adolescent-specific for several reasons, namely adolescents are much more involved in SNS and take more risks due to cognitive and socio-emotional differences compared to their emerging-adult peers. Such behaviors are believed to peak during middle school in which peer pressure and lack of forethought are often reasons for misguided actions among youth, especially when online.

For example of emerging adult cross-cultural comparisons, in South Korea, one study [17] reported majority of college students, three of every four college students, personally knew someone who was an actual victim of cyberbullying and over half of the sample also knew a cyberbully. In the US, one study [18] examined the rate of occurrence of several types of online bullying among emerging adults minorities. The study included questions that identified perpetrators of bullying as well as self-identified victims.

Findings indicated that well over one-third of students personally knew a cyber victim (38%). Nearly a quarter of students self-identified as victims of bullying themselves (22%). In terms of gender or ethnic differences they did not find any significant differences between type or groups but reported significant correlations between witnessing bullying and all types of cyberbully measures. Finally in terms of perpetration, they found only about 9% of participants admitted to bullying others online, a significant decline compared to the study in South Korea and slightly less frequency than another US-based study [19] that reported 10% of their sample as self-reported cyber victims and 9% for cyberstalking. Despite the variance among measures of cyber aggression, the last decade or so of findings indicate a real concern among emerging adults as well.

Another study [20] based out of the mid-Atlantic US reviewed prevalence, impact and coping strategies among college students who were targeted online within the last year. Researchers reported a fairly low percentage of reported cyberbully victims (about 9% of a sample of 800 participants), while this low number may seem positive it is important to note that among those who did report recent attacks online, the psychological impact of said attacks are quite concerning. According to the study, higher amounts of psychological distress were found among this group than compared to their non-bullied counterparts in the sample. Analyses drawn from the symptom checklist (SLC-90-R) indicated significant differences between victims and non-victims with respect to increased rates of depression, higher levels of anxiety and feelings of paranoia.

With regard to how victims behave or think after online targeting Schenk and Fremouw [20] followed up with cyber victims about their experience and how it had impacted them, if at all. Close to half of the victims had reported feelings of frustration (46%), others felt stressed out (41%). Many victims also reported feeling sadness or being hurt (38%), some were angry about the attack (s) (34%) and some shared that they were struggled to concentrate on various tasks (24%). These types of feelings may lead not only to decreased levels of self-esteem, more anger, less trust, etc., but it may become a more serious situation as this study also reported nearly 6% (5.7%) had attempted suicide and a total of 10% reported that they were thinking about suicide. For comparison, the non-victim participants reported neither suicide attempts, nor any ideation about suicide.

Comparatively, (see 13) a study in Turkey measured college students finding that over half (55%) of college students (n = 666) had been cyber victims, while nearly one quarter (22.5%) had bullied others online at least once. Females reported more victimization than males. Interestingly, succorance (to solicit sympathy or affection from others) predicted behaving as a perpetrator (as did aggression). Among cyber victims, endurance (persistence to complete tasks) was the only significant predictor of cyberbullying exposure. The author suggested that these significant "needs" reveal "psychological characteristics related to cyberbullying" (p. 1319).

## 3. Theoretical approach in understanding cyberbullying victimization

Although cyberbullying studies are often atheoretical [16], there are studies available that have quite a range of different lenses to use theory to provide a framework in which to better understand the internalized struggles in individual's psychological and behavioral processes, but also social and relational factors with peers-to-peer relationships, familial relationships and even workplace environments. Some examples of seldom used theories include intergroup emotion theory [21] which provides explanation among peer-groups and negative or intense emotions felt between a member of the group and members within the group. Within the context of cyberbullying, hateful or mean messages could elicit emotional responses. Choice theory [22] could provide another potentially helpful lens, as this theory suggests that perpetrators or victims are responsible for their own interpretations and maintain control of their own lives.

In terms of a more contemporary offering, Social dominance theory (SDT) was originally designed to uncover disparities in hierarchy and power [23]. This theory may be applicable in helping researchers to better understand victimization because this framework suggests that a cyberbully's goal is typically to inflict feelings of hurtfulness, fear, or helplessness, in other words, to harass someone and force them into submission [24]. Because cyberbullies cannot see their target's immediate reaction, they will be even more aggressive and callous to ensure harm to the victim, ultimately, ensuring dominance over the victim. If cyber victims realize they are being attacked, but do not allow attackers to see or sense their reactions, perhaps by ignoring them, this may inhibit a sense of domination and counteract the threat. On the other hand, at-risk youth in particular, have a difficult time ignoring directly harmful messages and could be at a greater risk for becoming dominated by a bully which could lead to misguided decisions.

Another lens that helps with understanding cyber victimization is routine-activities theory (RAT). Cohen and Felson [25] originally created the framework emphasizing necessity for a motivated perpetrator, an identified target and lack of surrounding safeguards (e.g., lack of monitoring, authority figure). This study has been applied to cyber aggressive research more often than most frameworks [26–29]. Even attempts to explain motivation for cyberstalking [30] or importance parental influence [31] have been explored. RAT helps to identify where victims are being targeted, methods used by cyber victims as well as to help find risk factors among victims, patterns that prevention specialists can identify and warn others with. Understanding differences in lifestyle choices between victims and non-victims may help expose risk and rate of victimization. As found in one study [32], researchers were able to determine why some targets are selected as well as why some cyber victims respond so different from others. Stemming from some types and differences of internet activities leads to increased rates of victimization. Social media being the leading cause followed by sharing personal information online.

## 4. Perspectives of negative coping from the perpetrator

Many studies on cyber aggression tend to focus on behaviors and responses from cyber victims after attacks, often anonymous and repetitive. Few tend to explore motives from a standpoint of the perpetrator, those that do often presume it is a revenge-seeking behavior primarily [8]. For example, in Argentina, researchers examined several emotional issues and personality types among cyberbullies [33]. These differences were compared to traditional bullies and other peers (n = 898) not involved as in either type of perpetrator. Eight percent identified as cyberbullies and only 4% as both traditional and cyberbullies. Interestingly, cyberbullies actually reported lowered amounts of depression or anxiety than traditional bullies reported. Cyberbullies were also less neurotic and more agreeable than traditional bullies. Perhaps the face-to-face nature of traditional bullying has higher stakes in terms of internal and external impact than online bullying in which perpetrators may not be able to see if their messages even reach their target.

Another article that wanted to understand more from the perspective of a perpetrator focused on revealing possible characteristics that are commonly found among cyberbullies [34]. One additional element the study first noted was that emerging adults, often moving away from home for first time are subject to little or no monitoring of their time or online behaviors and may be more likely to engage in or receive more online harassment [35].

### 4.1 The association between perpetration and victimization

The findings of the study (see [34]) just discussed only include cyberbullies who were involved in a minimum of four online attacks. Under this condition, only about 8% of participants (n = 799, 57% female) qualified as cyberbullies. A more selective process would theoretically increase likelihood of identifying important differences between perpetrators from others. Comparing this group of perpetrators to those who also reported as being both a cyberbully and a cyber victim, significant increases of psychological symptomology were found, especially when both of those groups were compared to the non-bully group that had significantly lower amounts of symptomology. These findings included increased reports of suicidal ideation (especially for those most heavily involved in bullying and being targeted).

In addition to exploring how those involved internalize this online phenomenon, the study also explored aggression, specifically proactive and reactive aggression. It turns out that both the cyberbullies and the bully-victims group (both cyberbullies and cyber victims) reported significantly higher levels of aggression compared to the non-involved group. So those who do not self-identify as cyberbullies or as cyber victims report significantly less aggressive behaviors. Moreover, the authors measured acceptance levels of theft, violent acts, and drug use. The group of participants that were both bullies and victims endorsed crime the most, followed by cyberbullies, both of which also significantly higher than those not involved in cyberaggression at all.

An additional study in Turkey by Aricak et al. [36] measured similar internalized responses from involvement in negative online behaviors. Although Turkey shares similarities with westernized cultures there are still significant differences in expected public and private behaviors. This could also mean significantly larger differences in how victimization is felt and/or reported. However, what this study found seems comparable to others in that one-in-five college students within the study self-reported engaging in cyberbullying and just over half at least once in the past year. Over one-third (37%) reported as being only cyber victims from unwanted online attacks. Comparatively, and uniquely high compared to other studies, is that nearly 18% of the participants identified as being a cyberbully and cyber victim. Two key takeaways from this particular study is that one, the majority of cyberbullies pretended to be someone else to mask their identity; second, that higher levels of hostility towards others and psychoticism significantly predicted involvement in cyberbullying. From the studies discussed so far, it is apparent that something is psychologically wrong with individuals who are recipients of cyberbullying as well as a perpetrator of said phenomena.

Another Turkish study [37] surveyed emerging adults and found close to 23% of their participants (n = 666) bullied others online at least one time. One of the unique findings from this study was that it was found that soliciting attention or sympathy from others predicted cyberbully behaviors; same was true for higher rates of aggression. This particular finding may suggest that narcissism or other attention-seeking behaviors may draw attention to oneself, but not necessarily in the way originally attended which may lead to lashing out or other aggressive behaviors.

A study in Portugal [13] (reviewed in depth below) assessed group-level differences between the non-victims, cyberbully-victims and cyberbullies, researchers found elevated levels of fear, sadness for cyber victims as discussed earlier but physical fights were highest among cyberbullies as well as having an easier time making new friends. Adolescent youth, particularly true for males, have long used aggressive behaviors against peers for their social gain [38] and this could explain motivation behind perpetration online as well as in person [39]. Those who engage in aggressive motives also lack empathy [40] often.

### 4.2 Digital self-harm

In the US, a study by Patchin and Hinduja [41] explored the act of cyberbullying oneself anonymously among a nationally representative sample of 12–17 year olds. Over 6% admitted that they had anonymously posted something mean about themselves. Just over one-third (35%) did this a few times and over 10% reported posting mean things about themselves multiple times. Moving beyond simply posting mean things about oneself, 5% of the sample reported actually self-cyberbullying. Of those who did self-cyberbully, 18% did so many times with males being significantly more likely to do so than their female counterparts. By means of open-ended questioning, the authors were able to identify reasoning first, for posting mean things about oneself and also explore reasoning for actually the cyberbullying of oneself. Over 30 reported it was due hating themselves, some shared it was an attempt at seeking attention. While more individuals reported it was just to be funny or joking around when bored, 15 individuals shared depressive symptoms and suicidal feelings.

In 2019, another exploratory study conducted in New Zealand [42] presented findings centered on extent of prevalence of self-harm. The study defined digital self-harm as "anonymous online posting or sharing of mean or negative online content about oneself" (p. 1). Self-cyberbullying has seldom been considered (see [43]) as an area of concern prior to this exploratory study but due to narcissistic behaviors often connected to selfie-taking culture [44], it is wise to explore this phenomena.

Among their randomized sample of just over 1000 adolescents (13–17), they reported 6% of New Zealand teens have participated in digital self-harm within the last year. Further, that those who did participate in this behavior, nearly two-thirds (65%) did so more than one occasion. Younger teenagers were more likely to engage in this phenomenon of self-harm compared to older teens. Some of the motivations behind digital self-harm uncovered were that individuals wanted to simply make a self-deprecating joke to entertain others, others wanted to prove or show their own resilience to receiving negative feedback. Teenagers were also motivated to do this as an attention-seeking behavior as a means of amassing sympathy from friends, to receive their reassurance of peer-support and friendship.

In terms of other unique differences that may help shield some light on this are gender differences that were revealed specifically about motivation. Girls tended to focus on aspect of showing resilience, reassurance from peers (as discussed) whereas boys were more likely to share reasoning from perspective of simply making a joke. Perhaps to be expected, those who did not participate in digital self-harm believed their peers engage in the behavior to gain attention and sympathy. Just over one-third of those who did the behavior however, reported achieving the desired outcome from engaging.

### 4.3 Perpetration by sexism

In 2019, a study conducted among university students in Spain also took a different approach into trying to understand perspectives of a cyberbully [45]. By examining dating relationships through mobile phone and online means of communication, this study sought to identify if cyberbullying by via acts of sexism was a significant factor among males towards their female counterparts. Indeed preliminary data revealed males engaged in higher levels of cyberbullying directed towards their girlfriends, significantly more than girlfriends did to their male counterparts. When considering sex and attitude as a contributing factor it was found that male hostile beliefs predicted cyberbullying toward their girlfriends through both mobile phone and the internet.

A qualitative study in Australia [46] by means of a focus group with adolescent youth sought to explore their understanding of sexting and cyberbullying. The researcher provided video clips to start conversation which covered the topic of slut-shaming. While participants understood slut-shaming as a form of sexism and even cyberbullying, some within the focus group justified the label as deserved in some cases. Interestingly, the study found that girls shared concern of being bullied because of nude or partial-nude images that may not even actually have been their own. An added area of concern was reported that individuals could be cyberbullied even if images or messages were shared without consent.

### 4.4 Drug and alcohol use

Another important consideration for researchers in understanding how cyberbullies behave should involve exploration of drugs and alcohol. Understanding how cyberbullies may cope with their own issues or engage in risky behaviors may provide important answers in learning how to prevent cyberbullying in the future as well as lower risky behaviors that may cause endangerment to self or other innocent people.

Recently, a study explored drug and alcohol use with a nationally representative sample of adolescents in Portugal [13]. Significant differences were found in consumption of alcohol and drug consumption. Cyberbullies did report a larger consumption of drugs, however it was the cyberbully-victims (both a victim and perpetrator of bullying) that most significantly used alcohol, even more than victims-only group. Researchers also explored peers' perspective of school-involvement and found cyber victims remained more connected to school whereas cyberbullies were less connected and also had lower well-being. Perhaps social/cultural connections are more constrained among cyberbullies for whatever reason, but there are clear differences among these group comparisons.

## 5. Motivation of a perpetrator

In a meta-analysis exploring an expansive body of work involving traditional bullying, traditional victimization, cyberbullying, and cyber victimization) researchers conducted a forest plot (see **Figure 1** below) which displayed predictor and outcome relationships in regard to cyberbullying ([3]. Strength (and direction) of correlations are available at the bottom of the figure. As this chapter has discussed, the figure illustrates quite clearly areas of concern among cyberbully perpetrators, their lack of empathy, low self-esteem, connection to victimization and traditional bullying, as well as a myriad of other negative internalized and externalized coping methods (e.g., lonely) or behaviors (e.g., spending time online).

In greater detail, those experiencing cyber victimization was strongly (positively) related to also being a perpetrator. The same was true of traditional bullies thus indicating the comorbid nature of bullying in person or online as suggested by previous works [1, 16]. Other, more moderate findings from the body of work presented in the findings were positive associations with acceptance of aggression and moral disengagement. Online risky behaviors were not as strongly correlated with cyberbullying but were significant; the same was true of narcissistic behavior, or feelings of anger. Increased level of cyberbullying perpetrations were also inversely correlated with safety, empathy and parental monitoring. By combining the works of several studies these findings provide a larger picture of the state of mind of cyberbullies and is useful for those interested in helping cyberbullies learn to cope more positively with past negative interactions, in person or online. Low parental monitoring and personal beliefs about aggression may be especially important to address particularly among youth and adolescents. By teaching digital citizenry early and assertively, they may develop better, more healthy coping skills.

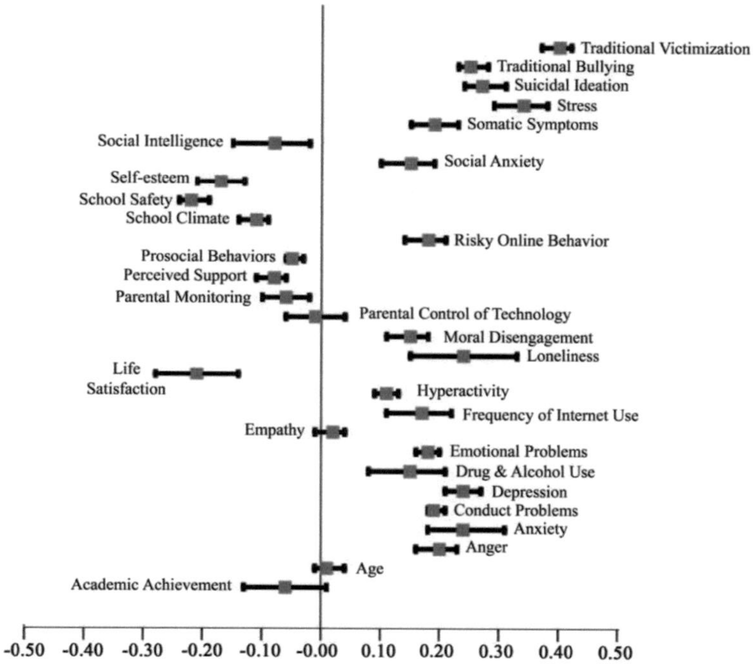


**Figure 1.**
*Forest plot for meta-analytic correlates of cyberbullying perpetration. Permission to share this original figure [3] granted from American Psychological Association.*

### 5.1 Motivation and reasoning in hiding behind the screen

In 2008, a qualitative study by Vandebosch and Van Cleemput [47] included over 50 focus groups comprised of youth and adolescents from 10 to 18 years of age. Within these groups the authors explored how youngsters interpreted cyberbullying behaviors, more specifically, the motivation in hiding behind a screen and aim of the perpetrator. Some findings from the focus groups indicated a clear understanding that cyberbullies want to cause actual pain and are sometimes motivated by revenge from traditional bullying during school. Some also cyberbullied anonymously because of arguments or disagreements they had face-to-face and wanted to get back at them. Boredom was also shared as a reason for engaging in cyberbullying as well as a feeling or sense of power and skill, while also understanding the importance of not divulging who they were.

Researchers were able to find that one common theme among those who admitted to cyberbullying others was that they were disguising themselves largely because their targets knew who they were in real life. Their targets were also considered weak for some or stronger for others and so motivation of bullying had some range. Weaker targets were also traditionally bullied, but stronger targets were chosen to empower the cyberbully, to feel like they could have some strength that otherwise would not get in a face-to-face situation. Individuals also shared that in some cases (friends or past friends), they were willing to give up their anonymity after some time.

Through a path model analyses, another study [48] was able to show the importance of anonymity as a predictor for cyberbullying. Anonymity was found to mediate sending IMs (instant messages) and cyberbullying. Being anonymous also served as a moderator between positive attitude toward acting as a perpetrator and frequency of attacking others. Thus, once anonymity is thought to be achieved, consequences of punishment are lowered and cyberbullying is more likely to occur. Use of e-mail was negatively related to anonymity and positive attitude towards cyberbullying, most likely to due to difficulty of keeping email from being identifiable. These findings are important to understand given the nature of new and ever-changing SNSs and applications. Apps that come out, even those designed for younger children may have talking, messaging, or direct messaging features and if permitted, the ability to remain anonymous will predictably allow for cyberbullying.

## 6. Theoretical approaches in understanding perpetration

General strain theory (GST) may serve as one of the superior frameworks for understanding motivation behind cyberbullies. Originally, this theory was used to explain the gap between feelings of aspiration and expectation [49]. In the 1930s, Merton suggested that the American dream was difficult to achieve and for those who felt the pressures of success but did not reach their expectations, they were more likely to engage in deviant, even criminal behaviors in order to help themselves reach their aspirations. Today, GST suggests that as individuals are pressured or rather, strained and pushed up against a wall, this will eventually result in negative feelings and ultimately towards deviant or risky behaviors. In the context of the internet and social media, individuals that are not as popular, or are bullied at school because of a power imbalance, could turn to cyberbullying as a means of coping or seeking revenge.

One study [50] applied GST in order to explain adolescent youth engaging in two forms of bullying (traditional/face-to-face and cyberbullying). The researchers were able to find support for GST by means of a direct relationship both types of bullying and strain. In other words, those who did feel increasingly more strain were more likely to engage in bullying in face-to-face situations but also cyberbullying. Negative emotions (e.g., anger, frustration) were correlated to bullying and these may serve as vehicle of strain pushing these youth to turn to perpetration. Moreover, negative copings methods may also lead to an increase of feelings of strain that may also lead towards deviant behaviors or potentially, self-harm.

In 2010, researchers actually applied GST to explore how strain may be built up among cyber victims, leading to self-harm [51]. GST is usually thought of as a lens for going on the offensive, committing crimes or attacking others; however, it does make sense to explore victims' responses when on the receiving side of bullying. Results from a survey involving over 400 adolescents found that traditional bullying victimization and cyber victimization were positively related to self-harm and thoughts about suicide. Similar to the aforementioned study, negative emotions are connected to feelings of strain. One additional element important to the scope and nature of feelings of strain was that one parenting style (authoritative-parents that are firm but fair) and having a high level of self-control removed any harmful effect from bullying.

Another theoretical lens that serves to explain motivation of perpetrators may be that of deindividuation theory (DT). Zimbardo [52, 53] created experimental conditions in which individuals could inflict pain anonymously. Indeed, those who were anonymous did shock confederates for a longer period of time. As the Stanford Prison Experiment is famously remembered, a deindividuated state yielded increased acts of aggression in the prison setting and the study was canceled altogether. Today, this lens may be more helpful as it suggests why individuals that are hidden, anonymous, or at least feel/believe that they are will eventually drop

*DOI: http://dx.doi.org/10.5772/intechopen.91433*

their guard, lowering their self-awareness which eventually may lead to antinormative behaviors [54]. Such behaviors may include engaging in unwanted sexual solicitations, getting into arguments and eventually encouraging their targets to kill themselves as discussions escalate. Brandtzaeg and colleagues suggested that anonymity is not the only important element in choosing to bully others, but that a lack of self-awareness is necessary to allow oneself to forget who they are, what they may stand for and to freely attack others online.

In 2017 another study [55] explored how DT may help explain lack of remorse among a large sample of college student cyberbullies. Cyber victims were also surveyed about their feelings of anonymous attacks. Through chi-square analyses and a series of regression models they found partial support for DT. While anonymity should provide a cover for perpetrators, cyber victims from this study were somewhat confident in identifying who their anonymous attacker was. In terms of cyberbullies, they were able to find that indeed, feelings of anonymity enabled cyberbullying behaviors. One additional finding from responses suggest that while anonymity helps permit aggressive actions, simply being hidden and keeping one's true identity secret should not be considered cyberbullying.

Oblad et al. [55] also gathered qualitative data from a series of open-ended questions to further investigate DT. Three themes emerged when participants were asked about their perceived acceptance of cyberbullying and anonymity. Majority of respondents were not okay with it at any level and many recommended avoiding involvement at all costs. Another theme suggested that there are some acceptable behaviors as long as they do not cross just joking or teasing, several hundred responses indicated that even when joking it may be perceived as targeting and thus is a "gray area," especially if messages are received or posted anonymously. The last theme that emerged suggested that participating indirectly is also a form of cyberbullying, for example liking or sharing videos or hurtful messages and not reporting them crosses the line.

## 7. Conclusions

This chapter has reviewed ways in which cyber victims are impacted negatively when they are victimized online or through social media. Many cyber victims lose self-esteem, delete their social media profiles, feel more depressed or even attempt suicide. Other victims simply ignore the bullying or report it and have no negative coping methods. Theoretical frameworks are important to help understand why and how some cyber victims are more capable than others in coping methods and routine activities theory may provide that knowledge.

Cyberbullying research typically focuses on victimization and the impact among them; however, cyberbullies themselves suffer from a myriad of mental and emotional issues. Their aggressive behaviors and other risk-behaviors were discussed to provide some reasoning, signs of maladaptive behaviors and examples of negative coping methods for those interested in preventing individuals from intentionally harming others as well as themselves. This field has come a long way over the last 15 years and it is clear that our cognitive and social-emotional states are somewhat well-connected to our online presence. What remains unclear is the best way to maintain safe, positive digital citizenship and how to help individuals avoid falling into deindividuated states, leading to aggressive acts against others.

## Author details

Timothy Oblad
Texas A&M University-Kingsville, Kingsville, Texas, USA

*Address all correspondence to: timothy.oblad@tamuk.edu

## References

[1] Kowalski R, Morgan C, Limber S. Traditional bullying as a potential warning sign of cyberbullying. School Psychology International. 2012;**33**:505-519

[2] Oblad T. Cyberbullying among emerging adults: Exploring prevalence, impact, and coping methods. International Journal of Criminology & Sociology. 2019;7:45-54

[3] Kowalski R, Giumetti G, Schroeder A, Lattanner M. Bullying in the digital age: A critical review and meta-analysis of cyberbullying research among youth. Psychological Bulletin. 2014;**140**:1073

[4] Donegan R. Bullying and cyberbullying: History, statistics, law, prevention and analysis. The Elon Journal of Undergraduate Research in Communications. 2012;**3**:33-42

[5] Olweus D. Bullying at school. In: Aggressive Behavior. Boston, MA: Springer; 1994. pp. 97-130

[6] Ybarra ML, Mitchell KJ. Online aggressor/targets, aggressors, and targets: A comparison of associated youth characteristics. Journal of Child Psychology and Psychiatry. 2004;**45**:1308-1316

[7] Sabella RA, Patchin JW, Hinduja S. Cyberbullying myths and realities. Computers in Human Behavior. 2013;**29**(6):2703-2711

[8] König A, Gollwitzer M, Steffgen G. Cyberbullying as an act of revenge? Journal of Psychologists and Counsellors in Schools. 2010;**20**(2):210-224

[9] Campfield DC. Cyber Bullying and Victimization: Psychosocial Characteristics of Bullies, Victims, and *Bully-Victims*. 2006. (Doctoral dissertation). Retrieved from: http://etd.lib.umt.edu/theses/available/.../umi-umt-1107.pdf

[10] Sontag LM, Clemans KH, Graber JA, Lyndon ST. Traditional and cyber aggressors and victims: A comparison of psychosocial characteristics. Journal of Youth and Adolescence. 2011;**40**:392-404

[11] Vandebosch H, Van Cleemput K. Cyberbullying among youngsters: Profiles of bullies and victims. New Media & Society. 2009;**11**:1349-1371

[12] Powell J. 33 Million People in the Room: How to Create, Influence, and Run a Successful Business with Social Networking. Indianapolis, IN: Que Publishing; 2009

[13] Carvalho M, Branquinho C, Matos M. Cyberbullies, cybervictims and cyberbully-victims: Discriminant factors in Portuguese adolescents. Psicologia, Saude & Doencas. 2017;**18**:657-668

[14] Sleglova V, Cerna A. Cyberbullying in adolescent victims: Perception and coping. Cyberpsychology: Journal of Psychosocial Research on Cyberbase. 2011;**5**(2):1

[15] Hinduja S, Patchin JW. Cyberbullying fact sheet: Identification, prevention, and response. Cyberbullying Research Center. Retrieved from: http://www.cyberbullying.us/Cyberbullying_Identification_Prevention_Response_Fact_Sheet.pdf

[16] Oblad T. Understanding Cyberbullying in the Net Generation: A Meta-Analytic Review. doctoral dissertation; 2012

[17] Ismail T, Kim C. The prevalence and views on cyber-bullying and related

internet regulation among South Korean University students. American Association of Behavioral & Social Science Journal. 2010;**14**:89-103

[18] MacDonald C, Roberts-Pittman B. Cyberbullying among college students: Prevalence and demographic differences. Procedia—Social and Behavioral Sciences. 2010;**9**:2003-2009

[19] Kraft E, Wang J. An exploratory study of the cyberbullying and cyberstalking experiences and factors related to victimization of students at a public liberal arts college. International Journal of Technoethics. 2010;**1**:74-91

[20] Schenk A, Fremouw W. Prevalence, psychological impact, and coping of cyberbully victims among college students. Journal of School Violence. 2012;**11**:21-37

[21] Jones SE, Manstead AS, Livingstone AG. Ganging up or sticking together? Group processes and children's responses to text-message bullying. British Journal of Psychology. 2011;**102**(1):71-96

[22] Verecio RL. Applications of latent Dirichlet allocation algorithm of published articles on cyberbullying. International Journal of Applied Engineering Research. 2017;**12**(21):10878-10884

[23] Sidanius J, Liu JH, Shaw JS, Pratto F. Social dominance orientation, hierarchy attenuators and hierarchy enhancers: Social dominance theory and the criminal justice system. Journal of Applied Social Psychology. 1994;**24**:338-366

[24] Pellegrini AD, Long JD. A longitudinal study of bullying, dominance, and victimization during the transition from primary school through secondary school. British Journal of Developmental Psychology. 2002;**20**:259-280

[25] Cohen LE, Felson M. Social change and crime rate trends: A routine activity approach. American Sociological Review. 1979;**44**:588-608

[26] Arntfield M. Towards a cybervictimology: Cyberbullying, routine activities theory, and the anti-sociality of social media. Canadian Journal of Communication. 11 Aug 2015;**40**:371-388

[27] Beran T, Li Q. Cyber-harassment: A study of a new method for an old behavior. Journal of Educational Computing Research. 2005;**32**:265

[28] Holt T, Bossler A. Examining the applicability of lifestyle-routine activities theory for cybercrime victimization. Deviant Behavior. 2008;**30**:1-25

[29] Navarro J, Jasinski J. Going cyber: Using routine activities theory to predict cyberbullying experiences. Sociological Spectrum. 2012;**32**:81-94

[30] Reyns BW, Henson B, Fisher BS. Being pursued online: Applying cyberlifestyle–routine activities theory to cyberstalking victimization. Criminal Justice and Behavior. 2011;**38**(11):1149-1169

[31] Dehue F, Bolman C, Völlink T. Cyberbullying: Youngsters' experiences and parental perception. Cyberpsychology & Behavior. 2008;**11**(2):217-223

[32] Mesch G. Parental mediation, online activities, and cyberbullying. Cyberpsychology & Behavior. 2009;**29**:387-393

[33] Resett S, Gámez-Guadix M. Traditional bullying and cyberbullying: Differences in emotional problems, and personality. Are cyberbullies more Machiavellians? Journal of Adolescence. 2017;**61**:113-116

[34] Schenk AM, Fremouw WJ, Keelan CM. Characteristics of college cyberbullies. Computers in Human Behavior. 2013;**29**(6):2320-2327

[35] Walrave M, Heirman W. Cyberbullying: Predicting victimisation and perpetration. Children & Society. 2011;**25**(1):59-72

[36] Aricak T, Siyahhan S, Uzunhasanoglu A, Saribeyoglu S, Ciplak S, Yilmaz N, et al. Cyberbullying among Turkish adolescents. Cyberpsychology & Behavior. 2008;**11**(3):253-261

[37] Dilmac B. Psychological needs as a predictor of cyber bullying: A preliminary report on college students. Educational Sciences: Theory & Practice. 2009;**9**:1307-1325

[38] Archer J, Coyne SM. An integrated review of indirect, relational, and social aggression. Personality and Social Psychology Review. 2005;**9**(3):212-230

[39] Spears B, Slee P, Owens L, Johnson B. Behind the scenes and screens: Insights into the human dimension of covert and cyberbullying. Journal of Psychology. 2009;**217**(4):189-196

[40] Ang RP, Goh DH. Cyberbullying among adolescents: The role of affective and cognitive empathy, and gender. Child Psychiatry & Human Development. 2010;**41**(4):387-397

[41] Patchin JW, Hinduja S. Digital self-harm among adolescents. Journal of Adolescent Health. 2017;**61**(6):761-766

[42] Pacheco E, Melhuish N, Fiske J. Digital self-harm: Prevalence, motivations and outcomes for teens who cyberbully themselves. SSRN Electronic Journal; 1 May 2019

[43] Pacheco E, Melhuish N. New Zealand teens and digital harm: Statistical insights into experiences, impact and response. SSRN Electronic Journal; 5 Jun 2018

[44] Halpern D, Valenzuela S, Katz JE. "Selfie-ists" or "Narci-selfiers"?: A cross-lagged panel analysis of selfie taking and narcissism. Personality and Individual Differences. 2016;**97**:98-101

[45] Martinez-Pecino R, Durán M. I love you but I cyberbully you: The role of hostile sexism. Journal of Interpersonal Violence. 2019;**34**(4):812-825

[46] Dobson AS. 'The things you didn't do': Gender, slut-shaming, and the need to address sexual harassment in narrative resources responding to sexting and cyberbullying. In: Narratives in Research and Interventions on Cyberbullying among Young People. Cham: Springer; 2019. pp. 147-160

[47] Vandebosch H, Van Cleemput K. Defining cyberbullying: A qualitative research into the perceptions of youngsters. Cyberpsychology & Behavior. 2008;**11**(4):499-503

[48] Barlett CP. Anonymously hurting others online: The effect of anonymity on cyberbullying frequency. Psychology of Popular Media Culture. 2015;**4**(2):70

[49] Merton RK. Social structure and anomie. American Sociological Review. 1938;**3**(5):672-682

[50] Patchin JW, Hinduja S. Traditional and nontraditional bullying among youth: A test of general strain theory. Youth & Society. 2011;**43**(2):727-751

[51] Hay C, Meldrum R, Mann K. Traditional bullying, cyber bullying, and deviance: A general strain theory approach. Journal of Contemporary Criminal Justice. 2010;**26**(2):130-147

[52] Zimbardo PG. The human choice: Individuation, reason, and order versus

deindividuation, impulse, and chaos. In: Nebraska symposium on motivation. University of Nebraska press; 1969

[53] Zimbardo PG. Prison Life Study: General Information. Available from: www.prisonexp.org

[54] Brandtzæg PB, Staksrud E, Hagen I, Wold T. Norwegian children's experiences of cyberbullying when using different technological platforms. Journal of Children and Media. 2009;**3**(4):349-365

[55] Oblad T, Trejos-Castillo E, Massengale E. Exploring cyberbullying among college students: Perceptions of anonymity. In: Proceedings of the 97th Southwestern Social Sciences Association Conference; 2017

Chapter 4

# Musical Performance Anxiety (MPA)

*Sérgio de Figueiredo Rocha*

## Abstract

The musical practice is an extremely complex activity that involves a series of cognitive abilities and functions, among them are hearing, memory, motor coordination, attention, affection, mathematical calculation, and the association of all of these concomitantly, including situations of public exposure. Because of this, musical performance is particularly susceptive to anxiety symptoms. Musical performance anxiety (MPA) is defined as an experience of persistent and distressing apprehension and/or real prejudice of the performance abilities in a public context in an unjustifiable degree given the individual musical aptitude and preparation level. It prevails more commonly on the female gender in a 3:1 proportion and affects about 20% of the professional musicians. In the present chapter, its main etiologies and psychic mechanisms, evaluation instruments, as well as the current therapeutic strategies available will be presented.

**Keywords:** performance anxiety, musical performance anxiety, musicians, perceived causes, psychological intervention, drug therapies, optimal performance

## 1. Introduction

The musical practice is an extremely complex activity that involves a series of cognitive abilities and functions, among them are hearing, memory, motor coordination, attention, affection, mathematical calculation, and the association of all of these concomitantly, including situations of public exposure [1]. Because of this, musical performance is particularly susceptive to anxiety symptoms.

Anxiety in itself is, up to a certain point, something favorable to the performance [2], since it helps the performer to perceive what favors him and disregard what could hinder his performance. After a certain point, anxiety starts to influence negatively the musical performance efficiency, according to the Yerkes-Dodson curve (**Figure 1**).

Musical performance anxiety (MPA) is a term that encompasses many dimensions and started being described in 1990. It is the experience of a persistent and distressing apprehension and/or real prejudice of the performance abilities in a public context in an unjustifiable degree given the individual musical aptitude and preparation level [3].

In the musical environment, MPA has been called as "stage fright" although MPA encompasses something much bigger than that [4]. The reason is that MPA has three axes that complement each other in terms of subjective manifestations of this picture.

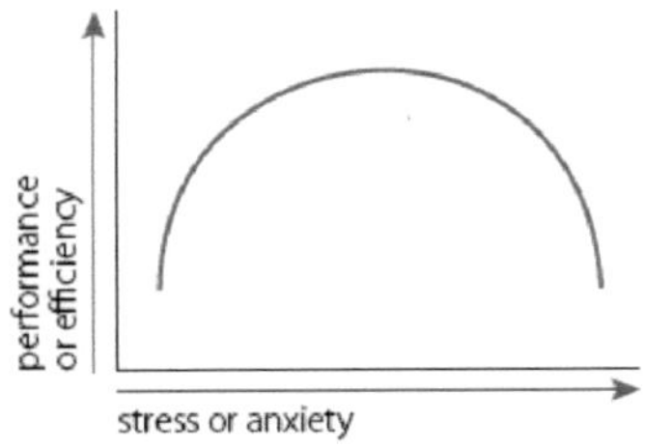


**Figure 1.**
*The Yerkes-Dodson curve.*

Performance anxiety affects equally music professional and students. There is a prevalence of around 18% [5]. The main reported symptoms are concentration decrease, tachycardia, tremor, sweating, and xerostomia, which are severe enough to negatively impact on the performance level [5, 6].

In the Diagnostic and Statistical Manual of Mental Disorders, 5th edition, or DSM-5, social anxiety disorder (SAD) is highlighted, in which the subject feels fear or anxiety in social interaction situations when he worries about the possibility of coming to be evaluated by the public [4].

In the present chapter, general aspects of MPA, its possible etiologies, its occurrence in the diverse age groups, the instruments of evaluation, and, at last, the therapeutic approaches will be approached.

## 2. MPA pathogenesis, susceptibility, and vulnerability

MPA is a complex phenomenon caused by the interaction of many factors, including genetics, environmental stimuli and individual experience, emotions, cognitions, and personal behavior.

Factors like age, gender, the kind of musical instrument, musical background, musical perception, perfectionism, and emotions compose the group of personal variables that can interfere more or less on the MPA levels [4, 7].

Although MPA can begin in childhood, the literary data are conflicting. While some studies suggest that in this age group there are no significant differences between the genders [8], others point out that there are significant differences in many parameters (physiological, cognitive, behavioral, and subjective perception) [9]. For example, the girls tend to show an anticipatory anxiety and also during the performance, while the boys only show anxiety during the performance. This profile seems to present itself gradually even more unfavorable to the female gender as age advances [10]. These data indicate that women are significantly less confident and more anxious and show less self-efficacy (attitude) in contexts such as jazz improvising learning. In women over 45 years old, the MPA prevalence is even bigger and can achieve up to 60% depending on the context [11]. However, there is a great relation between MPA and age increase among susceptible individuals, independently of the gender.

The way in which each individual processes his beliefs about the performance situation and how he perceives the way his somatic anxiety reactions affect his performance. This behavior is related to perfectionism. Perfectionism, a personality valence, is a complex and multidimensional construction that goes beyond the simple search for perfection. It concerns the fight for unreal self-imposed patterns, a fixed mentality, high levels of self-criticism, or expectation of high patterns of performance by a third party. This distorted expectation about one's own performance ends up influencing negatively self-confidence, and this, ultimately, can sabotage the performance quality.

Another important aspect that has been studied is the public impact over the performer [6]. In situations where the musicians are being judged in some kind of competition or selection, there is a significantly bigger incidence of symptoms such as tachycardia and anxiety observed compared to situations that do not involve judgment.

The three causes of MPA most commonly cited by musicians are pressure from self, excessive arousal, and inadequate preparation for performance [12]. Beyond personal impressions there seems to be a combination between genetic vulnerability and the learning environment [4, 7]. This learning environment is the result that builds a psychic pattern confrontation of the performance situations. This building is the sum of the situations that involve familiar experiences with teachers, colleagues, tests, and performances.

The *Barlow* model seems to be the most consecrated among the MPA scholars. It consists of an integrated group of three vulnerabilities: biological (genetics, endocrine, etc.) and psychological, that is, referring to the subject psychic formation and more specific psychological issues in which the environmental stimuli are processed according to the patterns learned by the individual [5, 13–15].

The psychological vulnerabilities are structured by elements like affection, cognition and its processing, attention, and personality traits [13, 15]. All these elements are processed together. For example, when attention is deviated from the performance priority objects, it can sabotage its own efficiency. The hyper-focus in a determined aspect of the performance can, equally, cause the performer to lose a systemic view of what is being presented.

The previous musical experiences and other experiences related to anxiety involved in personal and professional histories are also important in the MPA genesis [4].

Therefore, the most vulnerable profile to MPA can be identified. The subject that feels anxious only in the presence of the public and in front of them has unrealistic beliefs about his own potential is the most specific profile. This characteristic was also described in the DSM-5 new edition which "seems to represent a distinct subgroup of social anxiety disorder in etiology terms, initial age, physiological response, and treatment [16].

## 3. MPA in children and adolescents

Since the first childhood (up to 7 years old), MPA is rarely manifested, differently from adults/elderly ones [17]. On the contrary, children tend to show others their "feats" in a pleasurable way. The question is that this same subject, some years later, starts to develop a behavior opposite to this, avoiding to a maximum his own exposure to whoever it is.

The main factors that lead to this change in attitude are the innate temper, the trace of anxiety, the broadening of the integrated capacity of cognition, the auto-reflexive function, and the accumulation of the anxiogenic interpersonal experiences. The conjunction of these factors contributes for the formation of beliefs and emotions during performance in the adolescence [18].

The emotions that emerge in moments that precede the performance are positive as well as negatives. This occurrence of joint affections in general is uncomfortable. Therefore there is the need to work on recognizing this emotion/affection so that afterwards, there is a control of this situation. However, the reception given by the parents, teachers, and more experienced colleagues is fundamental for a better processing of these beliefs on behalf of the younger musicians, especially preadolescents.

It was observed that the students who started the musical practice after 7 years of age showed higher anxiety scores when compared to those who started at the age of 7 or less [19]. This has direct implications in the preventive strategies against MPA among children and adolescents. These strategies should privilege the recreation and in every opportunity minimize the negative aspects of the performance; in other words, the occurrence of some mistakes in the face of countless right ones does not matter.

## 4. MPA evaluation instruments

Currently, about 20 instruments validated in the English language[1] to evaluate MPA are available [3]. The majority of these scales is generic, that is, they are not specific for an instrument, although some are. There is the Piano Performance Anxiety Scale and the Stage Fright Rating Scale (specific for string musicians). Many of them are adaptations of the already existing scales for anxiety evaluation. These scales are aimed at the musicians' adult population. The *K-MPAI* and *perfAIM* scales will be highlighted as follows.

The *K-MPAI* is the MPA evaluation instrument that has more validations for other idioms in the world [20]. Its original version had 26 items, and the most recent one, published in 2009, has 40 items. The *Appel's Personal Report of Confidence as a Performer* (PRCP) and the *Performance Anxiety Inventory* (PAI) structured themselves having as their referential the three components of the *Barlow Theory* [3]; in other words, such scales encompass physiologic, cognitive, and behavioral aspects. In *K-MPAI* the people interviewed use a *Likert*-type scale of 7 points to answer each question, where zero represents no observed anxiety symptom and 6 represents extremely high levels of anxiety. Therefore, the score can vary from zero (Ø) to 240 points. A search to find a cutoff point has been made; however, the cut-off point concerning each test criteria vary, suggesting that the *K-MPAI* cutoff point depends on the clinical interest of each patient [20].

Another validated scale in 2011 was the *PerfAIM* [21]. The *PerfAIM* comprise 58 declarations divided into 34 items and 24 subitems. The possible scores vary from 58 to 290. Due to the normal standard distribution, the scale author suggested that the scores between 100 and 205 corresponded to the MPA normality band under stressful situations, whereas values above these are associated to extreme cases which would demand more attention. Besides, this reference interval can help to establish a level of comparison among the subjects, independently of the sample.

The *K-MPAI-A* is the correlative to *K-MPAI* for adolescents from 12 to 19 years old [8]. Despite being an instrument aimed at young ones in this age group, it was applied in other studies including 7-year-old children. Such as the version for the adult population, its structure also encompasses the physical, behavioral, and cognitive aspects; however, there are only 15 questions. The fulfilling scheme follows the *K-MPAI* for adults, so it is also the *Likert* type.

The main contribution of these scales is the assistance of the subjects and, together with other approach strategies, the structure of a continuous segmented project and, if necessary, subject treatment.

## 5. MPA management, treatments, and approach strategies

The MPA involves, in general, combined strategies. These strategies can be divided in therapies, medicinal intervention, and other approaches. The first

[1] Some of them are validated in more than 20 languages.

published studies that investigated the MPA non-pharmacological treatments are dated from the beginning of the 1980s, while the pharmacological studies started in the late 1960s decade [14].

### 5.1 Therapies

Among the therapeutic interventions, the main strategies pointed out in the literature are behavioral therapy, cognitive therapy, cognitive-behavioral therapy [14, 22–25], hypnosis [24–26], and, more recently, the Acceptance and Commitment Therapy (ACT) [27].

The cognitive and behavioral therapies have as their main objective to approach emotions and dysfunctional behaviors. The interest is in accessing thought patterns that form themselves and become more and more disabling if not treated. Therefore, these therapies aim at a change of faulty thought styles and their consequent inadequate behaviors [25].

The desensitizing process present in the cognitive-behavioral therapy allows, through guided images, the scene that generates anxiety to be gradually transformed in something more adaptive that does not involve anxiety. The reason is that learned answers can be substituted by more adaptive behaviors [25].

Hypnosis or hypnotherapy consists in inducing the patient to a state of sleepiness, easing the access to issues that involve the problems of nonadaptive behavior or dysfunctional thoughts. This access would allow an awareness to begin a change process in the way the subject deals with situations that generate MPA [25].

The Acceptance and Commitment Therapy is one of the most recent therapies of the *third wave* in which the dialectical behavioral therapy, the metacognitive therapy, and the depression therapy based on mindfulness are also part of it [27]. The focus of this therapy is the promotion of full attention and someone's emotional suffering acceptance instead of the symptom domain or control as in the conventional cognitive behavioral therapies.

### 5.2 Strategies and complementary therapies

Besides the classic therapies, there are MPA complementary control strategies. Among them expressive arts therapy (in which one is exposed to virtual reality [images] and music therapy), yoga, meditation, the Alexander technique, biofeedback, neurofeedback, and transcranial stimulation [23, 25] can be mentioned.

Image-guided therapy consists of employing internal images of the subjects to reveal and access internal conflicts that possibly relate themselves to the MPA genesis. This method is used frequently in sports performance [25, 28]. For this kind of strategy, the results show MPA level reduction, discomfort improvement, increase of self-confidence, and decrease of heart rate [23].

Music therapy, in turn, promotes a better musical and musicality perception and decreases the stress like distractibility [25].

There are few studies about the yoga impact on MPA [23]. In the few available studies, improvements of the MPA indicators, including humor, sleep and osteoarticular disturbances, and stress, were observed.

There are still no evidences that meditation alone can, in some unquestionable way, contribute to decrease the MPA indicators [23]. The few available studies only raise questions that speculate that meditation can be related to an improvement in some parameters such as heart rate.

The Alexander technique consists of closely observing the individual's attitude and, in the musical practice sphere, trying to check the more accurate possible causes of tension in the performer's body. Therefore, this technique can relieve muscle tensions and contribute to decrease the factors that impact, directly or indirectly, the MPA levels [29].

Biofeedback has been used for about 70 years in the experimental psychology and neurology fields [30]. It is a technique to accurately measure some organic data such as brain waves, heart rate, respiratory rate, muscle activity, and skin temperature. The main objective of this technique is to provide learning of the self-control of these functions. Thus, biofeedback can be part of a strategy to treat anxiety since it contributes to control part of the symptoms which are part of MPA. It is usually associated with other strategies [30, 31].

Neurofeedback is a kind of biofeedback that teaches individuals the self-control of brain functions, measuring the brain waves and providing a feedback signal. Neurofeedback usually does not provide an audio and/or video feedback. Positive or negative feedback is produced for desired goals or undesirable brain activities, respectively [32]. There are seven kinds of feedback, two of which are indicated for anxiety treatment, which makes this technique potentially suitable for treating MPA. The more frequent neurofeedback used is the frequency/power neurofeedback. It is used to alter the amplitude or velocity of specific brain waves in specific brain areas to treat TDAH, anxiety, and insomnia. This technique usually includes the use of two to four surface electrodes, sometimes called neurofeedback. There is a second modality called low energy neurofeedback system (LENS) which provides weak electromagnetic signal to alter brain waves on the patient while he is motionless and with his eyes closed. This kind of feedback has been used to treat traumatic brain injuries, TDAH, insomnia, fibromyalgia, restless legs syndrome, anxiety, depression, and irritability [33].

About 25% of the cases that involve anxiety are not responsive to conventional therapies and the psychopharmacological resources. The transcranial magnetic stimulation (TMS) is a noninvasive method created in 1985 [34]. TMS is based on the Faraday Law—electromagnetic induction—through which the electric activity of the brain tissue can be influenced by the magnetic field, therefore inducing an electrical current that depolarizes the neurons. In this context, TMS in its repetitive form, that is, rTMS, can modulate the cortical excitability besides the stimulation period in itself, originating its potential application as a clinical treatment for a variety of neurological and psychiatric disturbances, like the anxiety one [34, 35].

Other two noninvasive strategies of low cost are the physical activity and induction of the flow state. The regular physical activity, especially the aerobics modality, provides a decrease in anxiety levels [36, 37]. The literature data are robust in demonstrating the beneficial effect of the physical activity on anxiety scenarios. There are data which demonstrate that this evidence also applies to MPA [36].

On the other hand, the "flow state" is a state of awareness of the hyper-focus in which irrelevant details and intrusive thoughts about the performance are eliminated, resulting in the subject being fuller in the final activity which is the musical performance. In this context it would be a complete absorption in a determined task with enhanced performance skills [15, 26]. There seems to be an inverse relation between the flow sate and MPA [38]. From this relation a facilitator model was built for the flow state based on three factors: subject preparation, qualification of the teachers to deal with this focus, and the building of the flow experience [15]. These three axes are linked among themselves and necessarily need to access some valences such as learning/preparation that involves well-being, creativity, motivation, and musical skill mobilization [15, 26, 38].

### 5.3 Pharmacotherapy

MPA is limited to a determined situation that usually occurs on stage. Therefore, to do a medicament intervention, one must consider the need of using psychotropic or not. This will depend on, to a large extent, the frequency the subject is exposed to this situation and, certainly, its intensity.

Another important aspect is that the isolated use of drugs does not contribute for a change in the performer's attitude towards MPA. In this regard, the combined treatments involving countless psychotherapy alternatives and complementary therapies are highly recommended [25].

In the musical environment, the two most used drug types for the acute MPA treatment are the beta-blockers, mainly represented by the propranolol and benzodiazepines (BDZ) which have as their principal representatives alprazolam, diazepam, and bromazepam.

The use of BDZ is controversial. If, on the one hand, it has a relatively fast and well-tolerated beginning action, on the other hand, its long-term use can cause a dependency syndrome, becoming tolerant to the doses, which tends to cause an abusive and uncontrolled use [39]. Besides, the fact that they can cause sleepiness can compromise, in an import way, the musical performance. Therefore, the use of this drug must be very careful so that one uses the minimum possible.

In the cases where there is a prolonged and inadvertent use of these anxiolytic classes, employing combined strategies as a gradual discontinuation of the drug, followed by psychotherapeutic accompaniment and regular orientations about the collateral effects and commitment of the cognitive functions, is recommended.

The BDZ are usually prescribed in association with antidepressive drugs (these will be approached further on). The best answer taxes are around the sixth week of use [40]. The average daily doses found in the literature are, respectively, clonazepam 2.4 mg/day, bromazepam 21 mg/day, and alprazolam 4.2 mg/day.

The beta-blockers are very efficient in the containment of somatic symptoms, mainly the tremors and muscle tension; however, they do not have any action on the cognitive and behavioral symptoms [41].

Considering the most severe cases, there is always the possibility of comorbidity with other anxiety situations. This issue will be approached in the next topic.

The majority of the literary review studies about the strategies to handle MPA do not include psychotropic use [23]. However, basing on the recommendation that combined strategies are more efficient and considering that in the most severe cases the use of drugs will be necessary, one can, for example, adopt protocols to treat a social phobia [42] which, besides being a disorder of the common anxiety, is a situation that has the closest conceptual relations to MPA.

The psychotropic of the first-line choice are the selective serotonin reuptake inhibitors and dual serotonin-norepinephrine reuptake inhibitors (SNRIs) due to their efficacy and tolerability profile. The nonselective monoamine oxidase inhibitor, phenelzine, can be stronger than these two drug classes, but, due to its potential to interact with food and drugs, its use should be restricted to patients that do not respond to selective serotonin reuptake inhibitors or serotonin-noradrenaline reuptake inhibitors [40].

The initial alternatives include duloxetine, buspirone, hydroxyzine, pregabalin, or bupropion, in this order. If the response is unsatisfactory, the second recommendation is to try a different SSRI. If the answer to the second SSRI is unsatisfactory, the recommendation is to try a serotonin-norepinephrine reuptake inhibitor [43]. Other alternatives for SSRIs and SNRIs for patients resistant or intolerant to the treatment include tricyclic antidepressants, second generation of antipsychotics, and valproic acid.

There is less information available about the ideal treatment duration, although it has been observed that individuals who abandoned the treatment with less than 12–20 weeks have shown more relapses compared to the ones who continued making regular use of the medication [40–44]. The existing data suggest that it is reasonable to keep the treatment for at least 3 to 6 months after the situation has been stabilized, and this period can be even longer depending on the severity and individual characteristics of each subject [44].

In this context, other classes of drugs could be employed; however, there are no systematic reviews whose focus is the social phobia treatment. Nevertheless, the treatment protocols of other anxiety situations, such as generalized anxiety, can be considered. In this regard the following classes can be cited: (1) anticonvulsant drugs such as pregabalin for at least 24 weeks and (2) atypical antipsychotic of controlled release such as quetiapine, which reduce the chance of an anxiety upsurge [42]. Pregabalin, alternatively, can be employed in monotherapy in daily doses between 450 and 600 mg and is recommended as a first-choice agent for the social anxiety disorder [45]. Its beginning action is on the first week, and, in general, it shows less collateral effects than the BDZs.

Other still very recent pharmacotherapies can be cited as the use of botulinum toxin (BT) and cannabidiol. Recent studies indicate that the botulinum toxin injection on the glabella reduces the amygdala response with antidepressive effects [46]. If the BT effect in humor is, in part, due to the decrease in negative emotions in general, it is reasonable to suppose that other psychiatric disorders, such as social anxiety disorder, where negative emotions are highlighted, can respond to the BT glabellar injection.

Regarding cannabidiol, there is a growing evidence of studies in humans and animals that indicate this compound, the principal non-psychotomimetic phytocannabinoids present in *Cannabis sativa*, as an option to alleviate the anxiety in paradigms assessing fear. More recently, the effects of cannabidiol on learned fear have been investigated in clinical studies with relevance for clinical application in phobias [47]. In such studies the evidence shows that cannabidiol can be a useful option to treat social anxiety [48].

More recently the anxiolytic effect of melatonin was shown [49]. Melatonin is a hormone secreted by the pineal gland during the night. The melatonin receptors (MT2) seem to relate with mechanisms of decrease in anxiety levels. Besides, there is evidence that melatonin can stimulate the dopaminergic synthesis in the hippocampus, which contributes to suppress the induced stress behavior [50].

### 5.4 MPA prevention

Preventing MPA means to employ strategies in which the most vulnerable subjects can have access to a context in more favorable environments. Such strategies can be applied to the beginners as well as the professionals.

The learning/preparation process should involve well-being, creativity, motivation, and musical ability mobilization [15, 26, 38]. It is necessary to simulate the negative scenarios so that such situations can be trained in an imaginary way as well as a real one.

The exposition situation cannot be something new or unexpected for the performer. The oriented and repeated experience in stage situations allows the performer to become familiar with potentially anxiogenic stimuli. As these stimuli are faced without prejudice for the subject integrity, new situations must be created in order to develop handling and competence abilities to deal with them. This process needs to be regular and with a weekly frequency so that the situations can be assimilated and issues, such as attitude and creativity, can become part of a defense arsenal for each individual facing anxiogenic "scenes." There are many music graduation courses that structure activities of this nature, called performance workshop.

From the pharmacological strategies' point of view, it is important to detect the procedure as early as possible in the most severe cases, which have indication to use psycho-medicines.

### 5.5 MPA monitoring strategies

The early MPA detection is fundamental for a program of strategies for the subject's monitoring. The differentiated attention towards these individuals must include monitoring with screening tests, individual care, and the structuring of an activity plan that includes the gradual practice of public exposure.

The forming of vulnerable individual groups contributes for each one of them to perceive that their distresses are not exclusive or a rarity. The group can act as a facilitator of an encouraging experience.

The pedagogical, therapeutic, and medical dimensions must be shared. Each context requires that other dimension be known, even for creating a sharing environment where each one of the knowledge can intervene in determined situations. Thus, the pedagogical dimension needs to be in agreement with the therapeutic strategies, and the medical interventions need to know the context of the musical performance, the specificities and discomfort of each musician, as well as their routines and technical requirements [51].

## 6. Comorbidities

There are not many studies about comorbidities in MPA. The literature results indicate that the specific phobia, generalized anxiety disorder, panic disorder with/without agoraphobia, and major depression disorder (but not dysthymia) are the common comorbidities [3, 52].

Furthermore, one third of the subjects that show severe MPA also show a generalized anxiety disorder. There are studies that point to a prevalence of a 19 and 20% comorbidity of social phobia and depression, respectively [53]. This social phobia prevalence among musicians is about 10 times more prevalent than the general population.

On the other hand, more recent studies indicate that the generalized anxiety disorder is the strongest MPA predictor among all major DSM-5 anxiety types [54].

There is a model that proposes three MPA subtypes: MPA1, which is a variety restricted to the focus on the performance itself; MPA2, which establishes connections between (and with) social anxiety/social anxiety disorder; and MPA3 which establishes close relations with other nosologies in the anxiety spectrum such as panic disorder with or without depression [3, 55]. These relations configure a potential MPA worsening as other disorders manifest themselves, in a way that MPA will not necessarily convert itself in another anxiety disorder or establish a comorbidity but there is this potential.

## 7. Conclusion

These data indicate that MPA is complex and multifactorial. Probably the first symptoms are of an early start. Consequently, there is the importance of spreading the information about MPA, especially in the family level and the school/academic environment, contexts where the future professional musicians are formed.

Preventively, in the family environment as well as in the schools, one must build relationships that privilege the well-being, motivation, and reception of psychic distresses.

MPA has a worrying prevalence of about 20% among the professional musicians. This number can mean some million subjects! The preventive strategies, the qualitative and quantitative evaluation, and the management of the already installed situations are of upmost importance.

Currently there are countless strategies to approach MPA. They go from the traditional psychotherapy strategies (cognitive, behavioral, and cognitive-behavioral therapies) to the pharmacological resources. New approaches signal a new outlook in this area with the therapeutic use of cannabidiol, melatonin, botulinum toxin, neurofeedback, and transcranial stimulation.

## Acknowledgements

I thank the Music Post-graduation Program of the São João del Rei Federal University (PPGMUS/UFSJ) for the support in their teaching staff production.

## Conflicts of interest

The author declares that there are no conflicts of interest.

## Author details

Sérgio de Figueiredo Rocha
Federal University (UFSJ), São João del Rei, Brazil

*Address all correspondence to: sergiorocha@ufsj.edu.br

## References

[1] Kenny DT, Davis P, Oates J. Music performance anxiety and occupational stress amongst opera chorus artists and their relationship with state and trait anxiety and perfectionism. Journal of Anxiety Disorders. 2004;**18**:757-777. DOI: 10.1016/j.janxdis.2003.09.004

[2] Manning A. Instrument-specific music performance anxiety [thesis]. Hattiesburg: The University of Southern Mississippi; 2013

[3] Kenny DT. The Psychology of Music Performance Anxiety. 1st ed. Oxford: Oxford; 2011. p. 365. DOI: 10.1093/acprof:oso/9780199586141.001.0001

[4] Burin AB, Osório FL. Music performance anxiety: A critical review of etiological aspects, perceived causes, coping strategies and treatment. Archives of Clinical Psychiatry. 2017;**44**(5):127-133. DOI: 10.1590/0101-60830000000136

[5] Brugués AO. Music Performance Anxiety: A Comprehensive Update of the Literature. 1st ed. Newcastle: Cambridge Scholars Publishing; 2019. p. 240. ISBN (10): 1-5275-2251-2

[6] Taborsky C. Musical performance anxiety: A review of literature. Update. 2007;**26**(1):15-25. DOI: 10.1177/87551233070260010103

[7] Patston T, Osborne MS. The developmental features of music performance anxiety and perfectionism in school age music students. Performance Enhancement & Health. 2016;**4**:42-49. DOI: 10.1016/j.peh.2015.09.003

[8] Dempsey E, Comeau G. Music performance anxiety and self-efficacy in young musicians: Effects of gender and age. Music Performance Research. 2019;**9**:60-79. ISSN 7155-9219

[9] Ryan C. Gender differences in children's experience of musical performance anxiety. Psychology of Music. 2004;**3**(1):89-103. DOI: 10.1177/0305735604039284

[10] Wehr-Flowers E. Differences between male and female students' confidence, anxiety, and attitude toward learning jazz improvisation. Journal of Research in Music Education. 2006;**54**(4):337-349. DOI: 10.1177/002242940605400406

[11] Fernholz I, Mumm JLM, Plag J, Noeres K. Performance anxiety in professional musicians: A systematic review on prevalence, risk factors and clinical treatment effects. Psychological Medicine. 2019;**49**(14):2287-2306. DOI: 10.1017/S0033291719001910

[12] Matei R, Ginsborg J. Music performance anxiety in classical musicians – What we know about what works. BJPsych International. 2017;**14**(2):33-35. DOI: 10.1192/S2056474000001744

[13] Rodríguez-Carvajal R, Oscar L, Vilte LS, Moreno-Jiménez J, de Rivas S. Freeing the performer's mind: A structural exploration of how mindfulness influences music performance anxiety, negative affect and self-consciousness among musicians. MindRxiv. 2017:1-25. DOI: 10.31231/osf.io/657n8

[14] Kenny DT. A systematic review of treatments for music performance anxiety. Anxiety, Stress, and Coping. 2005;**18**(3):183-208. DOI: 10.1080/10615800500167258

[15] Li L. An investigation of relationships between flow theory and music performance anxiety [thesis]. Columbia: University of Missouri Columbia; 2019

[16] Nielsen C, Studer RK, Hildebrandt H, Nater UM, Wild P, Danuser B, et al. The relationship between music performance anxiety, subjective performance quality and post-event rumination among music students. Psychology of Music. 2018;**46**(1):136-152. DOI: 10.1177/0305735617706539

[17] Kenny DT, Osborne MS. Music performance anxiety: New insights from young musicians. Advances in Cognitive Psychology. 2006;**2**(2-3):103-112. DOI: 10.2478/v10053-008-0049-5

[18] Kaleńska-Rodzaj J. Pre-performance emotions and music performance anxiety beliefs in young musicians. Research Studies in Music Education. 2019:1-17. DOI: 10.1177/1321103X19830098

[19] Zarza-Alzugaray FJ, Orejudo S, Casanova O, Aparicio-Moreno L. Music performance anxiety in adolescence and early adulthood: Its relation with the age of onset in musical training. Research Studies in Music Education. 2018;**46**(1):18-32. DOI: 10.1177/1321103X19830098

[20] Kenny DT. Identifying Cut-off Scores for Clinical Purposes for the *Kenny Music performance anxiety inventory* (K-MPAI) in a populatIon of Professional Orchestral Musicians2015. pp. 1-22. DOI: 10.13140/RG.2.1.2481.2244

[21] Barbeau A-K. Performance anxiety inventory for musicians (PerfAIM): A new questionnaire to assess music performance anxiety in popular musicians [thesis]. Montreal: McGrill University; 2011

[22] Kenny DT, Halls N. Development and evaluation of two brief group interventions for music performance anxiety in community musicians. Psychology of Music. 2018;**46**(1):66-83. DOI: 10.1177/0305735617702536

[23] Burin AB, Osório FL. Interventions for music performance anxiety: Results from a systematic literature review. Archives of Clinical Psychiatry. 2016;**43**(5):116-131. DOI: 10.1590/0101-60830000000097

[24] Bissonnette J, Dubé F, Provencher MD, Moreno Sala MT. Evolution of music performance anxiety and quality of performance during virtual reality exposure training. Virtual Reality. 2016;**20**:71-81. DOI: 10.1007/s10055-016-0283-y

[25] Mcgrath CE. Music performance anxiety therapies: A review of the literature [thesis]. Urbana Champaign: University of Illinois; 2012

[26] Lockhart A. The anxious musician: Coping strategies used to combat music performance anxiety [thesis]. Lynchburg: Liberty University; 2019

[27] Juncos DG, Heinrichs GA, Towle P, Duffy K, Grand SM, Morgan MC, et al. Acceptance and commitment therapy for the treatment of music performance anxiety: A pilot study with student vocalists. Frontiers in Psychology. 2017;**8**:1-16. DOI: 10.3389/fpsyg.2017.00986

[28] Finch K. Music Performance anxiety and arousal imagery: Development of the musician's self-regulation imagery scale [thesis]. Waterloo: University of Waterloo; 2018

[29] Amos H. The effects of the alexander technique on the performance of music students [thesis]. Richmond: Eastern Kentucky University; 2016

[30] Zafeiri E, Kandylaki A, Zyga S, Zarogiannis I, Panoutsopoulos GI. The contribution of biofeedback brain boy method to the treatment of anxiety disorders. Materia Socio Medica. 2019;**31**(2):105-109. DOI: 10.5455/msm.2019.31.105-109

[31] Goessl VC, Curtiss JE, Hofmann SG. The effect of heart rate variability biofeedback training on stress and anxiety: A meta-analysis. Psychological Medicine. 2017;**47**:2578-2586. DOI: 10.1017/S0033291717001003

[32] Marzbani H, Marateb HR, Mansourian M. Neurofeedback: A comprehensive review on system design, methodology and clinical applications. Basic and Clinical Neuroscience. 2016;**7**(2):143-158. DOI: 10.15412/J.BCN.03070208

[33] Paes F, Machado S, Arias-Carrion O, et al. The value of repetitive Transcranial magnetic stimulation (rTMS) for the treatment of anxiety disorders: An integrative review. CNS & Neurological Disorders. 2011;**10**(5):610-620. DOI: 10.2174/187152711796234943

[34] Zandi-Mehran Y, Firoozabadi M, Rostami R. Improvement of neurofeedback therapy for improved attention through facilitation of brain activity using local sinusoidal extremely low frequency magnetic field exposure. Clinical EEG and Neuroscience. 2014;**46**(2):100-112. DOI: 10.1177/1550059414524403

[35] Paes F, Baczynski T, Novaes F, et al. Repetitive transcranial magnetic stimulation (rTMS) to treat social anxiety disorder: Case reports and a review of the literature. Clinical Practice and Epidemiology in Mental Health. 2013;**9**:180-188. DOI: 10.2174/1745017901309010180

[36] Rocha SF, Marocolo M, Vivas EN, et al. Physical activity helps to control music performance anxiety. Medical Problems of Performing Artists. 2014;**29**(2):111. DOI: 10.21091/mppa.2014.2022

[37] McDowell CP, Dishman RK, Gordon BR, et al. Physical activity and anxiety: A systematic review and meta-analysis of prospective cohort studies. American Journal of Preventive Medicine. 2019;**57**(4):545-556. DOI: 10.1016/j.amepre.2019.05.012

[38] Fullagar CJ, Knight PA, Sovern HS. Challenge/skill balance, flow, and performance anxiety. Applied Psychology. An International Review. 2013;**62**(2):236-259. DOI: 10.1111/j.1464-0597.2012.00494.x

[39] Guaiana G, Barbui C. Discontinuing benzodiazepines: Best practices. Epidemiology and Psychiatric Sciences. 2016;**25**:214-216. DOI: 10.1017/S2045796016000032

[40] Canton J, Scott KM, Glue P. Optimal treatment of social phobia: Systematic review and meta-analysis. Neuropsychiatric Disease and Treatment. 2012;**8**:203-215. DOI: 10.2147/NDT.S23317

[41] Steenen SA, van Wijk AJ, van der Heijden G, et al. Propranolol for the treatment of anxiety disorders: Systematic review and meta-analysis. Journal of Psychopharmacology. 2016;**30**(2):128-139. DOI: 10.1177/0269881115612236

[42] Perna G, Alciati A, Riva A, et al. Long-term pharmacological treatments of anxiety disorders: An updated systematic review. Current Psychiatry Reports. 2016;**18**(23):1-16. DOI: 10.1007/s11920-016-0668-3

[43] Abejuela HR, Osser DN. The psychopharmacology algorithm project at the Harvard South Shore Program: An algorithm for generalized anxiety disorder. Harvard Review of Psychiatry. 2016;**24**(4):243-256. DOI: 10.1097/HRP.0000000000000098

[44] Blanco C, Bragdon LB, Schneier FR, et al. The evidence based pharmacotherapy of social anxiety disorder. The International Journal of Neuropsychopharmacology.

2013;**16**(1):235-249. DOI: 10.1017/S1461145712000119

[45] Van Ameringen M, Patterson B. Refractory social anxiety disorder. Journal of Psychiatry & Neuroscience. 2017;**42**(1):1-2. DOI: 10.1503/jpn.160016

[46] Finzi E, Rosenthal NE. Botulinum toxin therapy of social anxiety disorder: A case series. Journal of Clinical Psychopharmacology. 2019;**39**(4):410-411. DOI: 10.1097/JCP.0000000000001066

[47] Jurkus R, Day HLL, Guimarães FS, et al. Cannabidiol regulation of learned fear: Implications for treating anxiety-related disorders. Frontiers in Pharmacology. 2016;**7**:1-8. DOI: 10.3389/fphar.2016.00454

[48] Masataka N. Anxiolytic effects of repeated cannabidiol treatment in teenagers with social anxiety disorders. Frontiers in Pharmacology. 2019;**10**:1-6. DOI: 10.3389/fpsyg.2019.02466

[49] Emet M, Ozcan H, Ozel L, et al. A review of melatonin, its receptors and drugs. The Eurasian Journal of Medicine. 2016;**48**:135-141. DOI: 10.5152/eurasianjmed.2015.0267

[50] Spasojevic N, Stefanovic B, Jovanovic P, et al. Anxiety and hyperlocomotion induced by chronic unpredictable mild stress can be moderated with melatonin treatment. Folia Biologica. 2016;**62**:250-257. DOI: 10.1590/0001-3765201520130400

[51] Burin AB, Barbar AEM, Nirenberg IS, et al. Music performance anxiety: Perceived causes, coping strategies and clinical profiles of Brazilian musicians. Trends in Psychiatry and Psychotherapy. 2019;**41**(4):348-357. DOI: 10.1590/2237-6089-2018-0104

[52] Dobos B, Piko BF, Kenny DT. Music performance anxiety and its relationship with social phobia and dimensions of perfectionism. Research Studies in Music Education. 2019;**41**(3):310-326. DOI: 10.1177%2F1321103X18804295

[53] Barbar AEM, Crippa JAS, Osório FL. Performance anxiety in Brazilian musicians: Prevalence and association with psychopathology indicators. Journal of Affective Disorders. 2014;**152-154**:381-386. DOI: 10.1016/j.jad.2013.09.041

[54] Wiedemann A, Vogel D, Voss C, et al. Music performance anxiety and its anxiety correlates. PsyArXiv Preprints. DOI: 10.31234/osf.io/cev7u

[55] Stein MB, Stein DJ. Social anxiety disorder. Lancet. 2008;**371**:1115-1125. DOI: 10.1016/S0140-6736(08)60488-2

Chapter 5

# Students Anxiety Experiences in Higher Education Institutions

*Nabila Y. AlKandari*


## Abstract

Students studying at higher education institutions face many challenges. Students who attempt to overcome these challenges may alter their behaviors. This may negatively affect their psychological state and cause them to feel anxiety. Anxiety is most prominent among college students. Many students face anxiety when they think they cannot achieve their academic or non-academic purposes; however, sometimes anxiety can encourage students to think more critically about how to achieve their goals. Students cope with anxiety in different ways, but some may struggle. This probably causes many symptoms that affect their mental health. Therefore, they should alleviate the anxiety to keep their mental health and persist in the institution.


**Keywords:** anxiety, symptoms, factors, faculty members, colleges' students

## 1. Introduction

College students' mental health plays a very important role in their success and persistence at their institution [1]. When the students can manage their anxiety, they feel less pressure. If the students remain anxious, they may not follow through with their academic studies. Also, anxiety could complicate their physical and psychological states and persist after graduation, and it may negatively affect their capacity to work in the future [2]. Therefore, it is important to understand the factors that cause students' anxiety at higher education institutions.

## 2. Methods

To achieve the purposes of the study which focused to present the factors that cause students' anxiety in higher education institutions and find the solutions to this issue, a literature review was used to describe students' perception of anxiety feelings while they study in higher education institutions. Many studies that described students' perceptions from different countries were used to present this issue.

### 2.1 Data analysis

The researcher collected the researches that focus on students' anxiety and grouped them in different subcategories and explained each category based on the availability of recent researches that belong to the topic and the experience of the researcher. Although there were many factors that may cause students' anxiety, the researcher focused on some critical factors that presented in most higher education institutions in recent years.

## 3. The factors that cause students' anxiety at higher education institutions

### 3.1 Studying a new language

Studying a new language is a major factor that causes anxiety among many students, especially those who follow their studies in a non-native language. Most students in higher education institutions study English as a foreign language or as a second language. Some of them may learn English before college. However, they may not able to meet the high level of English proficiency required at the college level. They face anxiety because if they cannot pass successfully, they may not be able to graduate from the institution.

Tian [3] indicates Korean students face language anxiety when they must make presentations in class, and they lack language proficiency. Moreover, they feel anxiety because of their peers' negative feedback. Charoensukmongkol [4] also indicates Thai students face language anxiety because they lack proficiency in the English language. Tsai and Lee [5] found Taiwanese students have anxiety when reading English because they do not understand the English vocabulary, the topics, or the long and complicated text structures, and they fear they will make mistakes when answering questions.

Jawas [6] found Indonesian students also have English language anxiety because they lack proficiency in writing, and the instructors present them with class essay assignments that probably increase their anxiety because of the limited time in class to finish the assignment with the appropriate answer. Also, some Indonesian students have anxiety when giving a presentation. Some of them may not prepare well and do not like when someone asks them difficult questions about the presentation [7].

Abdala and Elnadeef [8] also indicate that Saudi Arabian students feel anxious about learning the English language specifically when they make mistakes in the class and lack writing proficiency. They are scared when they hear unwanted comments and jokes from their classmates while they are speaking. Some other students face anxiety in learning the Chinese language [9]. The Chinese language is not easy to learn, specifically in speaking and writing. Also, some Hispanic students have difficulties when studying Spanish, specifically in writing, spelling words, and using conjunctions [10].

### 3.2 The curriculum difficulty

Curriculum difficulties are also considered a factor that causes students' anxiety in most higher education institutions. Some students cannot understand the curriculum and struggle to answer questions in the classroom, do assignments, and write research papers or reports. Some students may hesitate to ask the instructors for help; therefore, they become anxious because they are unable to meet the course requirements. Some difficult curriculums include mathematics [11–13], biology [14, 15], statistics [16], chemistry, physics, history [17], and law [18]. In addition, there are several medical specialization classes that cause students' anxiety, such as dental and medical [19], medical and engineering [20], dentistry and veterinary [21], and pharmacy [22].

### 3.3 The difficulty in exams

Some students face anxiety with midterm and final exams because they are not well prepared. Some students may not understand the exam questions and write the wrong answers as a result [17]. More importantly, sometimes there is not enough time to answer the exam questions. Some faculty members do not know the differences in the students' abilities, and they make exams that do not fit with some students' intelligence. As a result, students may fail the exams. Exam anxiety is widespread among college students [23, 24] in different majors like math, history, geography, chemistry, physics, engineering, arts, and music. For example, some students specializing in music have anxiety in exams where they must use a musical instrument [25]. Also, some pharmacy students have anxiety about their clinical exams [22].

Some students also face anxiety about online exams because some faculty members make the exams with a time limit, and some students may need more time. Also, the computer may not work well or Internet services may shutdown while students are taking the online exam. As a result, some students may not prefer online exams.

### 3.4 Financial pressure

Financial anxiety is considered an issue many students face when studying at higher education intuitions because they are responsible for paying for their studies, especially those at private institutions. Some of them may be in debt. This financial pressure leads students to feel anxiety, which causes them psychological distress [26] that results in a lower grade point average (GPA). Some students who face difficulties in understanding difficult subjects depend on costly private instructors. Students also need money for daily expenses such as food and transportation. When students feel they do not have enough money, they may be anxious and ask friends for money, which negatively affects students' feelings, leading to stress and anxiety.

### 3.5 Culture shock

Many international students suffer from alienation and culture shock when they seek to continue studying in other countries. This shock causes them psychological crises such as anxiety because of the distance from their family and country, the difficulty of a new language and speaking with others, and the difficulty of adapting to the new culture, which requires patience.

### 3.6 Family responsibilities

Some university students have many family problems that cause them anxiety while they are studying. One of these problems is the illness of a family member, such as a parent, which requires the student to remain close to the patient. If the students are they have responsibility of the children and the husband. These problems affect the student academically because it hinders him in preparing well for tests, performing academic duties, and attending lectures, which causes him concern about how to balance his family and academic responsibilities.

### 3.7 Illness

Some students who suffer from a chronic illness have anxiety [27]. For example, a student who suffers diabetes is required to take daily insulin injections and go to the health center, and some may experience dizziness while at the university campus. Diabetes may hinder a student if his health condition relapses, and he may be absent from the university. Other illnesses include cancer, anemia, heart problems, asthma, and obesity. These diseases may negatively affect the academic level of the students, which causes them anxiety.

### 3.8 Employment

Some students who attend higher education institutions work off campus part or full time. Some of them may not be able to attend classes, specifically if they work in the mornings and their classes are scheduled for the same time. Some of them face anxiety if they cannot manage their time. They may fail their courses because of their absences or fail exams because they do not prepare well. As a result, they receive a lower GPA and an academic warning.

### 3.9 Discrimination

Discrimination is a concern that many students face at higher education institutions. The institutions gather students and staff from different backgrounds, nationalities, ethnicities, religions, colors, cultures, and levels of intelligence. Some students feel anxiety because of unfair treatment from classmates, friends, and staff and faculty members. When the students feel they are not welcome and they are treated badly, this causes them to feel anxiety [28, 29].

### 3.10 Disabilities

Some disabled students enter higher education institutions to further their studies, despite the challenges they face. Some disabled students have anxiety because they are unable to major in some specializations they may need. Some specializations such as geology and biology need students to participate in course activities using labs and instruments, which is difficult for some disabled students. Also, they may not be able to socialize with other students and may prefer isolation. Some students are visually impaired and require specific resources like certain textbooks, handouts, and software [30]. However, these resources are not available for some courses. Also, some students may have psychiatric disabilities [31] and need special attention from the mental health center to help them succeed academically. Some students who have autism spectrum disorder have anxiety when trying to achieve success in their academic studies [32].

## 4. Anxiety symptoms

When students have anxiety, it affects their mind and body and causes several symptoms: cognitive, physical, and emotional.

### 4.1 Cognitive symptoms

Many students could experience symptoms along with their feelings of anxiety. They may have many negative and painful experiences, such as insomnia and other sleep disorders. Anxiety also negatively affects students' memories. They may become unable to think correctly and make decisions; therefore they cannot participate in classroom discussions and cannot share their opinions and ideas with other classmates and faculty members. Some of them feel sadness, fear, and panic. As a result, their academic achievements are negatively affected.

### 4.2 Physical symptoms

Students with anxiety can experience significant pain with symptoms like breathing problems, stomachaches, headaches, joint and muscle pain, and fatigue. These symptoms could make them unable to come to the university. Some students may fear from the faculty, so they upsent from the institution. Some students become fatigued when they have a lot of academic work to do on campus and feel anxious because they do not know how to manage this work. This academic anxiety badly affects students' health; however, they should cope with anxiety. Some students have sensitive behaviors, which play a role in their tendency to become overwhelmed with anxiety. This needs change for students to cope with academic life.

### 4.3 Emotional symptoms

Some students who suffer from anxiety experience painful emotional symptoms such as depression, sadness, nervousness, anger, and loneliness. Students may feel unhappy about coming to a university or become very nervous around people, such as friends and peers. Others feel worried and sad when they cannot overcome the challenges they face, such as having a low GPA. Some of them like to be alone when they have stressful feelings, which can lead to depression. Sometimes, these students may have negative thoughts about withdrawing from college, especially when their friends are successful and have good GPAs. Some students may feel tired from studying, the tough curriculum, and attending the university. They may have expected to be happy with university life but instead found it to be the opposite of what they wanted.

## 5. Alleviating students' anxiety

Mental health problems are a social phenomenon that requires attention in many societies [33]. Anxiety is an aspect of a college student's mental health. Attention must be paid to the means that help prevent students from falling into anxiety and reducing its severity and psychological impact on the students continuing their studies.

### 5.1 Improving relationships between faculty members and students

Having human relationships between faculty members and students is very important. Communication between these groups plays an important role in reducing students' anxiety. The faculty members should ask students if they need help to understand the curriculum, do assignments, and write reports. The faculty can design class activities related to the curriculum to make sure the students understand the content. For example, in teaching a language, the faculty should encourage group work in class to help students participate in communication to improve their speaking and their relationships with classmates to reduce the anxiety. Also, video games online can improve communication among students, increase students' confidence, and reduce their anxiety [34]. Collaborative work among students can also reduce students' anxiety, and they should be encouraged to use the strategies they prefer in learning [6].

The faculty members can encourage students to answer questions, whether they are right or wrong, to reduce students' fear. They should provide students with steps to do the assignments, write reports, and create projects. The faculty members should also understand that students differ in abilities and intelligence when they design exam questions. The exams should meet different students' abilities to reduce their anxiety. Hull et al. [35] indicate the importance of changing evaluation tools and improving students' self-efficacy.

The faculty members have important roles in guiding students and giving them advice related to academic decisions, such as selecting a college or selecting a major, and helping them manage their time for studying multiple curriculums. In helping them deal with anxiety, adapt to the challenges, and improve their thinking, faculty members can reduce anxiety's psychological side effects on students' bodies and minds.

### 5.2 Using mental health services

Many institutions provide students with mental health workers to help them cope with their negative feelings while they pursue their studies. To provide students with efficient mental services, the institutions should hire workers who specialize in psychology and counseling. This will provide students with effective strategies to reduce their anxiety. These mental health workers should be available to meet students on campus and, most importantly, give students a trusted and secure setting in which to improve their self-confidence when they seek help. They should provide students with a socialized atmosphere to reduce their isolation and fear, specifically students with psychiatric disabilities and autism spectrum disorder. These students need to manage their social emotions to adapt to university life [32]. Online social networks should be improved to help them socially [36].

Also, it's important to provide international students with mental health workers who can deal with their culture shock, speak different languages to meet various students' needs, and provide them with social support and a friendly relationship. Different social and cultural activities on campus can help students communicate with others and reduce their anxiety as well. Shelton, Wang, and Zhu [37] indicate that cultural orientation is an appropriate way to keep students mentally healthy.

### 5.3 Improving academic services

To reduce students' academic anxiety, institutions should provide students with effective academic services like a writing center, which helps students write in many subjects and improves their efficiency in using vocabulary and grammar. Tutorial services are also important in helping students reduce their anxiety. The tutorial should be provided by an effective staff specializing in the curriculum to help students understand the content of the courses, specifically in language courses, mathematics, statistics, and biology.

Improving library services can help students do research and experiments. According to Grandy [38], some adult students have library anxiety because they are unable to use the library services. Therefore, these students should be provided with information literacy courses to reduce their anxiety about using library resources, technology resources, and searching strategies.

### 5.4 Physical exercise and relaxation activities

Many students who suffer from anxiety can manage their negative feelings through exercises like walking, swimming, and playing tennis. Some students join sports clubs, which results in an improvement in their positivity and happiness. Taking part in physical activities can greatly reduce the negative psychological health impacts on a student's body and mood [17], reduce mental difficulties, and improve their health well-being [39]. Other students may prefer to reduce their anxiety by reading books about mental health and dealing with anxiety to be aware of how they can manage their symptoms. Some of them may also read novels and magazines for relaxation [17].

## 6. Discussion

Students at higher education institutions face many kinds of challenges that affect negatively their psychology feeling, causing them anxiety. Its effects vary among students in how to deal with it, overcome its symptoms, and find solutions. The study found that the most important factor that causes anxiety is related to academic study. For example, many students who study a new language face challenges in understanding language words, speaking, and writing. This issue was found in many students in different countries such as Korea, Thailand, Indonesia, China, and Saudi Arabia, which reflect that this issue is widespread internationally among higher education institutions. This finding needs a special issue from the faculty members to dedicate efforts in helping students understand a new language without the feeling of anxiety.

The finding also highlights that students in different colleges and specialization face anxiety. This finding may reflect that some students may have low academic competency to study in a specific specialization and not qualify to study high level of curriculum contents. However, some faculty members may not spend adequate time to explain to students the curriculums' contents, which may affect negatively students' feeling in searching and understanding. As it known that students vary in competencies, therefore the faculty members should focus in insuring that students understand the curriculum and how doing the assignments.

In addition, most students in higher education institutions face anxiety of midterm and final exams in most specialization. This issue needs faculty members' attention to focus on preparing students for exam and reduce their anxiety. As it is known, students attend the university or college to get knowledge and improve their abilities, not to feel anxiety and have a psychological sickness.

Besides academic factors, some students feel anxiety because of financial pressure and not being able to pay the tuitions and fees. This issue is widely spread among students specifically who study in a private institution. Actually the institution should consider the students' financial level before admitting them in the institution to insure their ability to pay to reduce their anxiety.

Some students feel anxiety because of illness and not being able to attend class daily and doing assignments and preparing for exams. The medical staff in the institution should consider students with illness and disabilities and follow their health situations to insure their capability to follow their study and provide them with support services to reduce their anxiety. Most importantly some students hesitate to inform the support staff with their illness or disability situation; as a result they may not able to deal with the problems that they might face, and as a result they feel anxiety.

Because the anxiety have several negative cognitive, physical, and emotional symptoms which negatively affect students' mental health. Several solutions were suggested to alleviate students' anxiety through developing human relationship between students and faculty members, which is an important factor in helping students reduce their anxiety feelings. It is important that faculty members recognize the importance of helping students in gaining knowledge and understanding curriculum contents to help them become qualified graduates in the work market with well body and mental health. As several researchers indicated, the negative effects of anxiety could have a continuous side effect on the students when they graduate and join the workforce. The workforce needs healthy and qualified graduates who can work without anxiety and stress.

## 7. Conclusion

Most students studying at higher education institutions face many challenges that give them a negative feeling and lead them to have anxiety. The most important factor that affects students is the academic challenges which are related to their persistence or retention in the institutions. Some of these academic factors include difficulty of studying new language, midterm and final exams, and curriculum. Some other students also face anxiety related to different reasons such as being ill or disabled students. Also some students feel discrimination which affects them negatively. International students also face culture shock anxiety which affects their persistence in the institutions. Students should learn managing this feeling to prevent their mental health from unwanted symptoms which may negatively affect their psychological behaviors. Also, students should understand how to improve their thinking and mind to adapt to the different challenges they face in their academic life. More importantly the university and college leadership should consider the importance of providing students with academic environment that encourage students' learning and persistence at the institution and protect them from an unwanted anxiety feeling which probably may change students' behaviors and attitudes negatively after graduation.

## Author details

Nabila Y. AlKandari
Kuwait University, Kuwait

*Address all correspondence to: nabilah.alkandari@ku.edu.kw

## References

[1] VanderLind R. Effects of mental health on student learning. Learning Assistance Review. 2017;**22**(2):39-58

[2] Basudan S, Binanzan N, Alhassan A. Depression, anxiety and stress in dental students. International Journal of Medical Education. 2017;**8**:179-186. DOI: 10.5116/ijme.5910.b961

[3] Tian C. Anxiety in classroom English presentations: A case study in Korean tertiary educational context. Higher Education Studies. 2019;**9**(1):132-143

[4] Charoensukmongkol P. The role of mindfulness in reducing English language anxiety among Thai college students. International Journal of Bilingual Education and Bilingualism. 2019;**22**(4):414-427

[5] Tsai Y-R, Lee C-Y. An exploration into factors associated with reading anxiety among Taiwanese EFL learners. TEFLIN Journal: A Publication on the Teaching and Learning of English. 2018;**29**(1):129-148

[6] Jawas U. Writing anxiety among Indonesian EFL students: Factors and strategies. International Journal of Instruction. 2019;**12**(4):733-746

[7] Djumingin S, Weda S, Juanda. Anxiety in classroom presentation in teaching-learning interaction in English for students of Indonesian study program at higher education. International Journal of Education and Practice. 2019;**7**(1):1-9

[8] Abdala AHEH, Elnadeef EAE. English language anxiety and stress among Saudi students in the first year at college of sciences and arts in Dharan Aljanoob. International Journal of Linguistics, Literature and Translation. 2019;**2**(1):270-275

[9] Basith A, Musyafak N, Ichwanto MA, Syahputra A. Chinese learning anxiety on foreign students. European Journal of Educational Research. 2019;**8**(4):1193-1200

[10] Torres KM, Arrastia-Chisholm MC, Tackett S. Perception of writing anxiety and self-efficacy among Spanish heritage language learners. Journal of Hispanic-Higher Education. 2020;**19**(1):84-98

[11] Alghazo Y, Al-Wadi H. English language anxiety and its effect on students' mathematics achievement. International Education Studies. 2019;**12**(12):130-140

[12] Cumhur M, Tezer M. Anxiety about mathematics among university students: A multidimensional study in the 21st century. Cypriot Journal of Educational Sciences. 2019;**14**(2):222-231

[13] Núñez-Peña M, Bono R. Academic anxieties: Which type contributes the most to low achievement in methodological courses? Educational Psychology. 2019;**39**(6):797-814

[14] England BJ, Brigati JR, Schussler EE. Student anxiety in introductory biology classrooms: Perceptions about active learning and persistence in the major. Public Library of Science One. 2017;**12**(8):e0182506. DOI: 10.1371/journal.pone.0182506

[15] England BJ, Brigati JR, Schussler EE, Chen MM. Student anxiety and perception of difficulty impact performance and persistence in introductory biology courses. CBE Life Science Education. 2019;**18**(2):ar21. DOI: 10.1187/cbe.17-12-0284

[16] Baloglu M, Abbassi A, Kesici S. Multivariate relationships between statistics anxiety and motivational beliefs. Education. 2017;**137**(4):430-444

[17] AlKandari NY. Female college students anxiety. Psychology and Education. 2017;**54**(1/2):44-54

[18] Flynn AM, Li Y, Sánchez B. The mental health status of law students: Implications for college counselors. Journal of College Counseling. 2019;**22**(1):2-12

[19] Quek TT-C, Tam WW-S, Tran BX, Zhang M, Zhang Z, Ho CS-H, et al. The global prevalence of anxiety among medical students: A meta-analysis. International Journal of Environmental Research in Public Health. 2019;**16**(15):2735. DOI: 10.3390/ijerph16152735

[20] Balaji NK, Murthy PS, Kumar DN, Chaudhury S. Perceived stress, anxiety, and coping states in medical and engineering students during examinations. Industrial Psychiatry Journal. 2019;**28**(1):86-97. DOI: 10.4103/ipj.ipj_70_18

[21] Knipe D, Maughan C, Gilbert J, Dymock D, Moran P, Gunnell D. Mental health in medical, dentistry and veterinary students: Cross-sectional online survey. British Journal of Psychiatry Open. 2018;**4**(6):441-446. DOI: 10.1192/bjo.2018.61

[22] Longyhore DS. Pharmacy student anxiety and success with objective structured clinical examinations. American Journal Pharmaceutical Education. 2017;**81**(1):7. DOI: 10.5688/ajpe8117

[23] Lowe PA. The test anxiety measure for college students: Examination of its psychometric properties using an online survey with a Canadian sample. Canadian Journal of School Psychology. 2018;**33**(4):279-296

[24] Lowe PA. Exploring cross-cultural and gender differences in test anxiety among U.S. and Canadian college students. Journal of Psychoeducational Assessment. 2019;**37**(1):112-118

[25] Umuzdas M, Tök H, Umuzdas S. An examination of the performance anxiety levels of undergraduate music teaching students in the instrument exams according to various variables ("case of Tokat Province"). International Journal of Higher Education. 2019;**8**(4):221-230

[26] Cadaret MC, Bennett SR. College students' reported financial stress and its relationship to psychological distress. Journal of College Counseling. 2019;**22**(3):225-239

[27] Mullins AJ, Gamwell KL, Sharkey CM, Bakula DM, Tackett AP, Suorsa KI, et al. Illness uncertainty and illness intrusiveness as predictors of depressive and anxious symptomology in college students with chronic illnesses. Journal of American College Health. 2017;**65**(5):352-360

[28] Badiee M, Andrade E. Microsystem and macrosystem predictors of Latinx college students' depression and anxiety. Journal of Hispanic Higher Education. 2019;**18**(4):422-434

[29] Shadowen NL, Williamson AA, Guerra NG, Ammigan R, Drexler ML. Prevalence and correlates of depressive symptoms among international students: Implications for university support offices. Journal of international students. 2019;**9**(1):129-148. DOI: 10.32674/jis.v9i1.277

[30] Stone BW, Kay D, Reynolds A. Teaching visually impaired college students in introductory statistics. Journal of Statistics Education. 2019;**27**(3):225-237

[31] McEwan RC, Downie R. Patterns of academic success and engagement among college students with psychiatric disabilities. Journal of College Student Psychotherapy. 2019;**33**(3):257-272

[32] Ward D, Webster A. Understanding the lived experiences of university students with autism spectrum disorder (ASD): A phenomenological study.

International Journal of Disability, Development and Education. 2018;**65**(4):373-392

[33] Marcotte J, Lévesque G. Anxiety and well-being among students in a psychoeducation program: The mediating role of identity. Journal of College Student Development. 2018;**59**(1):90-104

[34] Horowitz KS. Video games and English as a second language: The effect of massive multiplayer online video games on the willingness to communicate and communicative anxiety of college students in Puerto Rico. American Journal of Play. 2019;**11**(3):379-410

[35] Hull K, Lawford H, Hood S, Oliveira V, Murray M, Trempe M, et al. Student anxiety and evaluation. Collected Essays on Learning and Teaching. 2019;**12**:23-35

[36] Lei J, Ashwin C, Brosnan M, Russell A. Developing an online tool to measure social network structure and perceived social support amongst autistic students in higher education: A feasibility study. Journal of Autism and Developmental Disorders. 2019;**49**(9):3526-3542

[37] Shelton AJ, Wang CDC, Zhu, W. Perceived social support and mental health: Cultural orientations as moderators. Journal of College Counseling. 2017;**20**(3):194-207

[38] Grandy R. Investigating the effectiveness of a credit-bearing information literacy course in reducing library anxiety for adult learners. Communications in Information Literacy. 2019;**13**(1):23-42

[39] Velten J, Bieda A, Scholten S, Wannemüller A, Margraf J. Lifestyle choices and mental health: A longitudinal survey with German and Chinese students. BMC Public Health. 2018;**18**:632. DOI: 10.1186/s12889-018-5526-2

## Section 2

# The Psychopathology of Anxiety and Some Other Syndromes

Chapter 6

# Anxiety Disorders

*Hülya Kök Eren*


## Abstract

Anxiety disorders are the most common of all psychiatric illnesses and result in significant functional impairment and distress. In DSM 5, anxiety disorders are divided into eleven subgroups. Anxiety, which we consider normal (mild and moderate anxiety), plays an important role in the development of the individual. However, if the level of anxiety increases, it may lead to mental problems. A high level of anxiety, long duration, and intensification of anxiety symptoms may cause anxiety disorders. These are; separation anxiety disorder, selective mutism, panic disorder, agoraphobia, specific phobia, social anxiety disorder, generalized anxiety disorder, other unspecified anxiety disorder, anxiety disorder related to another medical condition, anxiety disorder caused by substance or medication, anxiety disorders caused by substances and medication are unspecified anxiety disorders. Treatment methods used in anxiety disorders are individual psychotherapy, cognitive therapy, behavioral therapy, systematic sensitization, exposure, and psychopharmacology.


**Keywords:** anxiety disorders, panic disorder, phobia, social anxiety disorder, generalized anxiety disorder, selective mutism

## 1. Introduction to anxiety disorders

### 1.1 Anxiety concept

Anxiety is a feeling that individuals experience at different levels throughout their lives. Anxiety is a healthy, normal response to perceived threats or unique experiences, and it is a necessary motivating force for survival. Mild anxiety is a driving force necessary for adaptation and advancement to the higher stage of spiritual development. However, when the anxiety level increases too much, it, on the contrary, serves as a hindering function [1].

### 1.2 Anxiety and fear

Anxiety and fear are emotions that people are usually confused about. Fear is a response to a known threat. However, anxiety can be defined as fear, tension, uneasiness, or restlessness expected from an unidentified or unknown source. We can evaluate anxiety as a cognitive state of fear [2]. Physical symptoms of anxiety include palpitations, difficulty breathing, rapid breathing, tremors in the hands and feet, and excessive sweating. Psychological symptoms, on the other hand, include distress, excitement, sudden feeling, and fear that something terrible will happen [3].

Anxiety, which we consider normal (mild and moderate anxiety), plays an important role in the development of the individual. However, if the level of anxiety increases, it may lead to mental problems. A high level of anxiety, long duration, and intensification of anxiety symptoms may cause anxiety disorders. Anxiety can be evaluated as pathological when it begins to have an impact on social and occupational actions, achievement of desired goals, and emotional state [4].

In short, anxiety can be deemed pathological if the following situations occur:

a. When anxiety is not proportional to the situation that creates anxiety,

b. When anxiety inhibits social, occupational, and other important functional areas.

Example: Ms. M., who was involved in a serious traffic accident a month ago, refuses to drive even to places in short distances. Her father has to take Ms. M. whenever she needs to go somewhere. Ms. M., who constantly refuses to drive, has even had to quit her job because of her anxiety about driving.

### 1.3 Epidemiology

Anxiety disorders are the most common of all psychiatric illnesses and result in significant functional impairment and distress [5, 6]. Its prevalence per year is reported as 17.7%. This rate is 30.5% for women and 19.2% for men, and the frequency decreases with the increase in socioeconomic level [7]. In a study conducted by Özcan et al. (2006), anxiety disorder was found to be the most common diagnosis among 950 psychiatric patients, and it was mostly observed in women, housewives, married people, and people with a low education level [8].

## 2. Etiology of anxiety disorders

### 2.1 Biological factors

In twin studies conducted, it was concluded that genetics was a huge factor. Structural neuroimaging studies in patients with panic disorder indicate pathological involvement in the temporal lobes, especially in hippocampus [9].

Although many neurotransmitters are effective in the pathophysiology of anxiety disorders, disorders in serotonin, norepinephrine, and gamma-aminobutyric acid (GABA) appear to be the most important. GABA has an important place among the causes of anxiety disorder. As the drugs used in the treatment of anxiety disorders increase GABA, it is thought that the insufficiency and imbalance in GABA are directly related to the anxiety experienced [3, 5]. Serotonin is another neurotransmitter linked to anxiety disorder. Deficiency or an imbalance of serotonin in the amygdala is observed in anxiety-related disorders. It is known that there is imbalance in the regions related to norepinephrine in anxiety disorders.

It has been revealed that the CRF (Corticotropin-Releasing Factor) system plays an important role among the biological causes of anxiety disorders [1].

### 2.2 Brain areas affected in anxiety disorders

The brain areas affected by anxiety disorders and the symptoms they cause are listed below:

- Amygdala: Fear, which is especially important in panic and phobic disorders.

- Hippocampus: Depends on memory which is related to fear responses.

- Locus coeruleus: Vigilance
- Brain stem: respiratory movement, heartbeat
- Hypothalamus: activation of the stress response
- Frontal cortex: Cognitive interpretations
- Thalamus: Integration of sensory impulses
- Basal ganglia: Tremors [10]

## 3. Psychological theories

**Psychodynamic Theory:** According to the psychodynamic view, anxiety is a state of tension that emerges in the self as a result of threats originating from within and outside the individual. Starting from childhood, repressed emotions, desires, impulses, experiences occasionally disturb the individual's self in the following years. A conflict arises between the self (ego), lower self (id), and upper self (superego), which creates anxiety in the individual. Anxiety is a harbinger of danger to the self, and the self tries to reduce anxiety by using self-defense mechanisms [11].

Freud argued that the child experiences anxiety specific to each period during the development process. These are superego anxiety, castration anxiety, fear of losing love, separation anxiety, annihilation anxiety, and disintegration anxiety.

**Behavioral Theory:** According to this theory, anxiety is an emotional experience developed based on the urge to escape from congenital pain or suffering. This theory suggests that if an individual experiences intense fears and stressful events in early periods of life, s/he is likely to experience high levels of anxiety in his/her later life. Fear responses acquired through conditioning, observation, and social learning cause "escape" and "avoidance" behaviors to be triggered, thereby reducing anxiety. The escape and avoidance behaviors are thus reinforced, and when any kind of anxiety is experienced, they come into play and the anxiety is prevented from fading. Thus, the continuity of anxiety is ensured in this way [11].

**Cognitive Theory:** In Beck's theory, how we interpret and perceive events determines our emotions; in other words, it is the meaning attributed to them rather than the events themselves that trigger our emotions. This interpretation depends on the characteristics of the environment in which the event occurs, the mood at the time of the event, and the past experiences of the individual. Individuals experience anxiety due to their false reasoning and irrational beliefs [1, 3].

## 4. Classification of anxiety disorders

In DSM 5, anxiety disorders are divided into eleven subgroups. These are:

- Separation anxiety disorder,
- Selective mutism,
- Panic disorder,

- Agoraphobia,
- Specific Phobia,
- Social anxiety disorder,
- Generalized anxiety disorder,
- Other unspecified anxiety disorder,
- Anxiety disorder related to another medical condition,
- Anxiety disorder caused by substance or medication,
- Anxiety disorders caused by substances and medication are unspecified anxiety disorders [12].

### 4.1 Separation anxiety disorder

Separation anxiety disorder can be defined as experiencing fear and anxiety that is more than expected and repetitive in terms of developmental level resulting from separation from home or someone the person is attached to for at least four weeks in children, and for at least six months or longer in adults. It is seen that individuals with separation anxiety disorder do not want to go to school or elsewhere because of the fear of separation. The main feature of separation anxiety disorder is excessive anxiety caused by leaving the mother, father, home or familiar environment. It is seen equally in boys and girls.

*Etiology:* According to the psychodynamic approach, children who are attached ambivalently are very busy with the care of their caregivers, which reduces their exploration behaviors of their environment and thus causes separation anxiety to develop. Stressful events such as parental divorce, illness, loss are important risk factors for separation anxiety disorder. In a study, it was found that the depressive, cyclothymic, irritable and anxious temperament scores of the mothers of children with separation anxiety disorder were higher than the control group [13].

Symptoms in separation anxiety disorder differ according to the developmental period. In children aged 5-8 years, the fear of a bad event and rejection of school, intense distress during separation at the age of 9-12, school refusal in adolescents aged 13-16, and physical complaints appear as symptoms.

*Comorbidity:* Frequently, depression, bipolar disorder, hyperactivity disorder, personality disorders and other anxiety disorders are seen together.

*Treatment:* In the treatment of separation anxiety disorder, the most important point is planning to include the family, school and child. Cognitive therapy is one of the effective methods. Antidepressants, selective serotonin reuptake inhibitors, are used in drug therapy. One study suggested that vilazodone can be used in the treatment of separation anxiety disorder [14].

### 4.2 Selective Mutism

The most important feature of this disorder is that although the individual can speak in other situations, s/he constantly does not speak in certain specific social situations (when s/he meets people s/he does not know, etc.) where s/he is expected to speak. The disorder must last at least one month and affect the person's education, work success, and social life. It usually occurs in the preschool period.

*DOI: http://dx.doi.org/10.5772/intechopen.93952*

*Etiology:* In the etiology of the disorder, there are reasons such as delay in language development, communication defects, lack of communication, presence of psychiatric disorders in the family, and overprotection of the family.

*Comorbidity:* Social phobia, obsessive-compulsive disorder, speech and language disorders are among the disorders accompanying selective speech disorders.

*Treatment:* Behavioral treatments, pharmacological treatments, group and family therapies are effective in treatment. It has been stated that the cognitive-behavioral approach especially encourages verbal and non-verbal forms of communication. In family therapy, it is important to identify healthy and dysfunctional family relationships and to raise awareness of family members about unhealthy communication patterns and behaviors. Selective serotonin reuptake inhibitors are preferred in pharmacological treatment.

### 4.3 Panic disorder

In the Diagnostic and Statistical Manual of Mental Disorders, Fifth Edition (DSM-5) [American Psychiatric Association (APA)] it is stated that at least four of the following symptoms must be present to determine the presence of a panic attack. These are:

- Palpitations, pounding heart or accelerated heart rate
- Sweating
- Shaking or trembling
- Feeling short of breath or smothering
- Choking sensation
- Chest pain or discomfort
- Nausea or abdominal distress
- Feeling dizzy, lightheaded, unsteady or faint
- Chills or hot flushes
- Paresthesias (tingling and numbness sensations)
- Derealization (unreal feelings) or depersonalization (feelings of being detached from oneself)
- Fear of losing control and going crazy
- Fear of dying [12]

Panic disorder, which is a very old disease, is a syndrome characterized by sudden and extreme anxiety with unreasonable and unpredictable panic attacks. Its most important feature is that it is accompanied by intense physical discomfort. Panic attacks can occur only once, or frequently, on a weekly, monthly or even annual basis. Panic attack disorder is usually seen in the 20s. The panic attack is an unreasonable and severe state of anxiety. During panic attacks, symptoms such as palpitations, accelerated heart rate, sweating, trembling/shaking, shortness of breath, feeling of choking, breathlessness, chest pain, fainting, fear of losing control or going crazy, numbness, tingling, chills or hot flushes can be seen.

The presence of a medical drum that may cause anxiety should first be investigated in a patient presenting with panic attack. All the drugs used by the individual should be questioned, and the side effects of the drugs should be considered. Below are some medical conditions that cause symptoms similar to panic attacks.

**Certain medical conditions that produce symptoms similar to panic attacks**

- Alcohol Withdrawal Syndrome
- Substance Withdrawal Syndrome
- Cardiac arrhythmias
- Hyperthyroidism
- Hypoglycemia
- Asthma
- Cushing's Disease

The majority of patients have challenging life events before the first panic attack occurs. Low socio-economic level, delay in treatment, presence of additional diagnoses cause a negative course in panic disorder.

Comorbidity: Depression is seen with social phobia, specific phobia, traumatic stress disorder and alcoholism.

Treatment: Specific serotonin reuptake inhibitors should be the first choice in the treatment of panic disorder. If the patient does not respond to treatment, switching to other specific serotonin reuptake inhibitors is recommended. If there is no response to two specific serotonin reuptake inhibitors and there is severe tolerance, it is recommended to switch to SNRI. Alprazolan is also highly effective. Drug treatment should last at least a year. Behavioral-cognitive psychotherapy is an effective method in panic disorder. This method attempts to change the patient's perception of physical symptoms. It will be useful to teach breathing exercises to the patient [15].

### 4.4 Agoraphobia

Agoraphobia, which is shortly defined as the fear of open space, is the fear of being deprived of help or being in places where it is difficult to escape.

*Treatment:* Combination of pharmacotherapy and psychotherapy (behavioral, cognitive, virtual therapies) is recommended in its treatment. Benzodiazepines, SSRIs, tricyclic and tetracyclicantidepressants are recommended as diocological [15].

### 4.5 Social phobia (social anxiety disorder)

It is a disorder characterized by blushing, sweating, and trembling of the hands when one believes that s/he is perceived negatively by others while sitting or talking in public. The individual is afraid of social or performance situations where embarrassment can occur and firmly believes that s/he will be subject to possible reproach by others [12]. The onset of the symptoms of this disorder often occurs in late childhood or early adolescence and becomes chronic and sometimes continues throughout life. It is equally prevalent in males and females (Puri & Treasaden, 2011). The disorder affects social or occupational functionality or causes significant distress.

*Treatment:* In its treatment, the combination of psychotherapy and pharmacotherapy has an advantage over the individual application of both treatments. The drug groups to be used in the treatment of social phobia similar to other anxiety disorders are SSRIs, benzodiazepines, venlafaxine and busprone. MAO inhibitors such as phenelzine and moclobemide have been shown to be successful in severe cases [15].

### 4.6 Specific phobia

It is an excessive, illogical and meaningless fear of a specific object (snake, dog, etc.) or a situation (injection, darkness, etc.). Exposure to phobic stimulus produces compelling panic symptoms, including palpitations, sweating, dizziness and difficulty in breathing. Phobias can begin at any age. People can be phobic towards almost any object or situation. Those that start in childhood often disappear without treatment. But those that start in adulthood or are persistent often require therapeutic support. The disorder is diagnosed more often in females than in males [16]. The specific classification of simple phobias is given in **Table 1**.

*Treatment:* It is not enough to use drugs alone in the treatment of specific phobias. Behavioral therapy, insight-oriented therapy, virtual therapy and pharmacotherapy are at the forefront in its treatment [17]. The main principle of treatment should be exposure to the feared situation. When the phobia is accompanied by panic attacks, beta-adrenergic receptor antagonists or benzodiazepines can be used. The combined use of pharmacotherapy and psychotherapy may also be effective.

### 4.7 Generalized anxiety disorder

It is an anxiety disorder characterized by being chronic and unrealistic, and extreme anxiety that must last at least 6 months. Symptoms can cause distress to the person in social, professional and other important areas. Individuals with this disorder are constantly worried. Restlessness, excessive excitement, fatigue, sleep disturbance and muscle tension are significant symptoms. Anxiety often results in difficulty in making self-decisions, and the person seeks constant approval from those around him. They always feel like they are going to get bad news. It usually starts in childhood and adolescence [2].

*Comorbidity:* It is seen with depression and other anxiety disorders.

*Treatment:* Cognitive-behavioral, supportive and insight oriented therapy and pharmacotherapy have a role in its treatment. The main drug groups used in the

| Clinical name | Feared object or situation |
| --- | --- |
| Acrophobia | Heights |
| Agoraphobia | Open spaces |
| Claustrophobia | Closed spaces |
| Hematophobia | Blood |
| Zoophobia | Animals |

**Table 1.**
*Specific classification of simple phobias.*

treatment are benzodiazepines, SSRI, buspirone and venlafaxine. Benzodiazepines in treatment should be started with the lowest dose of the therapeutic range to be used and the dose should be increased in case of unresponsiveness [1].

### 4.8 Anxiety disorder associated with another medical condition and substance/ medication-induced anxiety

Symptoms associated with these disorders are evaluated directly as a physiological consequence of another medical condition or directly due to substance intoxication or deprivation or exposure to the drug. Many medical conditions are related to the development of anxiety symptoms. Some of these include cardiac conditions such as myocardial infarction, congestive heart failure and mitral valve prolapse, endocrine conditions such as hypoglycemia, hypo/hyperthyroidism and pheochromocytoma, respiratory conditions such as chronic obstructive pulmonary disease and hyperventilation, and complex partial seizures, neoplasms and encephalitis [12].

## 5. Treatment methods in anxiety disorders

### 5.1 Cognitive - behavioral therapy

It is a widely used, successful and easy method in the treatment of anxiety disorders. This short-term treatment method focuses on changing the patient's thoughts and behaviors. This treatment includes emotional and behavioral changes to help the person to adapt to the environment perceived to be dangerous, as well as the initial definition and restructuring of cognitions related to anxiety in the form of unreal interpretation of danger [9, 18–20]. In their study, Andrews et al. (2005) also found that virtual reality practice therapy is effective in treating public speaking anxiety [21].

#### *5.1.1 Systematic desensitization*

In systematic desensitization, the patient is gradually exposed to the effect of phobia stimuli in real or imaginary situations. The concept was first introduced by Joseph Wolpe in 1958 and is based on the principles of behavior conditioning. Emphasis is placed on mutual inhibition or mutual conditioning [22].

*Mutual inhibition* is defined as limiting anxiety before trying to reduce avoidance behaviors. The rationale behind this concept is that individuals cannot be excited and relaxed at the same time, as relaxation is the opposite of anxiety [23].

There are two important elements in systematic desensitization by mutual inhibition:

1. Practicing relaxation techniques

2. Gradual exposure to fear stimuli in a relaxed state.

The individual is taught the art of relaxation by using techniques that are more effective for him/her (e.g. progressive relaxation, mental imagination, tension and relaxation, meditation). After the individual learns relaxation techniques, exposure to phobic stimuli is initiated. The patient is asked to rank hierarchically the situations that cause phobic stimuli from the most disturbing to the least disturbing. In case of maximum relaxation, the patient may be asked to visualize the phobic stimulus in his/her mind. First of all, the exposure focuses on the phobic stimulus that causes the least fear or anxiety. In subsequent sessions, the individual is exposed to the effects of increasingly more fearful stimuli. Sessions can be conducted in imaginary, real-life situations (live), or sometimes a combination of both [1].

#### 5.1.2 Flooding therapy

*Flooding* is the therapeutic process that involves the patient participating in real-life events or imaginary situations that s/he thinks to be extremely fearful for a long time. Relaxation training is not part of the technique. Such sessions should be given a long period because short periods can be ineffective and even harmful. The sessions are terminated when the patient reacts significantly less than s/he did at the beginning of the sessions [24].

#### 5.1.3 Relaxation exercise

Relaxation exercise is a method that effectively reduces tension and anxiety. It can be used alone or in conjunction with other cognitive-behavioral techniques [25].

### 5.2 Family therapy

Families have difficulties in understanding the symptoms of their relatives with anxiety disorders and may find it hard to tolerate, and this situation can disrupt the healthy family structure. It is important to remind family members of their roles in therapy and to emphasize that support is important. Besides, it is necessary to inform them about anxiety disorder symptoms and treatments [1]. In another study conducted, it was concluded that treatments aimed at reducing symptoms only were insufficient in the treatment of anxiety disorders and that programs for improving interpersonal relationships, communication skills and anger management of the individual should be added [26].

### 5.3 Psychopharmacology

*Anxiolytics:* Benzodiazepines are used successfully in the treatment of common anxiety disorders. It can be prescribed when the patient is particularly anxious. Alprazolam, lorazepam and clonazepam are particularly effective in treating panic disorder. In Benzodiazepine *treatment*, there are physical addiction and tolerance risks that can lead to addiction. This is because deprivation symptoms can be life-threatening, so patients should be warned against sudden termination of drug intake, and drug termination should be done with treatment. Due to potential for addiction, benzodiazepines, SSRIs, serotonin, and norepinephrine reuptake inhibitors (SNRs), and buspirone are the first-line therapy [27].

Buspirone, which as an anti-anxiety agent, is effective in approximately 60% to 80% of patients with a generalized anxiety disorder [3]. The only disadvantage of buspirone is the 10-14 day delay in relieving symptoms. However, the lack of physical addiction and tolerance disadvantage of buspirone makes it the drug of choice in the treatment of generalized anxiety disorders. The effects and side effects of anxiolytic agents are given in **Table 2**.

*Antidepressants:* Many antidepressants are as effective as anti-anxiety agents. Tricyclic, clomipramine and imipramine drugs are used successfully in patients with panic disorder. However, after the discovery of SSRIs, tricyclics are used less frequently because they tend to cause side effects when given in desired high doses to alleviate panic disorder symptoms [15].

| Anxiolytic agents | Effect | Side effects |
|---|---|---|
| Benzodiazepines | The GABA receptor increases the affinity of GABAA. | Sedation, dizziness, weakness, ataxia, decreased motor performance, addiction, withdrawal |
| SSRIs | Inhibiting serotonin reuptake at the presynaptic nerve end, increasing serotonin synaptic concentration. | Nausea, diarrhea, headache, insomnia, sleepiness, sexual dysfunction |
| SNRIs | Inhibition of neural serotonin and norepinephrine reuptake, mild reuptake of dopamine | Headache, dry mouth, nausea, drowsiness, insomnia, weakness, dizziness, constipation, diarrhea |
| Noradrenergic agents (propranolol, clonidine) | Propranolol: inhibits beta adrenergic receptor activity. Clonidine: stimulates alpha-adrenergic receptors. | Propranolol: bradycardia, hypotension, weakness, fatigue, impotence, gastrointestinal disorder, bronchospasm |
| Barbiturates | CNS depression also produces effects in the hepatic and cardiovascular systems. | Clonidine: dry mouth, sedation, fatigue, hypotension |
| Buspirone | 5-HT1A receptor partial antagonist | Drowsiness, agitation, confusion, ataxia, dizziness, bradycardia, hypotension, constipation |

**Table 2.**
*Anxiolytic agents.*

SSRIs are effective in treating panic disorders. Paroxetine, fluoxetine, and sertraline have been approved by the US Food and Drug Administration (FDA) for these purposes. The dosage of these drugs should be increased gradually, as patients with panic disorder are sensitive to overstimulation caused by SSRIs [1].

The use of anti-depressants in the treatment of generalized anxiety disorders is still under investigation. Some success has been reported with tricyclic, imipramine and SSRI drugs. The FDA has approved paroxetine, escitalopram, duloxetine and extended-release venlafaxine for the treatment of generalized anxiety disorders [28].

Beta blockers: Clonid and beta-blockers such as propranolol and atenolol are also used especially in maintenance treatment. These drugs are most effective in treating state anxiety [1].

## Author details

Hülya Kök Eren
Department of Mental Health and Diseases Nursing, Faculty of Health Sciences, Eskisehir Osmangazi University, Turkey

*Address all correspondence to: hulyakok2911@gmail.com

## References

[1] Townsend, M.C., Psychiatric mental health nursing: Concepts of care in evidence-based practice. 2014: FA Davis.

[2] Combs, H. and J. Markman, Anxiety disorders in primary care. Medical Clinics, 2014. **98**(5): p. 1007-1023.

[3] Sadock, B.J. and V.A. Sadock, Synopsis of psychiatry: Behavioral sciences/clinical psychiatry. Vol. 10. 2007, Philadephia: Lippincott Williams&Wilkins.

[4] Black, D.W. and N.C. Andreasen, Introductory textbook of psychiatry. 5 ed. 2011, Washington: American Psychiatric Publishing.

[5] Doğan, O., The epidemiology of anxiety disorders. Anatolian Journal of Psychiatry, 2012. **13**: p. 158-164.

[6] Baxter, A., et al., Global prevalence of anxiety disorders: a systematic review and meta-regression. Psychological medicine, 2013. **43**(5): p. 897.

[7] Erol, N., C. Kılıç, and M. Ulusoy, Türkiye Ruh Sağlığı Profili Araştırması, Ana Rapor. 1998, Ankara.T. C. Sağlık Bakanlığı.

[8] Özcan, M., F. Uğuz, and A.S. Çilli, Ayaktan psikiyatri hastalarında yaygın anksiyete bozukluğunun yaygınlığı ve ek tanılar. Türk Psikiyatri Dergisi, 2006. **17**(4): p. 276-285.

[9] Meier, S. and J. Deckert, Genetics of anxiety disorders. Current psychiatry reports, 2019. **21**(3): p. 2-8.

[10] Sevinçok, L., Yaygın anksiyete bozukluğunun nörobiyolojisi. Klinik Psikiyatri, 2007. **10**: p. 3-12.

[11] Köroğlu, E. and H. Türkçapar, Psikotrerapi Yöntemleri, Kuramlar ve Uygulama Yönergeleri. 2013, Ankara: HYB Basım Yayın.

[12] Association, A.P., Diagnostic and statistical manual of mental disorders (DSM-5®). 2013, Arlington: American Psychiatric Pub.

[13] Erermiş, S., et al., Ayrılma anksiyetesi bozukluğu olan okul öncesi yaş grubu çocukların annelerinin mizaç özellikleri. Türk psikiyatri Dergisi, 2009. **20**(1): p. 14-21.

[14] Schneier, F., et al., A randomized controlled pilot trial of vilazodone for adult separation anxiety disorder. Depression and Anxiety, 2017. **34**(12): p. 1085-1095.

[15] Reinhold, J. and K. Rickels, Pharmacological treatment for generalized anxiety disorder in adults: an update. Expert opinion on pharmacotherapy, 2015. **16**(11): p. 1669-1681.

[16] Varcarolis, E. and M. Halter, Psychiatric Mental Health Nursing. 2010, America: Tom Wilhelm.

[17] Işıklı, S., Z. Baran, and S. Aslan, Özgül fobilerde sanal gerçeklik teknolojisi uygulamaları ile tedaviye yardımcı araç geliştirme: Bir etkililik çalışması. Klinik Psikiyatri Dergisi, 2019. **22**(3): p. 316-328.

[18] Arch, J.J., et al., Longitudinal treatment mediation of traditional cognitive behavioral therapy and acceptance and commitment therapy for anxiety disorders. Behaviour Research and Therapy, 2012. **50**(7): p. 469-478.

[19] Fıstıkcı, N., et al., Sosyal anksiyete bozukluğunda bilişsel davranışçı terapi: Güncel kavramlar. Psikiyatride Güncel Yaklaşımlar, 2015. **7**(3): p. 229-243.

[20] Kaval, N.O. and S.T. Sütcü, Çocuk ve Ergenlerde Sosyal Anksiyete Bozukluğunun Tedavisinde Bilişsel-Davranışçı Grup Terapisinin Etkililiği:

Sistematik Bir Gözden Geçirme. Psikiyatride Güncel Yaklaşımlar, 2016. **8**(Ek 1): p. 3-22.

[21] Andrews, G., M. Davies, and N. Titov, Effectiveness randomized controlled trial of face to face versus Internet cognitive behaviour therapy for social phobia. Australian and New Zealand Journal of Psychiatry, 2011. **45**(4): p. 337-340.

[22] Obi, J. and A. Oguzie, Effects of systematic desensitization technique on generalized anxiety among adolescents in Enugu East Local Government. Enugu State, Nigeria. iJournals: International Journal of Social Relevance & Concern, 2019. **7**(5): p. 1-9.

[23] Bulantika, S., M. Wibowo, and M. Jafar, Group Counseling with Systematic Desensitization Techniques and Thought-Stopping Techniques to Reduce Social Anxiety. Jurnal Bimbingan Konseling, 2018. **7**(2): p. 106-112.

[24] Zbozinek, T. and M. Craske, The role of positive affect in enhancing extinction learning and exposure therapy for anxiety disorders. Journal of Experimental Psychopathology, 2017. **8**(1): p. 13-39.

[25] Zou, L., et al., Mindfulness-based Baduanjin exercise for depression and anxiety in people with physical or mental illnesses: a systematic review and meta-analysis. International journal of environmental research and public health, 2018. **15**(2): p. 321.

[26] Şahin, N.H., A.D. Batıgün, and C. Uzun, Anksiyete bozukluğu: Kişilerarası tarz, kendilik algısı ve öfke açısından bir değerlendirme. Anadolu Psikiyatri Dergisi, 2011. **12**(2): p. 107-113.

[27] Bandelow, B., et al., Efficacy of treatments for anxiety disorders: a meta-analysis. International clinical psychopharmacology, 2015. **30**(4): p. 183-192.

[28] Cuijpers, P., et al., Adding psychotherapy to antidepressant medication in depression and anxiety disorders: a meta-analysis. World Psychiatry, 2014. **13**(1): p. 56-67.

Chapter 7

# Prevalence and Comorbidity of Anxiety and Depressive Disorders in Studies of PRIME-MD and PHQ (Patient Health Questionnaire) in Japan

*Kumiko Muramatsu, Hitoshi Miyaoka, Kunitoshi Kamijima, Yoshiyuki Muramatsu, Katsuya Fuse, Fumitoshi Yoshimine, Ichiro Mashima, Yutaka Tanaka, Michio Hosaka, Kikuchi Toshiaki, Natsue Shimizu and Shigeji Baba*

## Abstract

We examine two studies on the prevalence and comorbidity of anxiety and depressive disorders in Japanese patients in primary care settings. The PRIME-MD study (Primary Care Evaluation of Mental Disorders) in Japan was conducted in seven primary care sites. The sample group included 601 adult patients (249 males, 352 females, mean age = 58.9 years, SD = 16.5). Of the 12.5% of patients diagnosed with mood disorders, 5.0% (n = 29) were major depressive disorder, and 6.7% (n = 40) were minor depressive disorder. The odds ratio for co-occurrence of major depressive disorder with generalized anxiety disorders and major depressive disorder with anxiety disorders (NOS) was 11.5 (95% CI: 2.17–18.45) and 8.00 (95% CI: 3.19–20.07), respectively. The PHQ (Patient Health Questionnaire) study in Japan was conducted in eleven primary care sites. A total of 1409 adult patients (611 males, 797 females; mean age: 56.2 years, SD: ±20.4) completed the PHQ in full. The prevalence of diagnosis of any mood disorder or any anxiety disorder was 25.0%. Of the 15.8% of patients diagnosed with mood disorders, 5.3% were for major depression and 8.4% for other depressive disorders. The odds ratio for co-occurrence of major depressive disorder with other anxiety disorders was 30.4 (95% CI: 13.19–70.28).

**Keywords:** anxiety, depression, comorbidity, PRIME-MD, PHQ

## 1. Introduction

Numerous epidemiological studies in Western countries have shown that anxiety and depressive disorders frequently occur together in [1–4]. Especially, comorbidity of anxiety and depressive disorders has been confirmed in patients presenting in primary care settings [3, 4].

The outcome of co-occurrence of anxiety and depressive disorders is more negative than each single occurrence. According to findings of a large cohort study in the Netherlands, clinically, comorbidity is associated with a greater severity of symptoms, an increased risk of suicide, a more reduced quality of life, and a lower level of functioning [2].

Despite the availability of studies and data examining anxiety and depressive disorders in patients in primary care settings in other countries, such studies are few in Japan. Consequently, recognition of the comorbidity of anxiety and depressive disorders in such patients in Japan remains a major clinical problem. With that issue in mind, here we examine two studies on the comorbidity of anxiety and depressive disorders in Japanese patients in primary care detected by PRIME-MD (Primary Care Evaluation of Mental Disorders) [5, 6] and the PHQ (Patient Health Questionnaire) [7].

## 2. The PRIME-MD Study in Japan

### 2.1 Objective

To define the prevalence and comorbidity of anxiety disorders and depressive disorders in primary care patients in Japan.

### 2.2 Materials and Methods

The PRIME-MD [5] was the first instrument designed for use in primary care as diagnostic criteria based on the Diagnostic and Statistical Manual of Mental Disorders, Revised Third Edition (DSM–III-R) [8], and the Diagnostic and Statistical Manual of Mental Disorders, Fourth Edition (DSM–IV) [9]. It is used in clinical settings and has been widely used in clinical research [10–12].

PRIME-MD is a two-step instrument consisting of a self-administered patient questionnaire and a structured clinical interview administered by the physician. The first step is a brief screening instrument in which the patient is required to complete answers in full. A structured interview is subsequently conducted if the result of the patient's screening suggests the presence of a psychiatric diagnosis, which allows for a DSM-IV diagnosis to be assigned if appropriate.

PRIME-MD was used to determine the presence of DSM-IV in the present study, which was conducted from 1998 to 1999. The sample group included 601 adult patients (249 males, 352 females, mean age = 58.9 years, SD = 16.5), who were selected randomly from seven primary care settings and assessed by twelve primary care physicians. Study protocol was approved by the Ethics Committee at the Niigata City General Hospital and the other participating institutions in accordance with the Ethical Principles for Medical Research Involving Human Subjects (Declaration of Helsinki).

### 2.3 Results

The percentage of patients with no psychiatric diagnosis was 61.3%, while those with a type of somatoform disorder was 15.5%, a markedly high rate. 12.5% of patients were diagnosed with mood disorders, 8.5% with anxiety disorders, and 2.2% with alcohol use (**Figures 1** and **2**).

We compared the results of our PRIME-MD study in Japan with a PRIME-MD study conducted in the USA [5]. The prevalence of any mood disorders in Japan is lower than that in the USA. In particular, the rate of major depression is far

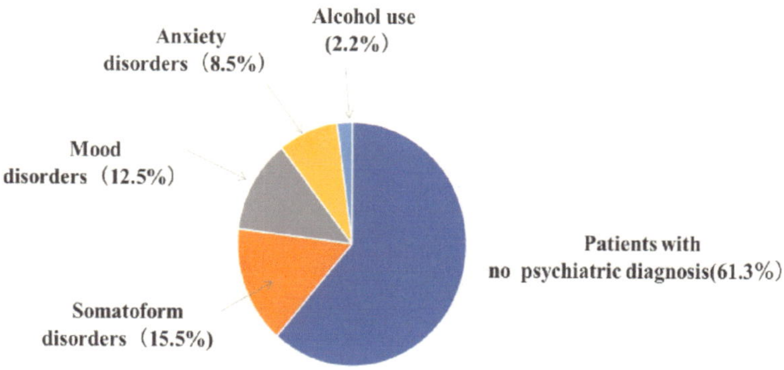


**Figure 1.**
*Prevalence of Mental Disorders Detected by PRIME-MD in Primary Care Patients in Japan (n = 601).*

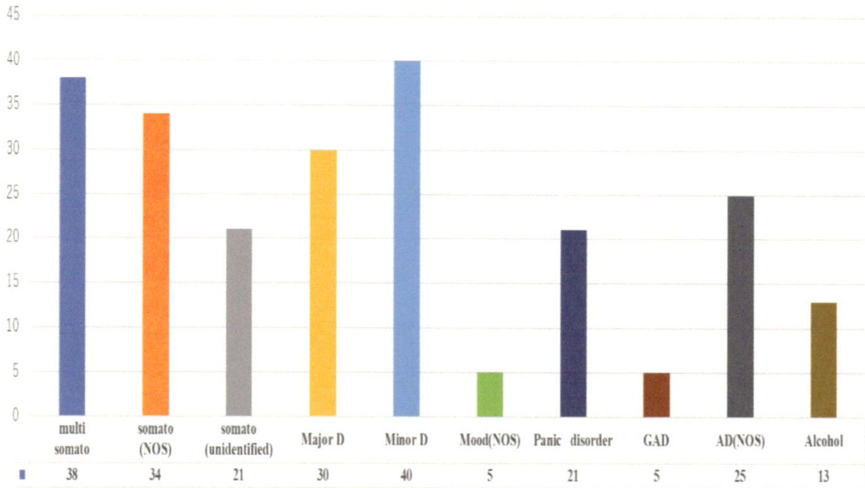


**Figure 2.**
*Breakdown of Mental Disorders Detected by PRIME-MD in Primary Care Patients in Japan (n = 601).*

lower in Japan. Minor depression, however, is almost as common in Japan as in the USA. Moreover, the rate of prevalence of any anxiety disorders in Japan is lower than in the USA, while figures for panic disorder are similar in both countries (refer to **Table 1**).

Of the 12.5% of patients diagnosed with mood disorders, 5.0% (n = 29) were major depressive disorder, and 6.7% (n = 40) were minor depressive disorder. 4.2% (n = 21) of patients were diagnosed with panic disorder, only 5 patients with general anxiety disorder (GAD), and 4.2% (n = 25) with anxiety disorders not otherwise specified.

As for diagnosis (n = 93) of somatoform disorders, 6.3% of patients (n = 38) were diagnosed with multisomatoform disorder, 5.7% (n = 34) with somatoform disorders not otherwise specified and 3.5% (n = 21) with identified somatoform disorders (refer to **Figure 3**).

The odds ratio for co-occurrence of major depressive disorder with generalized anxiety disorders, with anxiety disorders (NOS), and with panic disorders was 11.5 (95% CI: 2.17–18.45) and 8.00 (95% CI: 3.19–20.07), 6.33 (95% CI: 2.17–18.45), respectively (refer to **Table 2**).

**Table 3** shows the prevalence of mental disorder in women and men detected by the PRIME-MD study in Japan (n-601). With regards to major depression, a

| | PRIME-MD study (n-601) in Japan | PRIME-MD 1000 Study in USA |
|---|---|---|
| Patients with psychiatric diagnoses | 28.1% | 39% |
| Mood disorders(any) | 12.5% | 26% |
| Major depression | 5.0% | 12% |
| Minor depression | 6.7% | 6% |
| Dysthymia | 0.8% | 8% |
| Anxiety disorders(any) | 8.5% | 18% |
| Panic disorders | 3.5% | 4% |
| GAD | 0.8% | 7% |
| Anxiety disorders(any) | 4.2% | 9% |
| Somatoform disorders(any) | 15.5% | 14% |
| Multisomatoform | 6.3% | 8% |
| Somatoform NOS | 5.7% | 4% |
| Alcohol abuse | 2.2% | 5% |
| Binge eating | 0% | 3% |

**Table 1.**
*The comparison of PRIME-MD study in Japan and USA.*

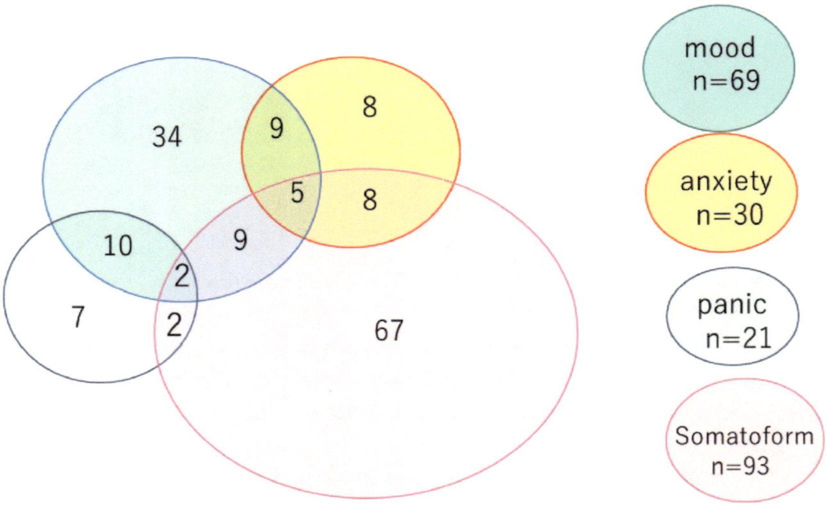


**Figure 3.**
*Comorbidity of mood disorders, panic disorders, anxiety disorders and somatoform disorders detected by PRIME-MD in Japan (n = 601).*

| Major Depression with Anxiety Disorders | OR | 95%CI | 99%CI |
|---|---|---|---|
| Generalized Anxiety Disorder | 11.5 | 2.17–18.45 | 1.55–25.80 |
| Anxiety Disorders (NOS) | 8.00 | 3.19–20.07 | 2.39–26.79 |
| Panic Disorders | 6.33 | 2.17–18.45 | 1.55–25.80 |
| *OR: odds ratio, CI: Confidence Interval.* | | | |

**Table 2.**
*Comorbidity of mood Disorders and anxiety Disorders by detected the PRIME-MD study in Japan (n = 601).*

| | Women n = 352 | Men n = 249 | OR | *P* |
|---|---|---|---|---|
| Any Prime diagnosis | 29.0% | 27.3% | 1.07 | ns |
| Mood disorders (any) | 11.9% | 10.8% | 1.07 | ns |
| Major depression | 6.5% | 2.8% | 2.41 | 0.0449 |
| Minor depression | 6.0% | 7.6% | 0.77 | ns |
| Anxiety disorders (any) | 8.5% | 6.0% | 1.44 | ns |
| Panic disorder | 1.4% | 6.4% | 2.32 | ns |
| GAD | 1.1% | 0.4% | 2.85 | ns |
| Anxiety disorders (nos) | 3.9% | 4.4% | 0.90 | ns |
| Somatoform disorders (any) | 16.4% | 14.1% | 1.21 | ns |
| Multisomatoform | 6.5% | 6.0% | 1.11 | ns |
| Somatoform (nos) | 6.5% | 4.4% | 1.52 | ns |
| Alcohol use | 0.3% | 4.8% | 0.56 | 0.0058 |

*GAD = generalized anxiety disorder, nos = not otherwise specified, OR = odds ratio.*

**Table 3.**
*Prevalence of Mental Disorder in Women and Men Detected by the PRIME-MD Study in Japan (n = 601).*

significantly higher odds ratio was observed in women than in men (p = 0.0449). Alternatively, the odds ratio for alcohol use in men far exceeds that for women (p = 0.0058) (**Table 3**).

## 3. The PHQ (Patient Health Questionnaire) Study in Japan

### 3.1 Objective

We defined the prevalence and comorbidity of anxiety disorders and mood disorders in primary care patients in Japan using the PHQ.

### 3.2 Background

The clinical usefulness of the PRIME-MD is limited due to its time-consuming procedures. The PHQ, which was developed from the original PRIME-MD, is a self-administered version used for making criteria-based diagnoses of mental disorders that are common in primary care. The diagnostic validity of the PHQ has been established in two studies involving 3000 patients in eight primary care clinics [7] and 3000 patients in seven obstetrics-gynecology clinics in the USA [6]. We examined the validation study of the Japanese version of PHQ in primary care settings [13].

The PHQ can be entirely self-administered by the patient. The clinician scans the completed questionnaire, verifies positive responses, and applies diagnostic algorithms that are abbreviated at the bottom of each page. The questionnaire assesses eight diagnoses, divided into threshold disorders (disorders that correspond to the following specific DSM-IV diagnoses: major depressive disorder, panic disorder, and bulimia nervosa), and subthreshold disorders (disorders whose criteria encompass fewer symptoms than are required for any specific DSM-IV diagnoses: other depressive disorder, other anxiety disorder, probable alcohol abuse/dependence, probable somatoform disorder, and binge eating disorder).

Major depression is diagnosed if five or more of the nine depressive symptom criteria have been present at least "more than half the days" over the last two weeks, and one of the symptoms is depressed mood or anhedonia. Other depression is diagnosed if two, three, or four depressive symptoms have been present at least "more than half the days" over the last two weeks, and one of the symptoms is depressed mood or ahendonia. One of the nine symptom criteria ("thoughts that you would be better off dead or hurting yourself in some way") counts if present at all, regardless of the duration. Panic disorder is diagnosed if the patient has had three of the anxiety attack symptoms in the last four weeks and also has experienced such anxiety attacks before, and during the last four weeks the patient had an anxiety attack in which at least four panic attack symptoms were present. Other anxiety disorder is diagnosed if the patient has been bothered by anxiety feelings, and if also at least three anxiety symptoms have been present "more than half the days" over the last four weeks [6, 7, 14]. A module for probable somatoform disorder is diagnosed on the PHQ as a severe form of DSM-IV undifferentiated somatization with a lower threshold [15].

### 3.3 Materials and Methods

The PHQ study in Japan was conducted from 2004 to 2005 at eleven primary care sites in Niigata, in addition to one site in Fukui, Nagano, and Tokyo. Patients coming in for a routine medical appointment with their physician or psychiatrist were approached for entry into the study. The purpose of the study was briefly explained to them and written informed consent was obtained. A total of 1409 adult patients (611 males, 797 females; mean age: 56.2 years, SD: ±20.4) completed the PHQ in full.

Here, results of the PHQ were analyzed to determine the presence of mood disorders and anxiety disorders. Moreover, the score obtained for the question related to difficulty in daily life was used to evaluate a patient's impairment in social and occupational functioning. The protocol for the study was approved by the Ethics Committee at the Faculty of Dentistry, Niigata University and the other participating institutions in accordance with the Ethical Principles for Medical Research Involving Human Subjects (Declaration of Helsinki).

### 3.4 Results

The prevalence of diagnosis of any mood disorder or any anxiety disorder was 25.0%. Of the 15.8% of patients diagnosed with mood disorders, 6.4% were for major depressive disorder and 9.4% for other depressive disorders. Anxiety disorders

| | Total Sample, NO (%) | PHQ study in the United States (n = 3000) |
|---|---|---|
| Any mood disorders | 223(15.8%) | 476(16%) |
| Major Depressive Disorders (MDD) | 90 (6.4%) | 292(10.0%) |
| Other Depressive Disorders (ODD) | 133(9.4%) | 184(6.0%) |
| Any anxiety disorders | 186(13.2%) | 317(11%) |
| Panic Disorders (PD) | 133 (9.4%) | 165(6%) |
| Other anxiety disorders(OAD) | 53 (3.8%) | 221(7%) |
| Any mood disorders or any anxiety disorders | 351 (25.0%) | |

**Table 4.**
*Prevalence of Mood Disorders and Anxiety Disorders Detected by PRIME-MD PHQ in Japan (n = 1409).*

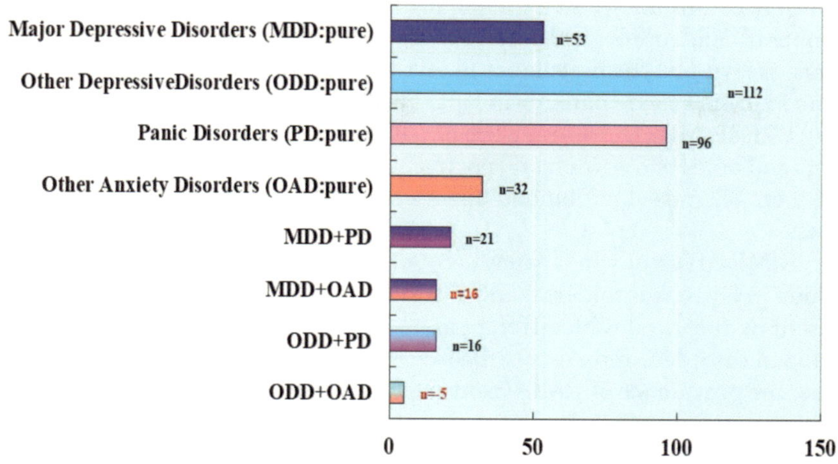


**Figure 4.**
*Comorbidity of mood disorders and anxiety disorders by detected by PHQ study in Japan (n = 1409).*

| Major Depressive Disorders with Anxiety Disorders | OR | 95%CI |
|---|---|---|
| Major Depressive Disorders with Other Anxiety Disorders | 30.4 | 13.19–70.28 |
| Major Depressive Disorders with Panic Disorders | 5.45 | 3.03–9.73 |

*OR: odds ratio CI: Confidence Interval.*

**Table 5.**
*Odds Ratios of Major Depressive Disorders with Other Anxiety Disorders or Panic Disorders Detected by PHQ in JAPAN (n = 1409).*

were diagnosed in 13.2% of patients, comprising 9.4% with panic disorder and 3.8% with other anxiety disorders with other anxiety disorders (refer to **Table 4**).

**Figure 4** shows the comorbidity of mood disorders and anxiety disorders. Co-occurrence of major depressive disorders with other anxiety disorders not specified was observed in sixteen patients, while overlapping of other depressive disorders with other anxiety disorders presented in five patients.

The odds ratio for co-occurrence of major depressive disorder with panic disorders and major depressive disorder with other anxiety disorders was 5.45 (95% CI: 3.03–9.73) and 30.4 (95% CI: 13.19–70.28), respectively, (refer to **Table 5**).

## 4. Discussion

### 4.1 The prevalence of anxiety, depression, and other mental disorders in Japan

The World Mental Health Japan Survey First (WMHJ1) was conducted from 2002 to 2006. A total of 4134 randomly selected residents aged 20 years or over (participation rate 55.1%) took part in the WMHJ1 from eleven areas throughout Japan. This was followed by the World Mental Health Japan Survey Second (WMHJ2), which was conducted from 2013 to 2015. The WHO Composite International Diagnostic Interview (CIDI) version 3.0 was used in WMHJ1, and a Japanese version of a computer-assisted personal interview derived from the WHO Composite International Diagnostic Interview (CIDI) version 3.0 was applied in WMHJ2 [16, 17].

Both were community-based mental health epidemiological studies. However, the number of epidemiological studies focusing on primary care in Japan is very few. Thus, we studied the prevalence of anxiety, depression, and other mental disorders in primary care patients in Japan using the PRIME-MD and the PHQ. Utilizing PRIME-MD, 12.5% and 8.5% of patients were diagnosed with mood disorders and anxiety disorders, respectively. With detection via the PHQ, 13.7% patients were diagnosed with mood disorders and 11.1% patients with anxiety disorders.

The PRIME-MD study in Japan was conducted from 1998 to 1999, however, the PHQ study in Japan was undertaken from 2004 to 2005. Despite being conducted in different decades and with different assessment instruments, the prevalence rate of mood disorders and anxiety disorders was similar in primary care patients. Likewise, the prevalence of CMD (common mental disorders), such as mood, anxiety, and substance-related disorders in Japan was relatively stable from the WMHJ1 in 2002 to the WMHJ2 in 2015. Similar trends are observed between the PRIME-MD of 1998 and the PHQ study in 2005. These findings suggest that the prevalence rate of mood disorders and anxiety disorders has remained relatively stable in primary care patients and the general population.

For an international comparison, we compared the prevalence rate in the PRIME-MD and the PHQ study between Japan and US. The prevalence rate of major depression is far lower in Japan. Minor depression, however, is almost as common in Japan as in the USA. Moreover, the rate of prevalence of other anxiety disorders in Japan is lower than in the USA, while figures for panic disorder are similar in both countries.

We compared the prevalence rate in the PRIME-MD and the PHQ study between Japan and Spain [4], and Japan and France [18]. Similarly, the rate of prevalence of any mood disorders and any anxiety disorders in Japan is lower than in Spain or France.

In 1995, the WHO concluded the largest international multicentric survey on Psychological Problems in General Health Care (PPGHC) [19]. The PPGHC investigated the psychological problems commonly seen in primary care settings. This research was comprised from the collaboration of fifteen centers in fourteen countries. The rate of current depression in Japan's Nagasaki research center was lower than in any other of the participating research centers.

Interestingly, according to results of studies in Japan detected by PRIME-MD, PHQ, WHMJ1, WHMJ2 and PPHGC, the rate of prevalence of major depressive disorders has been and continues to be lower in Japan than in other countries.

First, it remains possible that the diagnoses of the ICD and DSM do not accurately assess the intrinsic characteristics of depression that are unique to Japanese people. Kessler pointed out that there is no guarantee that the same good validity of the CIDI will be found in other parts of the world [20]. The DSM, in particular, only assesses symptoms at a cross-sectional level and does not capture cultural differences in the essential psychopathology of major depression.

Secondly, there are differences between Japanese and other nationalities, particularly Americans, in the way they perceive stressful events and in the emotional expression of depression. Recently, Vanderkruik and Whisman examined the associations between pleasant or reinforcing activities and depressive symptoms across cultures. Their results indicated that frequency, enjoyment, and obtained pleasure from pleasant events were significantly and negatively associated with depressive symptoms for both American and Japanese adults, and these associations were significantly greater in magnitude for American adults relative to Japanese adults [21]. Their findings suggest that there is a cross-sectional association between pleasant events and depressive symptoms in both the USA and Japan, and that this association is stronger in the USA.

In other words, Americans have more emotional ups and downs than Japanese in terms of how they perceive both pleasant and stressful events. Possibly, their results would support the findings of the present study, in which the rate of prevalence of major depressive disorders is lower in Japan than in other countries.

Third, epidemiological differences in depression and anxiety between Japan and other western countries may be related to genetic factors such as serotonin-related factors. Tsuchimine et al. reported that there was no association between a polymorphism in the serotonin receptor 2B (HTR2B) gene and personality traits in healthy Japanese subjects [22]. On the other hand, the prevalence of panic disorder in PRIME-MD and PHQ Study in Japan is similar with those in the USA. Recently, Ohi et al. investigated and suggested that transethnic polygenetic features are shared between Japanese panic disorder patients and European patients with psychiatric disorders by conducting polygenic risk score (PRS) analyses [23].

Genetic research about cultural differences between Japan and other countries and their potential relationship with depression and anxiety is underway, but at this point, many questions remain unanswered. Although some studies have been conducted on this subject, much greater investigation is required. Consequently, we did not address the issue in detail here.

In addition, with regards to major depression, a significantly higher rate was observed in women than in men detected by PRIME-MD in Japan, as with PRIME-MD in USA and Spain [4, 24, 25], and in the WHMJ1 and WHMJ2.

### 4.2 Comorbidity between depression and anxiety detected using PRIME-MD and the PHQ in Japan

Co-occurrence of major depressive disorder with generalized anxiety disorders and major depressive disorder with anxiety disorders (NOS) were detected using PRIME-MD (n-601) in Japan. The co-occurrence of major depressive disorder with generalized anxiety disorders had a far higher odds-ratio than major depressive disorder with anxiety disorders (NOS), along with panic disorders.

In addition, the findings of co-occurrence of major depressive disorder with other anxiety disorders and major depressive disorder with panic disorders were observed in the PHQ (n = 1409) study in Japan. Results showed a higher odds-ratio in the co-occurrence of major depressive disorder with other anxiety disorders than in major depressive disorder with panic disorders.

The results of the PRIME-MD and PHQ studies in Japan suggest that major depressive disorder is more likely to be comorbid with generalized anxiety disorder and other anxiety disorders than with panic disorder in Japanese primary care settings.

The comorbidity between depressive and anxiety disorders was not analyzed in detail in the WMHJ1 or WMHJ2. The Netherlands Study of Depression and Anxiety (NESDA) reported that 67% of subjects had a current and 75% had a lifetime comorbid anxiety disorder diagnosis and similarly, of those with a primary anxiety disorder diagnosis, 63% had a current and 81% a lifetime depressive disorder diagnosis [2]. In separate studies, Hirschfeld and Wittchen et al. reported that comorbidity rates in community samples are slightly lower the rates reported in NESDA [3, 25].

Using data from a previous WHO study of mental disorders in general medical and primary care settings in fourteen countries [19], Goldberg et al. [26]

revealed a high correlation between anxious and depressive symptoms. Moreover, their analysis showed that anxious depression is much more common in primary care settings than "comorbid generalized anxiety and depression," where the individual meets the diagnostic requirements of both a depressive episode and generalized anxiety disorder and a duration requirement of 6 months for anxiety symptoms.

The findings of NESDA, Goldberg et al., and other studies in Western countries are in line with the results achieved in the PRIME-MD and PHQ studies in Japan. Goldberg and Silverstone and von Studnitz proposed that the revised primary care classification for ICD-11 Mental and Behavioral Disorders (ICD-11 PHC) should consider anxious depression to be an important form of depressive episode in general medical practice [27, 28].

Whiteford et al. pointed out that in spite of the prevalence and importance of the comorbidity of depression and anxiety in primary care and its substantial contribution to disability [29], rates of identification and treatment remain very low, with less than half of all depressive episodes correctly identified even in high-resource primary care.

From a clinical viewpoint, Weitz and Kleiboer [30] and Cuijpers et al. [31] learned via meta-analysis that comorbid symptoms decreased during treatment of the more clinically significant disorder. This holds true for treating depression with psychotherapy regarding anxiety symptoms [30] and treating anxiety disorders with cognitive behavioral therapy regarding depressive symptoms [31].

Kalinin proposed a new concept, the comorbidity of anxiety and affective disorders as neuropsychiatric and evolutionary problems. He suggested a potential mechanism for comorbidity development based on neuropsychiatric and evolutionary data [32]. Stein et al. mentioned that the research of anxiety disorder will require the integration of nosological, epidemiological, and psychobiological viewpoints utilizing methods such as genomic data, physiological markers, and experiential sampling from a wider community and clinical survey. [33] Future research from their perspective is also needed.

There are very few studies on the comorbidity of depression and anxiety in Japan, therefore, data from these PRIME-MD and PHQ studies contribute to consideration of clinical treatment for depression and anxiety in primary care settings in Japan.

## 5. Conclusion

We detected the prevalence of anxiety, depression, and other mental disorders in primary care patients in Japan using the PRIME-MD and the PHQ. There were findings of comorbidity of depression and anxiety as seen in other countries.

## Acknowledgements

The PRIME-MD study and the PHQ study were supported partially by an educational grant from Pfizer US Pharmaceutical Inc. Moreover, these studies were also supported by grants from Niigata Seiryo University.

## Conflict of interest

The authors declare no conflict of interest.

**Author details**

Kumiko Muramatsu[1*], Hitoshi Miyaoka[2], Kunitoshi Kamijima[3], Yoshiyuki Muramatsu[4], Katsuya Fuse[5], Fumitoshi Yoshimine[6], Ichiro Mashima[4,9], Yutaka Tanaka[7], Michio Hosaka[3,8], Kikuchi Toshiaki[9], Natsue Shimizu[10] and Shigeji Baba[11]

1 Department of Clinical Psychology, Graduate School of Niigata Seiryo University, Niigata, Japan

2 Department of Psychiatry, Kitasato University School of Medicine, Sagamihara, Japan

3 Showa University School of Medicine, Tokyo, Japan

4 Kohdo Hospital, Niigata, Japan

5 Uonuma City Koide Hospital, Niigata, Japan

6 Niigata Prefectural Tokamachi Hospital, Niigata, Japan

7 Niigata University Graduate School of Medicine and Dental Sciences, Niigata, Japan

8 Katsuyama Medical Clinic, Yamanashi, Japan

9 Department of Respiratory Medicine and Infectious Diseases, Niigata University Graduate School of Medical and Dental Sciences, Niigata, Japan

10 Joetsu General Hospital, Niigata, Japan

11 Baba Medical Clinic, Tokyo, Japan

*Address all correspondence to: muramatu@n-seiryo.ac.jp

## References


[1] Kessler RC, Petukhova M, Zaslavsky AM (2011b): The role of latent internalizing and externalizing predispositions in accounting for the development of comorbidity among common mental disorders. Current Opinions in Psychiatry.2011;24. 307-312.

[2] Lamers F, van Oppen P, Comijs HC, Johannes HS, Spinhoven P et al: Comorbidity patterns of anxiety and depressive disorder in a large cohort study: the Netherlands Study of Depression and Anxiety (NESDA). J clin Psychiatry 2011;72(3): 341-348. doi:10.4088/JCP.10m06176blu

[3] Hirschfeld RMA : The comorbidity of major depression and anxiety disorders:recognition and management in primary care. Prim Care Companion J ClinPsychiatry. 2001;3(6): 244-254.

[4] Roca M, M. Gili M, Garcia-Garcia M, Salva J, Vives Ma, Garcia Campayo J, Comas A: Prevalence and comorbidity of common mental disorders in primary care. J. Affect. Disord.2009; 119 : 52-58.

[5] Spitzer RL, Williams JBW, Kroenke K, Linzer M, de Gruy FV, Hahn SR, et al. Utility of new procedure for diagnosis mental-disorders in primary-care: the PRIME-MD 1000 Study. JAMA. 1994; 272:1749-1756.

[6] Spitzer RL, Williams JBW, Kroenke K, Hornyak R, McMurray J. Validity and utility of the PRIME-MD Patient Health Questionnaire in assessment of 3000 obstetric-gynecologic patients: the PRIME-MD Patient Health Questionnaire Obstetrics Gynecology Study. Am J. Obstet. Gynecol. 2000; 183:759-769.

[7] Spitzer RL, Kroenke K, Williams JBW. Validation and utility of a self-report version of PRIME-MD — the PHQ primary care study. JAMA 1999;282: 1737-1744.

[8] American Psychiatric Association. Diagnostic and statistical manual of mental disorders. 3rd ed., rev 1987. Washington, DC.

[9] American Psychiatric Association. Diagnostic and statistical manual of mental disorders DSM-IV. 4th edition. 2000. Washington, DC.

[10] Baca E, Saiz J. Validation of the Spanish version of PRIME-MD: A procedure for diagnosing mental disorders in primary care. Actas Españolas de Psiquiatria. 1999; 6: 375-383.

[11] Boyer P, Bisserbe B, Falissart R, Spitzer R: Validation of the French version of PRIME-MD: a primary care evaluation of mental disorder. European Neuropsychopharmacology. 1996: 6 (Suppl. 3):210.

[12] Loerch B, KohnenA., The primary care evaluation of mental disorders: PRIME-MD (German). A comparison with CIDI. Journal of Psychiatric Research.2000. 34, 211-210.

[13] Muramatsu K, Miyaoka H, Kamijima K, Muramatsu Y, Yoshida M, Otsubo T, et al. The patient health questionnaire, Japanese version: validity according to the mini- international-neuropsychiatric interview-plus. Psychol Rep. 2007;101: 952-960.

[14] Kroenke K, Spitzer RL, Williams JBW. The PHQ-9: validity of a brief depression severity measure. J Gen Intern Med. 2001;16:606-613.

[15] Kroenke K, Spitzer RL. The PHQ-9: a new depression diagnostic and severity measure. Psychiatry Ann. 2002;32:509-515.

[16] Ishikawa H, Kawakami N, Kessler RC, World Mental Health Japan Survey Collaborators. Lifetime and 12-month prevalence, severity and

unmet need for treatment of common mental disorders in Japan: Results from the final dataset of World Mental Health Japan Survey. Epidemiol. Psychiatr. Sci. 2016; 25: 217-229.

[17] Ishikawa H, Tachimori H, Takeshima T et al. Prevalence, treatment, and the correlates of common mental disorders in the mid 2010's in Japan: The results of the World Mental Health Japan 2nd Survey. J. Affect. Disord. 2018; 241: 554-562.

[18] Joanna N, Guilhem De R, Boulenger JP, Ritchie K, Mann A et al. Use of the PRIME-MD Patient Health Questionnaire for estimating the prevalence of psychiatric disorders in French primary care: comparison with family practitioner estimates and relationship to psychotropic medication use. Gen. Hosp. Psychiatry. 2007;29: 285 – 293.

[19] Sartorius N and Ustün T B and World Health Organization. Mental illness in general health care : an international study/edited by T. B. Ustün, N. Sartorius. Chichester : Wiley; 1995. https://apps.who.int/iris/handle/10665/3693

[20] Kessler RC. Psychiatric epidemiology: Challenges and opportunities. Int. Rev. Psychiatry 2007; 19: 509-521

[21] Vanderkruik R and Whisman MA. A cross-cultural examination of pleasant events and depressive symptoms. J.Clin. Psychol. 2021;1-10. https://doi.org/10.1002/jclp.23111

[22] Tsuchimine S, Taniguchi T, Sugawara N, Kaneda A, Yasui-Furukori N. No Association between a Polymorphism in the Serotonin Receptor 2B (HTR2B) Gene and Personality Traits in Healthy Japanese Subjects. Neuropsychobiology.2013;68:59-62. https://doi.org/10.1159/000350998

[23] Ohi K, OtowaT, Shimada M, Sugiyama S, Muto Y et al. Shared transethnic genetic basis of panic disorder and psychiatric and related intermediate phenotypes. European Neuropsychopharmacology. 2021;42,:87-96.

[24] Linzer M, Spitzer R, Kroenke K, Williams JB, Hahn S et al. quality of life, and mental disorders in primary care: results from the PRIME-MD 1000 study. Am. J. Med. 1996; 101:526-533.

[25] Wittchen HU, Kessler RC, Beesdo K et al. Generalized Anxiety and Depression in Primary Care: Prevalence, Recognition, and Management. J. Clin. Psychiatry.2002;63 (suppl 8):24-34.

[26] Goldberga DP, Prisciandaro J J, Paul Williams P. The primary health care version of ICD-11: the detection of common mental disorders in general medical settings.Gen. Hosp. Psychiatry.2012; 34: 665-670.

[27] Silverstone PH, Studnitz E. Defining Anxious Depression: Going Beyond Comorbidity.Can J Psychiatry. 2003; 48:675-680.

[28] Goldberg DP, Reed GM, Roblesd R, Minhase F, Razzaquee B et al. Screening for anxiety, depression, and anxious depression in primary care: A field study for ICD-11 PHC. J. Affect. Disord. 2017; 213 :199-206.

[29] Whiteford HA, Degenhardt L, Rehm J, Baxter AJ, Ferrari AJ et al.Global burden of disease attributable to mental and substance use disorders:findings from the Global Burden of Disease Study 2010. Lancet. 2013; 382: 1575-1586. doi: 10.1016/S0140-6736(13)61611-6.

[30] Weitz E, Kleiboer A. van Straten A, Cuijpers P. The effects of psychotherapy for depression on anxiety symptoms: a meta-analysis. Psycho.Med.2018;48: 2140-2152.doi:10.1017/S003329171700362

[31] Cuijpers P, Cristea IA, Weitz E, Gentili C, Berking M. The effects of cognitive and behavioural therapies for anxiety disorders on depression: a meta-analysis. Psychol Med. 2016;46:3451-3462. doi10.1017/S0033291716002348.

[32] Kalinin V. Comorbidity of Anxiety and Affective Disorders as Neuropsychiatric and Evolutionary Problem (A New Concept), Anxiety Disorders, Edited by Kalinin V. 2011.InTech.

[33] Stein DJ, Scott K M, Jonge P, Kessler RC, PhD Epidemiology of anxiety disorders: from surveys to nosology and back. Dialogues in Clinical Neuroscience. 2017;19 (2): 127-136.

Chapter 8

# De Clerambault Syndrome: Current Perspective

*Tulika Ghosh and Minkesh Chowdhary*

## Abstract

De Clerambault syndrome is a psychological condition named after Gaetan Gatian De Clerambault in which the sufferer is under the delusion that a certain person is in love with him or her. This is a condition in which the patient, often a single woman, believes than an exalted person is in love with her although the alleged lover may never have spoken to them. Occasionally, isolated delusions of this kind are found in abnormal personality states. Erotomania may also be a feature of paranoid schizophrenia. Sometimes, schizophrenia may begin with a circumscribed delusion of a fantasy lover, and subsequently delusions may become more diffuse, and hallucinations may develop. This chapter will focus on the role of technological advancements in the origin of this syndrome in various age groups.

**Keywords:** De Clerambault syndrome, erotomania, delusion, paranoid schizophrenia

## 1. Introduction

De Clerambault syndrome, more commonly known as erotomania or fantasy lover's syndrome, is a psychological condition which was named after **Gaetan Gatian De Clerambault** who was a French psychiatrist. He was the first person to describe it as a distinct disorder in 1921. This disorder is one such condition in which the sufferer, who is very often a single woman, holds that a person of high repute is in love with her even though the claimed person may have never met or interacted with them [1]. Here, in this particular disorder, the sufferer's belief reaches to a delusional level with gradual passage of time in spite of having strong proofs against it.

De Clerambault, to his credit, distinguished a "pure" or "primary" erotomania (more or less approximating to Kraepelin's paranoia) from symptomatic erotomanias which could occur as part of other psychiatric disorders. Because of paranoia's virtual demise as a recognized diagnostic entity in the middle of the twentieth century and because, until recently, very few cases of erotomania were described in the literature, a great deal of confusion arose about the nature of the disorder, with some authorities insisting that it was always symptomatic of other conditions and denying that erotomania could exist as a primary illness [2, 3].

Erotomania as it is commonly known can originate instantaneously, and the manifestations are often enduring. The core of the delusions is frequently a renowned person, usually an elderly, or hardly accessible individual with a higher social position. This individual may have had little or no previous contact with the patient. The object of his or her obsession can be any fictional or deceased individual or it can be someone with whom the patient has never met. The sufferer of this condition may also believe that this particular person is interacting with them and are professing their love, by means of secret messages.

Occasionally, atypical delusions of this type are found in abnormal personality states. This particular condition may also be present in paranoid schizophrenia. Sometimes, it may begin with a restricted delusion of a fantasy lover. Later, the delusions may become more scattered gradually resulting in the development of hallucinations. A comparatively uncommon condition, this syndrome is most commonly seen in females who are having a demure personality, who get dependent quickly on others and who are sexually naive. It can be related to other psychiatric disorders, but sometimes it may also originate on its own.

Referential delusions are very common, as the sufferer very frequently perceives that the object of their love or the person whom they believe to be infatuated with them is sending them secret messages and are confessing about their love for them through some harmless cues like the green light at the traffic signal.

In secondary erotomania, the delusions can arise because of some other mental disorders such as bipolar I disorder or schizophrenia. The symptoms of this disorder may also get triggered by various substances like alcohol. It can also get accelerated by the use of antidepressants.

In this syndrome, there is a possible genetic element present as first-degree relatives of people with this particular syndrome had a family with history of psychiatric disorders. The famous psychoanalyst of Vienna, Sigmund Freud, made a commendable attempt to explain this atypical syndrome. As per Freud, this disorder is a defence mechanism which is employed by the sufferer to avert homosexual urges or instincts which in turn results in enduring feelings of paranoia, denial, displacement and projection.

Likewise, this particular atypical phenomenon was explained by some major theorists as having an instrumental role in coping with severe level of lonesomeness or a certain level of ego deficit which occurs after a major loss. This particular syndrome can be also associated with unfulfilled desires, wishes or urges. Sigmund Freud was of the notion that ungratified wishes or desires lead the sufferer towards homosexuality or narcissism. Some particular researches conducted in this area have found brain abnormalities to be present in patients with erotomania such as heightened temporal lobe asymmetry and greater volumes of lateral ventricles than those with no mental disorders.

## 2. Historical perspective

Initial references to this condition can be found in the work of Hippocrates, Freud (1911), De Clerambault (1942), Erasistratus, Plutarch and Galen. Bartholomy Pardoux (1545–1611), who was a Parisian physician, studied the concepts of nymphomania and erotomania. Jacques Ferrand referred to this syndrome as "erotic paranoia" in 1623 in a treatise known as "Maladie d'amour ou Mélancolie érotique". He also termed this condition as "erotic self-referent delusion" until the terms erotomania and De Clerambault syndrome came into common usage.

It was during the seventeenth century that this disorder which was known as "amor insanus" at that time was differentiated from nymphomania. Until recently, this disorder was thought to occur almost always in females, but now researches have proved that it is also found to affect males.

In the early eighteenth century, this disorder was conceptualized as a general disease, the causal factor of which was taken to be unrequited love. Later in the early eighteenth century to the beginning of the nineteenth century, this disorder was defined as showing excess of physical love. Gradually as the early nineteenth century came to an end and the twentieth century began, this syndrome was explained as an unrequited love which later gradually developed into a certain form of mental disease. The period of the early twentieth century introduced this definition of having a delusional belief of "being loved by someone else" which is continuing till date.

Later in the year 1971 and 1977, M.V. Seeman gave various terminologies for this syndrome such as "phantom lover syndrome", "psychotic erotic transference reaction" and "delusional loving". Emil Kraepelin and Bernhard have also contributed significantly in the development of this disorder; they wrote about erotomania. And more recently, Winokur, Kendler and Munro contributed to the knowledge available on this disorder. Berrios and Kennedy [4] described in *Erotomania: A Conceptual History* several periods of history in relation to this syndrome which resulted in significant changes in the definition of erotomania.

Thus, it is evident from the various definitions described above that this disorder had different connotations at different times.

## 3. Symptoms of erotomania

The chief feature of erotomania is a fixed, false and delusional belief that another person is deeply or obsessively in love with them. The other person may not even be aware of the existence of the person with erotomania. Often, there is no evidence of the other person's love. A person with this disorder might talk about the other person incessantly. They may also be obsessed with trying to meet with or communicate with this person so that they can be together. The behaviour associated to this disorder includes persistent efforts to make contact through stalking, written communication and other harassing behaviours.

The sufferer can also have this belief that their object of affection is sending secret, personal and affirming messages back. This belief can be precipitated by the targeted person making it known that the attention is unwanted. Individuals with erotomania can also act like a threat to their object of affection. Often, this threat is underestimated as a risk factor when the severity of this condition is evaluated. The following are the characteristics generally demonstrated by patients with erotomania [2, 5]:

1. The sufferer has this unshakeable belief that he/she is loved by a specific individual who is often of higher social status and sometimes is a well-known figure or even a celebrity.

2. Although the other person has had little (or absolutely no) previous contact with the patient, the latter usually believes that the other initiated the relationship.

3. The patient usually has strong erotic feelings towards the other person, although sometimes the "relationship" is regarded as platonic.

4. The other person is usually unattainable in some way, for example, because of marital status or high social visibility. In many cases the patient never makes any attempt to contact the love object, often writing letters but not mailing them or buying presents but never sending them. Even when given a chance to make real contact, the patient will frequently avoid doing so and will devise spurious explanations to account for this.

5. In those individuals who do make contact with the other person, reasons are found to explain the "paradoxical" (i.e. rejecting) behaviour which is naturally shown by the latter.

In some instances, there can be anger about this perceived rejection associated with acting out behaviour.

6. Sometimes the other person is believed to protect, watch over or follow the patient, and all kinds of behaviours are misinterpreted as evidence of passionate interest.

7. The onset of erotomania may be sudden or gradual.

8. Hallucinations may be present, and some individuals with tactile hallucinations may believe that they have been visited by a lover during the night, a phenomenon sometimes known as the "incubus syndrome" [6].

9. When the case is one of "pure" or "primary" erotomania, the accompanying features are those of delusional disorder. That is, it is a monodelusional disorder with relative preservation of normal personality features and often some capacity to remain functional in society. In these cases the patient not infrequently is able to conceal the abnormal belief from other people [7]. Thought disorder is virtually absent outside the delusional system.

Psychotic breaks: One more interesting aspect related to this disorder is that the course of erotomania is of two types. One is that it may happen over a long period of time and second, only in short episodes. These short episodes also come to be known as "psychotic breaks". Psychotic breaks are a common symptom of other mental health conditions. They involve an abrupt worsening of delusions or other psychotic features. They may occur in disorders such as schizophrenia, schizoaffective disorder, major depressive disorder with psychotic features, bipolar disorder or Alzheimer's disease.

**Aetiology:** Though the real cause behind this disorder is largely unknown, some studies have suggested that delusions may develop as a way of managing extreme stress or trauma. Genetics and personality patterns may also contribute to the development of this disorder.

One major factor which has been emphasized is the role of psychodynamic factors in the emergence of this disorder. Many authors have written about the psychodynamic aetiology of fantasy lover's syndrome and have said that this delusion acts as a gratification to the individuals' narcissistic needs. Every individual has this basic need to be loved. But when an individual is rejected by the society, he has to go through that perceived sense of rejection.

This, in turn, develops the fantasy that some other human being is in love with them. By developing such kind of a belief, they tend to feel important in their own eyes and are able to cope with the societal rejection. Kraepelin was of the view that it develops as a compensation for the disappointments of life. De Clerambault highlighted the idea of sexual pride. He elaborated this idea as when there is an absence of affective and sexual approval in an individual's life, this stimulates the development of erotomania in order to satisfy the individual's pride.

Another psychodynamic explanation which was given by Hollender and Callahan [8] says that this disorder develops as a result of an ego deficit. The sufferer feels that he/she is not attractive enough. Segal says that erotomanic delusion results from the patient's need for love. The sufferer relates his need for love as a way to gain approval. Taylor highlighted the idea that the individual's loneliness, isolation and extreme dependence on others also leads to the development of erotomanic disorder.

**Diagnosis:** Erotomania has flouted easy categorization for several years. De Clerambault syndrome or erotomanic delusion is a rare delusional disorder which makes the diagnosis of erotomania very challenging. Though Kraepelin and De Clerambault had discussed this syndrome in detail, it appeared officially as a diagnosis for the first time in DSM-III R as a subtype of delusional disorder. Erotomanic delusions may be a part of schizophrenia, schizoaffective disorders or mood disorders. Thus, much care should be taken before reaching to a confirm diagnosis because the treatment and management of the disorder is planned as per the diagnosis. Rudden et al. [9] conducted a study on 28 patients with erotomanic delusions and compared them to 80 patients with other delusions and found that erotomanic patients had significantly more manic symptoms than the comparison group and more affective diagnosis. The following conditions must be met before a stand-alone diagnosis of erotomania can be made:

1. Delusions should involve possible events, even if they are highly unlikely.

2. The delusion should be only applied to the relevant issue, with all other domains of the sufferer's life being functional and normal.

3. If depressive moods or manic episodes are present along with delusional disorder, then the duration of the delusional period should be longer than the depressive or manic episode.

4. Schizophrenia, mood disorders and substance use disorders should be excluded.

## 4. Differential diagnosis of erotomania

When an individual is recognized as having erotomanic delusions, the following disorders must be considered:

1. Delusional disorder, erotomanic subtype.

2. Schizophrenia, especially of the paranoid type. Here, there will usually be other delusions with a variety of themes, hallucinations and relatively widespread thought disorder. The personality is less well preserved, and obvious abnormalities of behaviour may occur [10–12].

3. Major mood disorders. Erotomania has been noted in association with unipolar and bipolar affective disorders [9, 13, 14], and there is a description based on one case which suggests that it can appear as a variant of pathological mourning [15].

4. Various organic brain disorders. There have been descriptions of erotomania occurring in epilepsy, as part of the after-effects of head injury and amongst the late effects of substance abuse [16, 17]. It has also been observed in senile dementia [18, 19] and apparently as a side effect of certain therapeutic drugs including oral contraceptives and steroids [16]. Signer and Cummings [20] have suggested that abnormalities of the left temporal lobe may be particularly likely to cause symptoms of erotomania.

5. Mental handicap. Callacott [21] and Ghaziuddin and Tsai [22] have reported erotomanic delusions in mentally retarded individuals. There is no reason why such persons cannot have delusions associated with a superimposed psychiatric illness, but it is possible that part of their erotomania may be due to a simple person's misunderstanding of another individual's intentions. However, in this context, one must be aware that mentally handicapped patients can sometimes be taken advantage of sexually by helpers or relatives and that sexually laden remarks made by the patient about others may have had a basis in fact.

6. Delusional misidentification syndrome (DMS). Erotomania has been described in association with DMS in a small number of cases [23, 24].

7. Shared psychotic disorder (folie a' deux). A sharing of the erotomanic beliefs with another individual (not the victim), and acceptance of these as truth by that individual, has been described [25]. This is hardly surprising since folie à deux has been shown to be relatively common in delusional disorder [26].

8. Non-delusional erotomanic beliefs. These have already been touched upon, and it does appear that certain people may have very powerful erotomanic emotions which are in the nature of over-valued ideas rather than delusions [15, 27]. It is important to make this distinction because, in such cases, psychotherapy rather than medication may be indicated.

## 5. Course and prognosis

The "pure" or monosymptomatic form of erotomania is the one which usually corresponds with the diagnosis of paranoia/delusional disorder. In the past this has been regarded as unremitting and associated with a poor prognosis, but there is no early evidence that, analogous to other subtypes of delusional disorder, the condition may respond well to neuroleptic treatment. When erotomania is a symptom of another psychiatric illness such as major mood disorder, schizophrenia or some form of dementia, the course of the phenomenon is that of the parent illness and the prognosis depends on the natural history and adequate treatment of that illness. It is also important to take into account the possible presence of mental handicap, and to consider that, at least in some cases, erotomania may be non-delusional in nature. All of this emphasizes, as always, the need for complete and detailed history-taking and mental status examination as well as careful physical examination. Unfortunately, as we already know, patients with delusional disorder are not always prepared to be cooperative in such investigations. In special circumstances, as, for example, in the forensic psychiatric field, where repeated harassment of one person by another, assault of a female by a male or statements about alleged sexual feelings or behaviours have occurred, great care must be taken with assessment. If the perpetrator has a subtle delusional illness, the facts may be very difficult to tease out, and his certainty may, as has been noted, in some ways seem more convincing than the victim's bewilderment and denial. Good collateral information is of the essence here, and the person doing the assessment should be aware that professionals in the past have themselves been drawn into a kind of folie a' deux situation when they have come to believe uncritically in the statements of a highly persuasive paranoiac, as well as being influenced by implied or overt threats of litigation.

**Complications of erotomania and comorbid conditions:** Erotomania can make the patients show risky and aggressive behaviour. Sometimes, this behaviour can also result in the person getting arrested for stalking or harassment. Very rarely, erotomania can also result in the death of either person. Erotomanic delusions may be a single symptom which is also known as primary or pure erotomania and classified as a delusional disorder as per the DSM-IV. It may also occur as a secondary or symptomatic erotomania as a part of an extensive psychopathology. It can occur in various mental disorders such as schizophrenia, mood disorder or organic brain disorder.

This syndrome has been described in both heterosexual and homosexual forms. Comorbidity with other rare psychotic conditions has been reported, particularly with the delusional misidentification syndromes, including Fregoli's syndrome. More cases of secondary in comparison to primary erotomania have been reported usually in the context of a schizophrenic illness. This disorder has been often associated with bipolar disorder. It has been found to be associated with other conditions like anxiety disorder, drug or alcohol dependence, eating disorders and attention deficit hyperactivity disorder.

## 6. Treatment and management

The prognostic factors vary from person to person, and the ideal treatment is not completely understood. Though it has been seen that those patients who are having this syndrome along with some major psychiatric disorder like schizophrenia show poor prognosis as the complexity of the symptoms of both the disorders makes it difficult for the patient to get treated. Simultaneously, the patients become drug resistant also as they have to take the medicines for a very long period of time. This results in the body getting adjusted to the drug, and very less improvement is noticed as a result. Researches have proved that treatment for this disorder gives the best results when they are tailored specifically as per the requirements of each individual. The most common modes of treatments are medication and therapy. Till recently, the mainline pharmacological treatments have been pimozide, which is a typical antipsychotic approved for treating Tourette's syndrome, and atypical antipsychotics like risperidone and clozapine.

Treating this disorder can be tough because those individuals who are affected are not likely, or even able, to see that their beliefs are tenuous. Comparatively, few of the affected people seek treatment by their own will, and they may find it difficult to engage successfully in therapy. Non-pharmacological treatments that have shown some degree of efficacy are electroconvulsive therapy (ECT), supportive psychotherapy, family and environment therapy, rehousing, risk management and treating underlying disorders in cases of secondary erotomania. ECT may help in the temporary remission of delusional beliefs; antipsychotics help attenuate delusions and reduce agitation or associated dangerous behaviours, and SSRIs may be used to treat secondary depression.

In this disorder, there is some evidence that pimozide has superior efficacy as compared to other antipsychotics. Psychosocial psychiatric interventions can help enhance the quality of life by allowing some social functioning, and treating comorbid disorders occupies a very important place during the treatment of secondary erotomania.

Other than pharmacological treatments, some non-pharmacological treatment methods are also there which prove to be important in the treatment of this syndrome. Amongst them, family therapy, adjustment of socio-environmental factors and replacing delusions with something positive may be beneficial to all. In maximum cases, harsh confrontation should be avoided. Structured risk assessment helps to manage risky behaviours in those individuals more likely to engage in actions that include violence, stalking and crime. For particularly troublesome cases, neuroleptics and enforced separation may be moderately effective. Priorities should focus on maintaining social function, minimizing the risk of problematic behaviour and improving the affected person's quality of life. It may also be helpful to provide social skills training and to provide practical help in dealing with any problems stemming from erotomania.

Apart from the classic modes of treatment, as the situations are changing and exposure to social networking sites is unavoidable, thus the treatment mechanisms should also employ the strategies needed to help people decrease their social media use. Clinicians should enquire about the pattern of social media use when taking the clinical history of the client, and immediate action should be taken to reduce the chances of such behaviour. Similarly, people should be made aware of the information which they should avoid revealing on social media. In addition, more research should be conducted in this area in order to explore the interplay between social media and erotomanic delusions.

Successful symptom management will focus on treating the underlying disorder and may include medications, therapy and hospitalization. Any or all of these approaches can be applied, depending on the person concerned and the underlying causes. Therapy should help the affected person to comply with an agreed treatment plan and to educate them about their illness.

Hospitalization may be needed if the affected person becomes a danger to themselves, to the object of their affection or to anyone else. Antipsychotic medication may control symptoms effectively and can be prescribed for the underlying disorder. Medication and psychotherapy can be used together. The role that social media plays in any problematic behaviour should be considered when developing a treatment plan.

**Current perspective:** Erotomania is a type of delusional disorder. Other types include delusions of persecution, grandiosity or jealousy. Recent researches have concluded that an extensive use of social media may potentially cause or exacerbate erotomania. Social media eliminates some of the barriers between unacquainted people and can easily be used to observe, contact, stalk and otherwise harass people who would previously have been completely inaccessible. Social media platforms can also reduce the level of privacy of individuals, which can make stalking behaviour much easier. A case study was reported by Faden et al. [28] of a 24-year-old male college student who used social media to stalk a female college student which resulted in his suspension from school and hospitalization. He was diagnosed with delusional disorder, erotomanic type. This case demonstrates that social media can act as a triggering factor of this disorder. Social networking has become a necessity nowadays; thus communication with the object of attention has become easier.

Many a times, girls in the adolescent phase go through different kinds of psychological and physiological changes. They experience attraction towards the opposite gender and want to experience affection from them. Nowadays, access to the Internet and social media has become very easy. Thus, it has led the teens to get information about the celebrity individuals, especially the movie stars very conveniently. When the teens are going through this tumultuous phase of change, the easy access to celebrity's lives can create a feeling of being in love with some celebrity very easily. Some adolescents tend to accept this as an infatuation and forget everything. But some are unable to pass through this phase and start believing that their love is real and mutual. Gradually, it reaches to the delusional level and ultimately ends up in erotomania.

**Forensic aspects of erotomania:** In general, women do not flamboyantly act out their erotomanic delusions, although a well-known American film of the 1970s, Play Misty for Me, describes in fictional terms the dangerous outcome of erotomania occurring in a female. Less dramatic but nonetheless disturbing instances do sometimes occur in real life, to the annoyance, alarm and distress of the object of the deluded individual's attention; nowadays, when male professionals are under so much moral pressure to guard against inappropriate sexual behaviour towards clients, it can be devastating if a deluded woman publicly declares that a doctor, a counsellor, a university teacher or someone else has been demonstrating strong erotic feelings towards her. If the deluded individual has a non-deteriorated personality, totally believes her own story and presents her claims as vehemently and persistently as such people do, it may be almost impossible to get the public to believe that what she is saying is untrue. Real unrequited love is bad enough: delusional unrequited love can be impossible. Taylor et al. [5] studied a group of males charged with antisocial behaviour, including persistent unwelcomed importuning of women, and were able to identify cases of erotomania amongst these. Often, they were initially diagnosed as schizophrenic, but closer examination sometimes suggested the presence of paranoia/delusional disorder. The same researchers noted that several patients exhibited quite grandiose behaviours, a common feature of delusional disorder which makes it especially difficult to engage in logical discussion with the person about his false belief or to persuade him to change his behaviour. None of these particular cases had behaved violently towards their victims, but their unremitting harassment often caused the women involved to feel threatened. Goldstein [29] has described cases of severely aggressive, erotomanic behaviour in males, some of whom gained widespread public notoriety. One of these was the young man who attempted to assassinate Ronald Reagan when the latter was President of the United States, apparently believing that this would gain the attention of a well-known female film star, towards whom he entertained erotic delusional feelings. Amongst the other cases Goldstein describes, murder, serious assault, kidnapping and severe harassment occurred. In these individuals the underlying diagnoses were varied but mostly fell within the categories of delusional disorder or paranoid schizophrenia. Goldstein proposes that the changing role of women in society and their higher public profile may act as a stimulus to male erotomania, possibly making the phenomenon more common, but that is hypothetical.

Although the origins of erotomania can be traced to the time of Hippocrates, and from that time onwards, many efforts have been done by different people to explain the nature and root cause of this disorder, but there is limited information about how this disorder, which was first described by De Clerambault, began its course and treatment.

## Author details

Tulika Ghosh[1]* and Minkesh Chowdhary[2]

1 Department of Clinical Psychology, SGT University, Gurugram, Haryana, India

2 Department of Psychology, SNS College, Motihari, Bihar, India

*Address all correspondence to: itstulika@yahoo.com

## References


[1] Kelly BD. Erotomania: Epidemiology and management. Review article. CNS Drugs. 2005;**19**:657-669

[2] Ellis P, Mellsop G. De Clerambault's syndrome—A nosological entity. British Journal of Psychiatry. 1985;**146**:90-93

[3] Signer SF. Erotomania. The Canadian Journal of Psychiatry. 1991;**36**(3):237

[4] Berrios GE, Kennedy N. Erotomania: A conceptual history. History of Psychiatry. 2002;**13**(52, pt4):381-400

[5] Taylor P, Mahendra B, Gunn J. Erotomania in males. Psychological Medicine. 1983;**13**(3):645-650

[6] Raschka LB. The incubus syndrome. A variant of erotomania. Canadian Journal of Psychiatry. 1979;**24**(6):549-553

[7] Munro A. Delusional Disorder: Paranoia and Related Illnesses. Cambridge: Cambridge University Press; 1989. ISBN: 0-521-58180-X

[8] Hollender MH, Callahan AS. Erotomania or de Clerambault syndrome. Archives of General Psychiatry. 1975;**32**(12):1574-1576

[9] Rudden M, Sweeney J, Frances A. Diagnosis and clinical course of erotomanic and other delusional patients. American Journal of Psychiatry. 1990;**147**(5):625-628

[10] El-Assra A. Erotomania in a Saudi woman. The British Journal of Psychiatry. 1989;**155**:553-555

[11] Hayes M, O'Shea B. Erotomania in Schneider-positive schizophrenia: A case report. The British Journal of Psychiatry. 1985;**146**(6):661-663

[12] Gillett T, Eminson S, Hassanyeh F. Homosexual erotomania. The British Journal of Psychiatry. 1989;**155**(1):128-129

[13] Remington G, Book H. Case report of de Clerambault syndrome, bipolar affective disorder, and response to lithium. American Journal of Psychiatry. 1984;**141**(10):1285-1287

[14] Wood BE, Poe RO. Diagnosis and classification of erotomania. American Journal of Psychiatry. 1990;**147**(10):1388-1389

[15] Evans DL, Jeckel LL, Slot NE. Erotomania—A variety of pathological mourning. Bulletin of The Menninger Clinic. 1982;**46**:507-520

[16] Lovett-Doust JW, Christie H. The pathology of love: Some clinical variants of de Clerambault Syndrome. Social Science and Medicine. 1978;**12**:99-106

[17] El-Gaddal YY. De Clerambault's syndrome (erotomania) in organic delusional syndrome. British Journal of Psychiatry. 1989;**154**:714-716

[18] Carrier L. Erotomania and senile dementia. American Journal of Psychiatry. 1990;**147**:1092

[19] Drevets WC, Rubin EH. Erotomania and senile dementia of Alzheimer type. American Journal of Psychiatry. 1987;**147**:1092

[20] Signer SS, Cummings JL. Erotomania and cerebral dysfunction. British Journal of Psychiatry. 1987;**151**:275

[21] Callacott RA. Erotomanic delusions in mentally handicapped patients: Two case reports. Journal of Mental Deficiency Research. 1987;**31**:87-92

[22] Ghaziuddin M, Tsai L. Depression-dependent erotomanic delusions in a mentally handicapped woman. British Journal of Psychiatry. 1991;**158**:127-129

[23] Signer SF, Isbister SR. Capgras syndrome, de Clerambault's syndrome, and folie a deux. British Journal of Psychiatry. 1987;**151**:402-404

[24] Wright S, Young AW, Hellawell DJ. Fregoli delusion and erotomania. Journal of Neurology, Neurosurgery and Psychiatry. 1993;**56**(3):322-323

[25] Pearce A. De Clerambault's syndrome associated with folie a deux. British Journal of Psychiatry. 1972;**121**(560):116-117

[26] Munro A. Paranoia revisited. British Journal of Psychiatry. 1982;**141**:344-349

[27] Seeman MV. Delusional loving. Archives of General Psychiatry. 1978;**35**:1265-1267

[28] Faden J, Levin J, Mistry R, Wang J. Delusional disorder, erotomanic type, exacerbated by social media use. Case Reports in Psychiatry. 2017

[29] Goldstein RL. More forensic romances: De Clerambault syndrome in men. The Bulletin of the American Academy of Psychiatry and the Law. 1987;**15**(3):267-274

Chapter 9

# What is Capgras Syndrome? Diagnosis and Treatment Approach

*Aslı Enzel Koc and Cicek Hocaoglu*

## Abstract

Capgras delusion is a complex psychopathological phenomenon that presents in a wide range of psychiatric and neurological disorders with differing patterns dependent on the main etiology. An underlying neurological disease should be suspected where the delusion concerns a spouse or inanimate objects and is associated with visual hallucinations, while a functional disorder is suggested by multiple imposters, strangers, additional delusions, and auditory hallucinations. Misidentifications in Capgras syndrome (CS) are fixed false beliefs and, therefore, represent true delusions. Even if when patients are confronted over and over with the illogical nature of the delusion, they keep their beliefs. Surprisingly, patients may show implicit or explicit awareness of their true situation. Some research suggests that a considerable number of patients with CS have some awareness of the bizarre nature of the misidentification delusions and therefore tend not to report them, especially during initial interviews when they are less likely to be confident with the clinician. Specific questions and interventions may assist clinicians in successfully identifying patients with CS. In a series of interviews with these patients, some focus on identifying CS, rather than a single interview which is likely to increase the detection of the delusional misidentification. The clinician should always be mindful of the risk of aggression and homicide in CS.

**Keywords:** Capgras syndrome, misidentification syndromes, psychotic disorder

## 1. Introduction

In delusional misidentification syndromes (DMSs), the individual everlastingly misidentifies persons, places, objects, or events. Capgras syndrome (CS) is the most common in the umbrella term DMS [1, 2]. Perhaps the best known form of DMS is the *Capgras syndrome*, originally described by Dr. Joseph Capgras and his colleague, J. Reboul-Lachaux, in the early twentieth century [3]. They first encounter this impressive phenomenon when their patient Madame M. insisted that all her friends, family, relatives, and neighbors were being replaced or constantly misperceived as being an imposter [4]. The term *l'illusion des sosies* (the illusion of doubles) was used to describe the case of a woman who strongly believes that various "doubles" had taken the place of people she knew [3]. It is an essential feature of the Capgras syndrome, the denial of identity of known persons and the delusional belief that this person has been substituted by a double [5].

CS is characterized by the delusional denial of identity of a significant other and the belief that they have been replaced by a double. Some patients with CS may deny the identity of the actual spouse and claim that there are two spouses, the actual and the imposter [6]. Therefore there are four conditions in patient with CS: the person is recognized, and the patient affirms the resemblance of the double to the misidentified significant other; no identity is attributed to the double, who has neither name nor existence; the double is an imposter, pretending to be the original they are replacing; the original has disappeared, his/her absence remaining unquestioned [7].

## 2. Features of Capgras syndrome: phenomenology, diagnosis, and epidemiology

The rareness of CS, as well as its impressive clinical manifestation as a colorful syndrome, has caused most publications to present case descriptions as scientific curiosities [8, 9]. CS has also attracted the attention of novelists in fictional literature. Dostoevsky provided a dramatic description of the phenomenon in his novel, *The Possessed* [6]. Sociocultural factors essentially shape the phenomena and thus mightily influence the establishment of definitions of this disorder [10]. Therefore, it may be necessary to mention. The meaning given to the terms 'change' and 'transformation' of physical identity has been called 'incarnations' or 'possessions' of other bodies in some cultures [10]. Possessions by an evil spirit have early origins within Paganism, Wicca, Haitian voodoo, Buddhism, Hinduism, Judaism, and Christianity [11]. There is a belief in some countries that people can be possessed by Satan and made to act in strange, immoral, and antisocial ways. In the United States, among European-American Catholics, there exists a belief that demons may possess a person. Possessing demons are presumed to cause experiences of proscribed feelings, thoughts, or behaviors in the person. Occasionally, solutions involve exorcism rituals [12].

It is generally being reported as single case studies in the literature. Although an uncommon psychiatric disorder, Capgras delusion has been central to the development of theories of delusions [6]. It is not dealt with particularly in the DSM-5 and may be classified as delusional disorder, suiting either the persecutory or the unspecified type [13]. With no consensual clinical criteria for this syndrome, it is usual to refer to their original description [7]. The basic manifestation was a false belief that real and familiar persons or oneself is replaced by strange, malicious imposters [14]. In fact, CS is a 'hypoidentification' of a person closely related to the patient [6]. CS is more frequent in women than men, with a sex ratio of approximately 2:1, but this result was not found across all studies [7]. Only a few reports have described this syndrome in patients during childhood [15].

The remarkable feature of Capgras delusion is that patients are able to recognize the close relation, the related person's face, but deny his or her identity and often use subtle misperceived differences in behaviour, personality, or physical appearance to distinguish between him or her and the imagined impersonator [16, 17]. Patients with CS find ways to defend their irrational beliefs [4]. Generally, the patients support their conviction in revealing detail. This sign may be a habit or a personality trait; small misperceived differences, for instance, in physical appearance and behaviour, may vary over time [7]. And these are frequently used to distinguish the imposter from the loved one [18]. Surprisingly, patients may show implicit or explicit awareness of their true situation [6]. Some research suggests that a considerable number of patients with CS have some awareness of the bizarre nature of the misidentification delusions and therefore tend not to report them, especially during initial interviews when they are less likely to be confident with the clinician [19].

Common to all DMS is the delusional denial of identity of objects having affective significance for the patient, and it is exceptional for there to be only one imposter, but these objects are limited in number. CS may be associated with other DMSs, and these frequently evolve from one another because of this relation and similarity [7, 20].

It sometimes occurs isolated, hereby justifying its autonomy as a 'delusion' [7]. CS may be accompanied by other delusions and thus may rarely exemplify a 'monothematic' delusion [6]. Erotomanic delusions and delusional jealousy [i.e., Othello jealousy] were identified in 9.1% and 6.4% of patients with CS, respectively [21, 22]. However, delusional misidentification syndromes uncommonly appear independent of comorbid pathology [23].

The absence of consensual clinical criteria makes the epidemiological data uncertain [7]. Thus, the prevalence of CS may be underrated. More than half of the patients of the registered cases suffered from mental disorders without any organic association, among which schizophrenia spectrum disorders were diagnosed in 6 of 10 patients with CS [21, 22]. The Capgras delusion has been reported in association with other psychiatric disorders in 60–75% of cases and in organic illnesses in 25–40% of cases [23]. The Capgras delusion has usually been recognized in the contextual relationship of psychiatric disorders and often occurs in conjunction with paranoia, derealization, and depersonalization [6]. The Capgras syndrome may represent a delusional evolution of the phenomena of depersonalization and derealization [24]. Nonspecific, derealization-depersonalization experiences are frequent, especially in psychotic disorders, and are considered a significant core symptom of CS [7]. Studies on the prevalence of this disease or comorbid disease show differences. A study has found that the prevalence of DMS in psychiatric populations was less than 1% [14]. Another study has found that its prevalence in all psychiatric inpatients is 1.3–4.1% [25]. It is around 3% for hospitalized psychotic patients [17]. In a recent prospective study of patients hospitalized for a first psychotic episode, it was found that CS was diagnosed approximately 1 in 10 of patients. The prevalence was maximal among patients presenting schizophreniform psychosis 50%, brief psychosis 34.8%, and unspecified psychosis 23.9%, and the prevalence was moderate for a major depressive episode 15%, schizophrenia 11%, or delusional disorders 11% [14]. The most common psychiatric diagnoses in CS have been paranoid schizophrenia, schizoaffective disorder, and bipolar affective disorder [23]. CS has been linked with multiple pathologies. It has been described in psychiatric as well as organic disorders. In the last few decades, reports have increasingly stressed the aetiologic importance of heterogeneity of conditions that have been found in the patients with misidentification syndromes like the Capgras delusion, including cerebrovascular disease, post-traumatic encephalopathy, temporal lobe epilepsy, postencephalitic Parkinsonism, viral encephalitis, migraine, vitamin B12 deficiency, hepatic encephalopathy, chronic alcoholism, hypothyroidism, pseudohypoparathyroidism, and dementia [23]. Schizophrenia remains the most common co-occurring mental disorder associated with case reports of Capgras delusion [25, 26]. Also, family history of psychosis is reportedly present in half of CS patients [20]. Medications and drug toxicity have also been reported to cause CS [27].

## 3. Explanations for Capgras syndrome

Since initial reports of CS involved patients with psychiatric illness, their close relations, and how they interacted with each other, early explanations of the delusion were predominately psychodynamic interpretations. There are several psychodynamic approaches. Consequently, these explanations included suggestions that CS might develop out of Oedipal issues in women as a defence against hostility or incestuous, guilty desires, or out of hidden homosexuality in men. Later attempts to account for CS resulted in hypotheses of anxiety-induced regression of cognitive and emotional functioning, pathological splitting of internalized object representations, insufficiently repressed conflicting or ambivalent feelings toward the implicated person, and the projection of negative emotions that come to light from these conflicting feelings [17]. In the psychodynamic theory, it is supposed that the delusion is a way in which the patient copes with the ambivalent emotions that he feels toward the close family member who is duplicated [15]. There are several explanations brought about by psychodynamic approaches of misidentification syndromes. Premorbid psychopathology, motivation, and loss of ego functions may be important in determining which vulnerable patients develop CS [6].

Capgras delusion can occur due to 'spatial disorientation, anatomic disconnection, memory and executive process impairment, and loss of ego' [4]. While psychodynamic theories consist of ambivalence theory, depersonalization theory, and regression theory, neurocognitive hypotheses focus on right hemispheric dysfunction, face-recognition processing abnormalities, and focal structural cerebral abnormalities [28]. There are two components of the visual recognition of a familiar face, one of which is responsible for conscious recognition of the face and the remembrance of associated semantic information, while the other is responsible for the limbic-mediated emotional arousal including the feeling of familiarity that accompanies the conscious recognition of a known face [9].

## 4. Psychodynamic proposals in Capgras delusion

Despite the sharp increase in the number of published cases accompanied by various suggestions regarding an organic etiology, to accurately explain the delusion, it is necessary to embrace the psychodynamic as well as the organic. Even if a specific neuropsychological lesion is found in the end, the psychodynamics of the individual will still be pertinent and remain substantial [29]. An association between CS and depersonalization has been thought to exist onward the time when the disorder was first described. Some authors put forward that depersonalization may be the basis of the disorder which may develop in some individuals. CS can be evaluated as a disorder of ego function which permeates the entire personality [29]. Some authors postulated that cerebral dysfunction leads to feelings of derealization and depersonalization which in turn may develop into Capgras' syndrome in the presence of paranoid ideation [29].

The psychodynamic conception of the Capgras phenomenon is basically a love-hate conflict that is resolved by reflecting ambivalent feelings onto a fictitious double [29]. On the one hand, there are a long-standing love and on the other hand a visible hatred. In those cases when it occurs, it is very substantial that before the onset of the delusion of doubles, the patient shows an increased love and sexual desire toward the object. This overreaction results from a desire for reassurance regarding the love of the object and fear of losing it simultaneously. Theories suggested that CS could arise out of an Electra complex and incest desires, Oedipal problems, and latent homosexuality. Personality disintegration coupled with an evolutionary regression to more primitive modes of cognitive and emotional functioning; division of internalized object representations; ambivalent feelings toward a familiar other that are not sufficiently suppressed; and the feelings of anxiety, guilt, and anger resulting from this struggle are reflected onto imagined imposter [20]. Instead of approving these demands, the object becomes even more repulsed and is unable to cover up these feelings that clearly aggravate the situation, and a vicious circle is established [29].

## 5. Face-recognition system in Capgras delusion

Usually, we do not strive for facial recognition. The ability to identify people who we met before is a headstone of our social interactions. Face recognition is a multi-stage process ending with the identification of a person. Prosopagnosia is defined as loss of familiarity to previously known faces and the inability to learn to recognize new faces. Although these patients fail to recognize faces, they are still able to show affective responses to these faces [30, 31]. Several studies have suggested that CS represents a 'mirror image' of prosopagnosia, thus suggesting different neural circuits for facial processing: a cognitive circuit (impaired in prosopagnosia) and an affective circuit (impaired in CS). In the affective circuit, the ventral route from the visual centers to the temporal lobes may be protected, also active in conscious face recognition; however, the dorsal visual track that gives the face its emotional significance is damaged. A brief disruption of the ventral visual pathway leads to prosopagnosia, whereas damage to the dorsal visual areas leads to an impaired sense of familiarity for known faces, as in CS [9, 17, 30, 32]. While the ability to identify that person is intact, patient with CS probably has a brain lesion that interferes with the patient's ability to sense a familiarity toward the significant other [15]. It has been suggested that the impairment seen in the Capgras delusion was linked to a disruption of pathways connecting face-sensitive regions to limbic cortex, which is involved in the accompanying emotional response [30]. Perhaps arising from the conflicting experience of recognizing a known face without any accompanying affective reaction, the patient can understand that the absence of this emotional arousal is to establish the belief that the person he is looking at is an imposter [9, 33]. In another connectivity study, posterior coupled with anterior right hemisphere dysfunction may have involved in the emergence of Capgras delusion [34]. Also, it has been suggested that CS results from the disconnection of the face processing regions in the inferior temporal lobe from structures in the limbic system, especially the amygdala, which is very important in assigning emotional value to familiar faces [34]. Common to the CS is a fixed false belief but infrequently transient [35]. However, anatomical disconnection models fail to efficiently consider the transient nature of the misidentification episodes [34]. Therefore, it has been suggested that CS may be associated with the 'kindling of subcortical structures'. Kindling refers to repeated subthreshold stimuli which may result in psychomotor outbursts or overt seizure activity [34]. Autonomic responses and eye movements are involved in face perception which may cause the patient believe that the person has been replaced by an imposter. Studies on patient with CS like other psychiatric disorders have shown abnormal scan paths to facial stimuli or abnormal skin conductance response (SCR) in face processing tasks [30, 33]. The absence of identity recognition, accompanied by a lack of SCR, stimulates the patient to explore unfamiliar faces, and identity recognition of familiar faces leads to a more detailed exploration in the eye region, and it results in gaze avoidance of the eye region [33]. Vision is important in accessing reserved knowledge in the etiology of CS. However, surprisingly CS has also been reported in a number of blind patients which suggests that it cannot have an exclusively visual basis [34]. Some theories assume that two deficits are necessary for delusions to occur in the case of Capgras delusion like other DMSs [32, 36]. This is also called 'two-hit' process [20]. The first one, the brain's ability to attach emotional emphasis, may be the lack of autonomic arousal which leads to the abductive inference that the person is an imposter [30]. The other deficit is an impaired ability to reassess beliefs [the global consistency-checking mechanism] which prevents the rejection of the bizarre belief. The second deficit leads to the persistence of that abnormal perception as a delusion resistant to reasoning, also related to the right anterior cortex of the second deficit [9, 30, 32, 36].

## 6. Cognitive domains in Capgras delusion: memory, executive impairment, and confabulation

Neuropsychological deficits in patient with CS were reported across multiple cognitive domains, including memory, executive functioning, and visuospatial processing. These studies suggest that memory was statistically more likely to be impaired than other cognitive domains. Therefore, the memory may be playing an important role in the development of these delusions [32]. The existence of confabulations may have a role in prognosis and predicted significantly longer delusion duration, once more supporting the importance of memory impairment in patients with CS [32]. To mention a little more about the confabulation, some authors are focusing on confabulation in these patients because they are thought to be confabulation and delusion are closely related. When asked how they can explain their beliefs, Capgras patients will often confabulate. Confabulation is a kind of false memory that occurs when patients produce stories that fill in gaps in their memories, whereas a delusion is a mental state, typically thought of as a belief. Confabulation and delusion cannot be completely the same [37, 38]. Some researchers suggested that CS comes out when right hemisphere dysfunction causes a memory disconnection that leads to a failure to put new information together with representations about a significant individual and to keep in reserved over time [17]. Against all of these, although many patients have subtle deficits in face recognition and memory for faces, they do not have difficulty in recognizing faces in everyday life [1, 2]. CS is distinguished by its delusional mechanism: it is neither a hallucination nor an illusion—the object is correctly recognized in its appearance. CS is not a memory disorder. The person is correctly recognized; people are memorized [7]. Language deficits may not be absent, because of the right hemispherical dominance of the lesions [32].

## 7. Neuroanatomical and neuropsychological impairments in Capgras syndrome

In 1971 a case of Capgras was described in a young man following a head injury, with no previous history of psychiatric disorder. Since then, many patients with CS have undergone more thorough neurological investigations [29]. Identification disorders like CS are very frequent in neurodegenerative diseases [7]. Regarding the organic conditions that occur in Capgras delusion, this appears mainly in various types of dementia like Alzheimer, Lewy bodies, and Parkinson [39]. The prevalence of CS in Lewy body dementia may be as high as 25% and 10% in Alzheimer-type dementia. Identification disorders are much rarer in other types of dementia, especially those associated with Parkinson's disease [7]. Nearly half of the cases in CS were associated with neurocognitive disorders, such as delirium, traumatic brain encephalopathy, cerebrovascular disease, dementia, meningioma, encephalitis, and multiple sclerosis [21, 22]. Although there is usually a delay in the presentation of Capgras delusion after cerebral events, there are also such cases of immediate presentation [31]. Psychotic disorders with CS tend to present in the late teens and early twenties. It reflects the long mean duration of the delusion in the functional group [26]. Those with neurological disorder associated with the onset of the delusion had a mean age of 60, in keeping with their presentation in middle to late adulthood, especially as Capgras delusion in dementia tends to occur in the later stages [26]. Therefore all individuals with Capgras should be examined for organic pathology [9]. In a literature review of patients with CS who had associated organic factors, there are several single case reports in patients with Capgras delusion which suggest structural and metabolic anomalies in mostly right-sided frontal, temporal, or parietal brain regions. But most of CS patients had bilateral lesions although, for those with unilateral lesions, right hemisphere lesions were much more likely [30]. Some studies give emphasis to the presence of two lesion sites, one in right frontal and the other in right temporal cortex [30]. The identity of the imposter is significantly associated with the reported underlying etiology. Capgras' delusion is reportedly due to functional psychiatric disorder, which is more likely to view their parent as an imposter, whereas the spouse is involved in those with suspected neurological etiology. There may be mentioned two reasons. The first one is may be because of the different mean age for the groups. The age of onset of Capgras delusion is different between those with organic disorders and those with neurological disorders [26]. The other reason is about Capgras delusion's feature. Capgras delusion is the phenomenon mostly specific to close relatives. This supports the role of intimacy [9, 26]. Selectivity for familiar persons is essential, though sometimes relative, and the syndrome can extend to persons who are simply known or famous [7]. Against this, the frequency with which strangers and multiple imposters are implicated in all cases of Capgras delusion can be up to 39% [26]. Multiple imposters are significantly more likely to occur in functional cases, while the involvement of inanimate objects would seem to suggest organic etiology [26]. The neuropsychological findings discussed may lead to some account of the possible mechanisms by which an abnormal experience may be generated in a subset of Capgras patients, but some researchers do not think in itself account for the formation of delusional belief [40]. Consequently, the explanation may offer a useful, helpful analysis of a certain step in the pathology of the CS in a subgroup of more neurological patients but could be unlikely to enlighten about delusions more generally or those with Capgras in the context of a functional psychosis such as schizophrenia or bipolar disorder [40].

## 8. Neuropsychological assessment for Capgras syndrome

The term CS does not demonstrate a well-defined mental disorder. Over the years various studies have suggested psychodynamic and neurophysiological interpretations for CS, and various aetiologies have been recommended for the condition's development [15, 17, 28].

Although frequently seen in psychotic cases, Capgras has also been associated with neurological disorders suggesting that the syndrome has an organic basis [14]. According to a study, CS patients were classified into groups according to whether or not they had evidence of neurological disorder. Some of the patients identified as having no neurological lesion might be found to have organic brain disease with more sophisticated imaging techniques or at post-mortem evaluation [41]. In another study, approximately one in five of patients with CS presented with organic mental disorders [1, 2]. Multiple hypotheses have been put forth regarding the underlying pathophysiology of CS. Some areas of the brain are responsible for the etiology of this disease. Results of structural and neuroimaging studies of CS provide support for an organic etiology [17]. Multiple studies and reports have remarked on CS in the setting of various neurological and neurodegenerative diseases [42]. There is a study that found more widespread bilateral frontal and temporal cortex atrophy in schizophrenia patients with CS than schizophrenia patients without the syndrome by using computerized tomography (CT) [17]. Likewise other studies using CT found global brain atrophy in combination with right hemisphere lesions in patients with dementia. There is also reported that positron emission tomography [PET] demonstrated abnormal brain glucose metabolism in paralimbic structures and temporal lobes of patients with Alzheimer's dementia comorbid with CS and other subcategories of delusional misidentification syndromes [17]. Numerous neuropsychological researches support an association between CS and right frontal and temporal lobe abnormalities, and also many study reports indicate that patients with CS tend to have inferior scores on neuropsychological tests of frontal lobe function [17]. Even though less well documented, regions of the prefrontal cortex are also associated within facial processing: projections from the face processing areas in the right ventromedial occipitotemporal regions to the ventromedial prefrontal cortex via the uncinate fasciculus as well as limbic-thalamic pathways are well established [34].

## 9. The association between Capgras delusion and schizophrenia

Some people with schizophrenia exhibit this syndrome, but it is not related directly to schizophrenia itself; there are people with schizophrenia who do not exhibit CS, as well as people with CS who do not exhibit schizophrenia. The mean age of schizophrenic patients with Capgras syndrome is older than the age at which schizophrenia alone is usually expected to occur. When brain abnormalities of people with schizophrenia affect certain areas, CS and schizophrenia will occur concurrently. Capgras delusion and schizophrenia seem to be statistically related, at least in the case of the paranoid subtype of schizophrenia. It has been claimed that right hemisphere damage is a characteristic of schizophrenia; perhaps the imperfect evaluation of beliefs, which we have suggested, occurs as an outcome of damage to a particular area of the right frontal lobe, which is necessary for the occurrence even of the persecutory and grandiose delusions that are common in paranoid schizophrenia. Accounting the association of Capgras delusion with paranoid schizophrenia, the same neuropsychological deterioration of belief assessment is required for both, and in cases of patients with persecutory or grandiose delusions where the neuropathology also has affected the track from face recognition to the autonomic nervous system, Capgras delusion will also be existing [43, 44]. CS in paranoid schizophrenia may improve with successful treatment. But recurrence of illness may be accompanied by a return of delusional material [44].

## 10. Differential diagnosis of primary and secondary Capgras delusions

It is important to note that the Capgras delusion can be either a primary condition that is part of a 'mental illness' or a secondary condition that is the direct result of an organic disease of the brain. Also, the primary and secondary versions differ significantly in their presentation. In primary Capgras syndrome, the patient is more likely to be furious or violent toward the imposter. In secondary CS, the imposters do not change over time. This is different from the situation in schizophrenia where the delusions can vary [45]. The mean age of onset of the delusion was earlier in primary Capgras (mean age 32 years) than in secondary Capgras (mean age 48.5 years). Primary cases are more likely to have a subtle onset which evolved gradually, whereas secondary cases are more likely to have sudden-onset delusions. Primary cases show associated psychotic symptoms, particularly paranoid thought, whereas psychotic symptoms are not very often of the secondary cases. The patients with CS without apparent organic cerebral dysfunction were more likely to have experienced other psychiatric symptoms prior to the onset of the Capgras delusion than those with organic cerebral dysfunction [41]. Patients with neurological impairments were more likely to regard the misidentification as benign or as due to illusory, whereas patients without evidence of neurological basis were more likely to appraise the delusions as being threatening [41]. Thus, hostility and violence are seen much more frequently in those patients diagnosed as schizophrenic than in other patients [46].

## 11. The role of Capgras syndrome in violence

Acting on delusions is a crucial clinical issue. There is a positive relationship between delusions and serious violent acts. Although the pathway from delusions to violent outcomes is not direct, the risk is greatly increased when symptoms are acute, especially at the time of initial presentation and if not treated [19]. And the risk also can be changed according to the etiology of delusions. There is a requirement to be concerned about the patient's tendency for violence and to evaluate for it thoroughly in Capgras delusion [45]. In patients with CS of an organic nature, violence may be associated with few or no affective manifestations (e.g., hostility, aggression, and auditory hallucinations), and may not be associated with paranoid elements [7]. Delusional symptoms in CS such as persecutory thoughts, threat-control symptoms, command auditory and/or visual hallucinations, and hallucinations of threatening content have all demonstrated to be significant predictors of violence act and aggressive behaviour [28]. If the patients are married, divorced, or separated, the most frequent doubles are the spouse. If the patients are single, the most frequent doubles are the siblings [19]. It should be noted that healthcare professionals may become the objects of delusional misidentification [42]. Because the double is usually assumed to have malicious, the CS could be characterized by hostility toward misidentified objects, and, later, it can lead to physical harm to others [19]. The assault associated with CS, the tendency to violence, cannot be attributed purely to the delusion's existence. Other factors are presumably to affect the possibility of violent act. A significantly higher tendency for interpersonal violence are men disclosed among male subjects, average age at 40 years old, with a history of aggressive behaviour and substance abuse; social withdrawal prior to the violent act is common, and the violence is usually well planned [19, 21, 22]. Persecutory paranoid motivations have been implicated as a key factor in acts of violence toward family members who constitute the majority of victims in CS [28]. Physical violence was expressed by 58.2% of patients with CS and 62.5% of patients with CS engaged in acts of interpersonal violence toward their close family members and caregivers [21, 22]. Mothers and spouses were the most frequently attacked group of relatives, respectively. Also, it was found that 1 of 10 Capgras patients attempted homicide [21, 22]. Most of the perpetrators were males suffering from mental disorders without organic association. A higher incidence of self-harm and suicide attempts, which is about 1 in 10 of patients with CS, was detected among females even in patients with psychiatric disorders and in patients with neurodegenerative disorders [21, 22]. Although in the usual cases, the misidentified object is a person, hence justifying the title of delusional identification of people, the CS is not restricted to person misidentification but can also involve other living or lifeless objects [7, 19]. Physical violence against objects was also common, such as setting fire to one else's estate [21, 22].

## 12. Differential diagnosis of Capgras syndrome

The differential diagnosis of patients who suffered CS is crucial. It is substantial to rule out the presence of brain disease in every patient with Capgras delusion [45].

Many patients with CS also present with medical illnesses of organic etiologies, associated with delusional misidentification; these patients may respond well to treatment of the medical condition underlying the onset of CS [47]. The syndrome should be differentiated from the quite common false recognitions which occur in confusional states and the transient misidentifications encountered in mania [8]. For this purpose, ending with a complete mental status examination, as well as thorough testing of cognition, is important. Neuropsychological testing and neuroimaging are often indicated. Clinicians should clarify the nature of the underlying psychiatric illness [45].

## 13. Key features and biomarker of Capgras syndrome

Low platelet monoamine oxidase (MAO) activity is a biochemical abnormality which is present in some psychiatric disease. Some authors suggested that the low platelet MAO activity might be proposed as a potential biochemical marker of CS. It is also thought that reduced *monoamine oxidase* activity in primary psychiatric patients with CS may give a piece of information to the pathogenetic mechanism underlying the reported cases of CS in organic patients without a primary behavioral disorder. However, study results show that platelet *monoamine oxidase* activity in patients with delusional misidentifications did not differ notably from that of schizophrenia and nonpsychiatric controls [41, 48].

The key features currently considered to be critical to the development of the Capgras delusion are as follows:

- There is an abnormal perceptual experience that is a prerequisite for the delusion.
- This perceptual experience is accompanied by a paranoid which leads to misattribution of the abnormal perceptual experience.
- The loss of normal response to known faces occurs in the context of more generalized derealization-depersonalization [41].

## 14. Treatment considerations

Delusion in CS should be treated timely because it can cause a dangerous condition [42]. However, there are no guidelines to assist clinicians to care for patients presenting with CS in selecting complementary examinations to be performed or in selecting treatment [7]. Likewise, the symptoms of DMS are very refractory to treatment despite various interventions including psychotherapy and pharmacotherapy approaches [19]. The CS like other DMSs is known to develop similar to the comorbid disorder that they accompany, disappearing after remission even though it is not unusual for them to continue after the disappearance of the comorbid disorder [7]. Thus, treatment of the underlying neurological or psychiatric conditions may not lead to remission of CS [27]. The presence of depersonalization, derealization or visual-perceptual disturbances, and other comorbidities may influence the treatment of CS [47]. The syndrome has been linked to dopaminergic overactivity, and serotonin abnormality has been implicated in some but not all studies. Similarly, reduced platelet monoamine oxidase activity has been noted by some but not by others [17]. According to the results of the case studies in the literature, CS patients are sometimes responsive to typical and atypical antipsychotics such as olanzapine, risperidone, quetiapine, sulpiride, trifluoperazine, and pimozide [19]. Pharmacological treatment of

CS is based on antipsychotics, antidepressants, anticonvulsant, and benzodiazepines considering patient needs and characteristics, but no control trials are available [49]. In the literature, there have been reported cases with a diagnosis of organic or functional delusional disorder associated with CS whose DMS responded well to pimozide that is well known for the treatment of monosymptomatic delusional disorders [49]. Experience with the new generation of atypical antipsychotics for the treatment of CS is quite limited. Although for patients manifesting any psychotic disorder, atypical antipsychotics are usually recommended because of the reduced risk of adverse effects [6, 47]. A crucial point of a case report is the positive outcome in response to antipsychotic medication [olanzapine] [49]. The combination of antipsychotic drug therapy and selective serotonin reuptake inhibitor (SSRI) may produce a positive outcome in patients with CS [15].

A case report also suggested the use of clorazepate which is benzodiazepine. In this case report, in addition to the antipsychotic properties of clorazepate, its anticonvulsant properties were also utilized in CS patient with the suggestion of some researches that found an over 90% incidence of electroencephalographic abnormalities in CS patients [26]. According to the results of the case studies, it showed a positive outcome in a patient with CS after treatment with mirtazapine that is also a serotonin 2A receptor antagonist, which could potentially afford its antipsychotic effects resulting in significantly decreasing the symptoms of CS [19, 27].

With patients who have progressive dementia, such as dementia with Lewy bodies, in which misidentification syndromes are common occurred, cholinesterase inhibitors have demonstrated benefit to reduce psychiatric symptoms [6].

Electroconvulsive therapy (ECT) has been reported to benefit either alone or in conjunction with antipsychotics, mood stabilizer, or antidepressant medication in patients with CS. It has been suggested that ECT provides permanent effective control of CS [42, 47, 49].

Psychotherapy may be beneficial in the treatment of selected patients with CS in order to reform the patient's relationship with his family. The psychoanalytic theories show that the emotions which the patient experiences in regard to the people with whom he is confronted are transferred to the imposters, and therefore, in this way from a safe delusional distance, the patient gives himself to refuse them without guilt, sometimes manifesting an aggressive behaviour toward them [21, 22]. It has been shown that group psychotherapy may also be beneficial by becoming less prone to feel hostile toward others, thereby weakening the delusional misidentification process for psychotic patients with DMS [40]. Cognitive behavioural therapy (CBT) may be a utilized form of psychotherapy intervention in some cases by assisting the patient to overcome the delusional beliefs [21, 22].

It is quite common in cases of delusion for his/her family members of the deluded person to be concerned about the delusion and to try to get rid of it by constantly challenging it [43]. It may be beneficial to know that just as an impairment in the interpersonal relationship between the patient and the object may occur before the onset of the delusion, an amelioration in this relationship is an essential factor in the amelioration of symptoms. Therefore treatment must include helping the partner or person implicated to gain insight and perhaps change their attitude toward the patient [29].

## 15. Conclusion

CS is a different neuropsychiatric symptom of interest to researchers over the past century. No approved questionnaires focus on CS. While noting that the Capgras syndrome has no formal place in recognized diagnostic systems, it should be emphasized that this is of significance. It is crucial to keep them in mind as a possibility and to pursue any possible clues. Capgras delusion is a complex psychopathological phenomenon that presents in a wide range of psychiatric and neurological disorders with differing patterns dependent on the main etiology. Misidentifications in CS are fixed false beliefs and, therefore, represent true delusions. Even if when patients are confronted over and over with the illogical nature of the delusion, they keep their beliefs. Specific questions and interventions may assist to clinicians in successfully identifying patients with CS. In a series of interviews with these patients, some focus on identifying CS, rather than a single interview which is likely to increase the detection of the delusional misidentification. The clinician should always be mindful of the risk of aggression and homicide in CS.

## Author details

Aslı Enzel Koc and Cicek Hocaoglu*
Medical School, Recep Tayyip Erdogan University, Rize, Turkey

*Address all correspondence to: cicekh@gmail.com

## References

[1] Breen N, Caine D, Coltheart M. Mirrored-self misidentification: Two cases of focal onset dementia. Neurocase. 2001;**7**(3):239-254. DOI: 10.1093/neucas/7.3.239

[2] Feinberg TE, Roane D. Self-representation in delusional misidentification and confabulated “others”. Cortex. 2017;**87**:118-128. DOI: 10.1016/j.cortex.2016.07.014

[3] Alam A. A Brief Overview of the Capgras Delusion Brooklyn College. Available from: https://www.academia.edu/33990249/Brief_Overview_of_Capgras_Delusion

[4] Lykouras L, Typaldou M, Mourtzouchou P. Neuropsychological relationships in paranoid schizophrenia with and without delusional misidentification syndromes: A comparative study. Progress in Neuro-Psychopharmacology & Biological Psychiatry. 2008;**32**:1445-1448

[5] Feinberg TE, Roane DM. Delusional misidentification. Psychiatric Clinics of North America. 2005;**28**(3):665-683. DOI: 10.1016/j.psc.2005.05.002

[6] Barrelle A, Luauté JP. Capgras syndrome and other delusional misidentification syndromes. Frontiers of Neurology and Neuroscience. 2018;**42**:35-43. DOI: 10.1159/000475680

[7] Christodoulou GN. The syndrome of Capgras. The British Journal of Psychiatry. 1977;**130**(6):556-564. DOI: 10.1192/bjp.130.6.556

[8] Hirstein W, Ramachandran VS. Capgras syndrome: A novel probe for understanding the neural representation of the identity and familiarity of persons. Proceedings. Biological Sciences. 1997;**264**(1380):437-444. DOI: 10.1098/rspb.1997.0062

[9] Currell EA, Werbeloff N, Hayes JF, Bell V. Cognitive neuropsychiatric analysis of an additional large Capgras delusion case series. Cognitive Neuropsychiatry. 2019;**24**(2):123-134. DOI: 10.1080/13546805.2019.1584098

[10] Rodrigues ACT, Banzato CEM. Delusional misidentification syndrome: Why such nosologic challenge remains intractable. Psychopathology. 2006;**39**(6):296-302. DOI: 10.1159/000095777

[11] Antonio V, Iris B, Fabiana R, Federica C, Vishal B. Delusion, possession and religion. Nordic Journal of Psychiatry. 2018 Sep;**72**(Suppl 1):S13-S15. DOI: 10.1080/08039488.2018.1525639

[12] Gaines AD. Culture-specific delusions. Psychiatric Clinics of North America. 1995;**18**(2):281-301. DOI: 10.1016/s0193-953x(18)30055-8

[13] Salvatore P, Bhuvaneswar C, Tohen M, Khalsa HM, Maggini C, Baldessarini RJ. Capgras' syndrome in first-episode psychotic disorders. Psychopathology. 2014;**47**(4):261-269. DOI: 10.1159/000357813

[14] Mazzone L, Armando M, De Crescenzo F, Demaria F, Valeri G, Vicari S. Clinical picture and treatment implication in a child with Capgras syndrome: A case report. Journal of Medical Case Reports. 2012;**6**:406. DOI: 10.1186/1752-1947-6-406

[15] Thiel CM, Studte S, Hildebrandt H, Huster R, Weerda R. When a loved one feels unfamiliar: A case study on the neural basis of Capgras delusion. Cortex. 2014;**52**:75-85. DOI: 10.1016/j.cortex.2013.11.011

[16] Bourget D, Whitehurst L. Capgras syndrome: A review of the neurophysiological correlates and presenting clinical features in cases

involving physical violence. The Canadian Journal of Psychiatry. 2004;**49**(11):719-725. DOI: 10.1177/070674370404901102

[17] Edelstyn NMJ, Oyebode F, Barrett K. The delusions of Capgras and intermetamorphosis in a patient with right-hemisphere white-matter pathology. Psychopathology. 2001;**34**(6):299-304. DOI: 10.1159/000049328

[18] Karakasi MV, Markopoulou M, Alexandri M, Douzenis A, Pavlidis P. In fear of the most loved ones. A comprehensive review on Capgras misidentification phenomenon and case report involving attempted murder under Capgras syndrome in a relapse of a schizophrenia spectrum disorder. Journal of Forensic and Legal Medicine. 2019;**66**:8-24. DOI: 10.1016/j.jflm.2019.05.019

[19] De Pauw KW, Szulecka TK. Dangerous delusions, violence and the misidentification syndromes. The British Journal of Psychiatry. 1988;**152**:91-96

[20] Edelstyn NMJ, Oyebode F. A review of the phenomenology and cognitive neuropsychological origins of the Capgras syndrome. International Journal of Geriatric Psychiatry. 1999;**14**(1):48-59. DOI: 10.1002/(sici)1099-1166(199901)14:1<48::aid-gps891>3.0.co;2-0

[21] Jariwala PC, Shah ND, Dave KR, Mehta RY. Delusional misidentification syndromes in patients of paranoid schizophrenia: Case series and review. Telangana Journal of Psychiatry. 2018;**3**(2):125-129

[22] De Pauw KW. Psychodynamic approaches to the capgras delusion: A critical historical review. Psychopathology. 1994;**27**(3-5):154-160. DOI: 10.1159/000284864

[23] Silva A, Leong GB, Weinstock R, Sharma KK, Klein RL. Delusional misidentification syndromes and dangerousness. Psychopathology. 1994;**27**(3-5):215-219. DOI: 10.1159/000284872

[24] Pandis C, Agrawal N, Poole N. Capgras' delusion - A systematic review of 255 published cases. Psycho-pathology. 2019;**52**:161-173. DOI: 10.1159/000500474

[25] Khouzam HR. Capgras syndrome responding to the antidepressant mirtazapine. Comprehensive Therapy. 2002;**28**(3):238-240. DOI: 10.1007/s12019-002-0033-9

[26] Sinkman A. The syndrome of Capgras. Psychiatry: Interpersonal and Biological Processes. 2008;**71**(4):371-378. DOI: 10.1521/psyc.2008.71.4.371

[27] Carabellese F, Rocca G, Candelli C, Catanesi R. Mental illness, violence and delusional misidentifications: The role of Capgras' syndrome in matricide. Journal of Forensic and Legal Medicine. 2014;**21**:9-13. DOI: 10.1016/j.jflm.2013.10.012

[28] Albonico A, Barton J. Progress in perceptual research: The case of prosopagnosia. F1000Research. 2019;**8**:765. DOI: 10.12688/f1000research.18492.1

[29] Enoch MD, Ball HN. Uncommon Psychiatric Syndromes. 4th ed. Arnold; Hodder Arnold Publication, CRC Press; 2001

[30] Darby R, Prasad S. Lesion-related delusional misidentification syndromes: A comprehensive review of reported cases. The Journal of Neuropsychiatry and Clinical Neurosciences. 2016;**28**(3):217-222. DOI: 10.1176/appi.neuropsych.15100376

[31] Ellis HD, Young AW. Accounting for delusional misidentifications.

The British Journal of Psychiatry. 1990;**157**:239-248

[32] Brighetti G, Bonifacci P, Borlimi R, Ottaviani C. "Far from the heart far from the eye": Evidence from the Capgras delusion. Cognitive Neuropsychiatry. 2007;**12**(3):189-197. DOI: 10.1080/13546800600892183

[33] Garcha M, Sivakumar K, Leary M, Yacoub HA. Transient Capgras syndrome secondary to bilateral ischemic stroke. Cognitive and Behavioral Neurology. 2018;**31**(2):96-98. DOI: 10.1097/wnn.0000000000000152

[34] Coltheart M, Langdon R, McKay R. Delusional belief. Annual Revues of Psychology. 2011;**62**:271-298

[35] Hirstein W. The misidentification syndromes as mindreading disorders. Cognitive Neuropsychiatry. 2010;**15**(1-3):233-260. DOI: 10.1080/13546800903414891

[36] Estrada-Bellmann I, Ulloa-Escobar Y, Barbosa-Flores SL, Pech-George RE, González-Treviño R, Conde-Gómez L, et al. Capgras syndrome as a psychiatric manifestation in Parkinson's disease: A case report and literature review. Medicina Universitaria. 2015;**17**(66):49-52. DOI: 10.1016/j.rmu.2014.07.002

[37] Bortolotti L, Broome MR. If you didn't care, you wouldn't notice: recognition and estrangement in psychopathology, Philosophy, Psychiatry, & Psychology. 2007;**14**(1):39-42

[38] Ullrich S, Keers R, Shaw J, Doyle M, Coid JW. Acting on delusions: The role of negative affect in the pathway towards serious violence. The Journal of Forensic Psychiatry & Psychology. 2018;**29**(5):691-704. DOI: 10.1080/14789949.2018.1434227

[39] Cipriani G, Vedovello M, Ulivi M, Lucetti C, Di Fiorino A, Nuti A. Delusional misidentification syndromes and dementia. American Journal of Alzheimer's Disease & Other Dementiasr. 2013;**28**(7):671-678. DOI: 10.1177/1533317513506103

[40] Spiegel DR, Laroia R, Samuels D. A possible case of Capgras syndrome after a right anterior cerebral artery cerebrovascular accident treated successfully with mirtazapine. The Journal of Neuropsychiatry and Clinical Neurosciences. 2008;**20**(4):494

[41] Breen N, Caine D, Coltheart M, Hendy J, Roberts C. Towards an understanding of delusions of misidentification: Four case studies. Mind and Language. 2000;**15**(1):74-110. DOI: 10.1111/1468-0017.00124

[42] Silva JA, Leong GB, Miller AL. Delusional misidentification syndromes. CNS Drugs. 1996;**5**(2):89-102. DOI: 10.2165/00023210-199605020-00002

[43] Coltheart M, Langdon R, McKay R. Schizophrenia and monothematic delusions. Schizophrenia Bulletin. 2007;**33**(3):642-647. DOI: 10.1093/schbul/sbm017

[44] Merrin EL. The Capgras phenomenon. Archives of General Psychiatry. 1976;**33**(8):965. DOI: 10.1001/archpsyc.1976.01770080083008

[45] Sharpless B. Unusual and Rare Psychological Disorders: A Handbook for Clinical Practice and Research. New York: Oxford University Press; 2017

[46] Jocic Z. Delusional misidentification syndromes. Jefferson Journal of Psychiatry. 1992;**10**:4

[47] Joseph AB. Delusional misidentification of the Capgras and intermetamorphosis types responding to clorazepate. Acta Psychiatrica Scandinavica. 1987;**75**(3):330-332. DOI: 10.1111/j.1600-0447.1987.tb02797.x

[48] Barton JL, Chaparala S, Barton ES, Jackson IV, Davis LG. Delusional misidentification and platelet monoamine oxidase. Biological Psychiatry. 1980;**15**(/2):275

[49] Torales J, Rodríguez H, Arce A, Moreno M, Riego V, Chávez E, et al. Olanzapine in the treatment of Capgras syndrome: A case report. International Journal of Culture and Mental Health. 2013;7(2):224-228. DOI: 10.1080/17542863.2013.775782

Section 3

# The Biological Mechanisms of Anxiety Disorders

Chapter 10

# Technologically Processed Highly Diluted Antibodies to S100 Protein in the Treatment of Neurotic Disorders: The Review

*Kristina Konstantinovna Khacheva,*
*Gulnara Rinatovna Khakimova, Alexey Borisovich Glazunov and Victoria Vyacheslavovna Fateeva*

## Abstract

Neurotic disorders (NDs) are among the most common mental diseases leading to a decrease in the quality of life, lack of socialization, and increased mortality. The diagnosis and treatment of all types of NDs are challenging. In the light of the ongoing search for an effective and safe therapeutic strategy influencing certain aspects of ND pathogenesis, technologically processed highly diluted antibodies to S100 protein (TP Abs to S100) seem to be a promising treatment option for patients with NDs. TP Abs to S100 possess stress-protective, anxiolytic, antidepressant, antiamnestic, and neuroprotective activities. In the current review, we describe the mechanisms of action and pharmacological effects of TP Abs to S100 demonstrated in nonclinical (preclinical) and clinical studies. Based on the data, we tried to evaluate the future prospects of the TP Abs to S100 as the drug of choice for ND treatment.

**Keywords:** neurotic disorder, anxiety, anxiolytic therapy, S100 protein, somatoform disorder

## 1. Introduction

Neurotic disorders (NDs) are among the most common mental diseases leading to a decrease in the quality of life, lack of socialization, and increased mortality [1]. Around 20–40% of primary care outpatients are diagnosed with NDs according to International Disease Classification (ICD)-10 or Diagnostic and Statistical Manual of Mental Disorders (DSM) V criteria [2].

ICD-10 classification of the NDs F40–F48 includes phobic anxiety disorders (F40), other anxiety disorders (AD, F41), obsessive-compulsive disorder (OCD, F42), reaction to severe stress, adjustment disorders (F43), dissociative and conversion disorders (F44), somatoform disorders (SD, F45), and other nonpsychotic mental disorders (F48). In the DSM V, the same disorders are classified as Anxiety

Disorders, Obsessive-Compulsive and Related Disorders, Trauma- and Stressor-Related Disorders, Dissociative Disorders, and Somatic Symptom Disorder [3, 4].

Phobias are present in 1.3–5.7% of all NDs [5]. Anxiety symptoms are thought to occur in every 14th person during the lifetime [6]. The prevalence of SD is 20–25%, but at least one medically unexplained symptom is found in 40–49% of patients [7, 8]. Around 10% of all psychiatric patients have dissociative disorder [9, 10]. A lifetime prevalence of OCD is 2.3%, and the rate of adjustment disorder is 1–2% [5].

The overlaps between AD, phobias, and SD were shown and considered a result of similarity of pathogenesis, which involves disturbances in hypothalamic-pituitary-adrenal axis (HPAA), cytokine levels, and changes in the state of receptors in the nervous system [11–15]. Continued and prolonged stress may disturb the HPAA to such an extent that the negative feedback mechanisms (glucocorticoid negative feedback, in particular) are disrupted, and the adaptive responses of the HPAA may then become maladaptive. Enhanced proinflammatory cytokine production and overactivation of the sympathetic nervous system contribute to a state of chronic low-grade inflammation.

NDs have a great social impact. A British survey (1993) reported that 8.3% of 10,000 responders had ND limiting their daily activities and 3.4% experienced severe "disabling" NDs, associated with a higher chance of being unemployed [16]. The cost of AD treatment in the European Union was approximately 41 billion € in 2004 and 66 billion € in 2010 [17, 18]. Taking into consideration the prediction of the growing influence of mental health problems on the economic output by 2030 [19], we expect the increasing burden of NDs.

The diagnosis and treatment of all types of NDs are challenging. More than 20% of AD patients are undertreated and continue to suffer from symptoms [11]. A study by Wang revealed a 2–3-year delay in the diagnosis of NDs [20]. Around 40–66% of SD cases are underdiagnosed in primary care [21]. The first line of treatment for most of NDs is selective serotonin reuptake inhibitors (SSRIs). Nevertheless, their efficacy and safety are still under consideration. The high placebo effect was shown in randomized controlled studies of SSRI in the treatment of phobic disorder, OCD, and generalized anxiety disorder (GAD) [22]. There are only 40–60% of responders to first-line therapy among OCD patients [23]. In the Cochrane review by Kleinstaeuber et al., low-quality evidence for the efficacy of new generation antidepressants in SD was obtained [24]. Adverse events such as insomnia, nausea, sexual dysfunction, and withdrawal are common for SSRI. Negative drug interactions are also limiting their use in patients receiving therapy for somatic diseases. Other antidepressant drugs such as tricyclic antidepressants (TCA) have been shown to be effective for the treatment of some NDs in several trials, although the Cochrane review did not reveal any significant differences in the comparison of tricyclic antidepressants (TCA) and other medications in SD [24]. The safety profile of TCA is more unfavorable than SSRI. The use of benzodiazepines in ADs is limited due to the sedation, myorelaxant effect, and negative impact on cognition they provoke in long-term use. Among nonpharmacological treatments, only cognitive behavioral therapy was shown to be effective with greater results in combination with medication [22].

In the light of the ongoing search for an effective and safe therapeutic strategy influencing certain aspects of ND pathogenesis, technologically processed highly diluted antibodies to the brain specific S100 protein (TP Abs to S100) seem to be a perspective substance for treatment.

In the central nervous system (CNS), the brain-specific S100 protein is synthesized mainly by astrocytes and then transported to neurons where it is involved in numerous processes. In particular, it was shown that S100 affects the differentiation and survival of neurons, the growth of dendrites, the integrity of cytoskeleton, and energy metabolism [25].

Increased level of S100 is considered a marker of blood brain barrier failure. S100 serum levels are elevated after stroke, subarachnoid hemorrhage, and brain trauma and correlate positively with patient outcome. However, the brain-specific S100 protein may be secreted peripherally, and its elevated serum levels are also found in heart diseases and infections. High serum levels of the brain-specific S100 protein are also found in patients with schizophrenia, depressive/bipolar disorders, and obesity, but which cells are the sources of S-100 protein in these conditions is unknown [25, 26].

A number of nonclinical studies of TP Abs to S100 efficacy, safety, and mechanisms of action using the commonly applied experimental *in vivo* and *in vitro* models preceded clinical investigation. While studying the drug's primary and secondary pharmacodynamics, it was shown that TP Abs to S100 exert stress-protective [27], anxiolytic [28–33], antidepressant [30, 31, 34], antiamnestic [35–37], and neuroprotective [38, 39] activities.

Target identification and mechanism-of-action studies revealed that the drug recruits serotonin-, dopamine-, GABA-, noradrenaline-, and glutamatergic systems [29, 30, 40–42] and thereby might be considered a player in various neurotransmitter-mediated processes. Moreover, TP Abs to S100 influence sigma$_1$ receptor [41] that in turn modulates the activity of almost all neurotransmitter systems and thereby possesses a spectrum of psychotropic activities [43, 44].

Data on the TP Abs to 100 mechanisms of action and identified pharmacodynamics of the drug are consistent with the literature data on the relationship between influencing certain neurotransmitter systems (their receptors) and observing subsequent psychotropic effects. For example, it is known that benzodiazepines mediate their anxiolytic activity and sedation via GABAA receptors [45, 46]. GABAB receptor agonists are known to attenuate the behavioral deficit-restoring effect of antidepressants [47, 48]. Ligands of 5-HT1A, 5-HT1B, 5-HT1F, 5-HT2a, 5-HT2B, 5-HT2C, and 5-HT3 receptors were shown to regulate aggression, anxiety, learning, addiction, locomotion, memory, mood, and so on [49]. Ligands of the glycine site of the NMDA receptor exhibit anxiolytic and antidepressant properties and impact memory-related processes [50–53, 80]. D3 receptor deficiency can result in chronic depression and anxiety [54]. Sigma$_1$ receptor ligands have a whole spectrum of psychotropic effects due to their modulating effect on all major neurotransmitter systems [43, 44], which also are in line with TP Abs to S100 mechanism of action.

More than 2000 patients with GAD (F41.1), SD (F45), adjustment disorders (AjDs) (F43.2), neurasthenia (F48.0), and anxiety accompanying somatic diseases (cardiovascular and gastrointestinal disorders) took part in phase III, IV, and post-marketing clinical trials (CTs) of TP Abs to S100, including two double-blind placebo-controlled randomized CTs and nine open-label comparative randomized CTs [55–57]. TP Abs to S100 were shown to be as effective as clonazepam 0.5–1 mg/day, bromdihydrochlorphenylbenzodiazepine 1.5 mg/day (for 7 days), and tofisopam 100 mg/day but causing less adverse events (AEs) [58–60].

The evidence on the safety of TP Abs to S100 was obtained in clinical and nonclinical trials. In CTs, TP Abs to S100 exerted less AEs typical for other anti-anxiety medications such as daytime sleepiness and muscle relaxation. No cases of withdrawal symptoms, addiction to TP Abs to S100, or negative drug interactions have been registered up-to-date. In nonclinical trials, no myorelaxant and toxic effects were observed.

In the current review, we describe the mechanisms of action and pharmacological effects of TP Abs to S100 demonstrated in nonclinical (preclinical) and clinical studies. Based on the data, we attempt to evaluate the future perspectives of the TP Abs to S100 as the drug of choice for ND treatment.

## 2. Preclinical trials of technologically processed highly diluted antibodies to S100 protein

### 2.1 Pharmacodynamics

*2.1.1 Biological activity*

*2.1.1.1 Antistress activity of TP Abs to S100*

Antistress activity of TP Abs to S100 was studied using three approaches.

*2.1.1.1.1 Effect on somato-vegetative manifestations of stress*

Negative emotions arising from stress caused by the anticipation of pain or other negative expectations (in particular, on the eve of surgical operations, educational tests, important meetings, etc.) are accompanied by anxiety and fear. Concurrently, a cascade of somato-vegetative manifestations of stress is initiated [61].

Modeling of a conditioned emotional reflex to unescapable electric pain stimulation was performed on outbred white male rats weighing 220–280 g [27]. This was followed by monitoring of animal behavior in a stressful situation (repeated placement in an experimental 'dangerous' camera) as well as emotional responses when stress was intensified by an additional negative provocation (approaching an unfamiliar object to the animal's head). Antistress activities of TP Abs to S100 and diazepam ('classical' benzodiazepine tranquilizer, positive control) were estimated by administering drugs one day after development of the conditioned reflex.

Rats in the control group (hereinafter, animals that received distilled water as a placebo) when they were subsequently placed in a "dangerous" chamber responded by freezing (45%) or actively trying to escape the chamber (35%) (**Table 1A**). Only 20% of rats showed calm behavior. At the same time, somato-vegetative manifestations of stress were observed in animals (especially with a passive reaction): increased frequency of breathing, urination, defecation, and squeaking. Both TP Abs to S100 and diazepam caused a decrease in the number of rats with a passive and active response to stress, as well as significantly (three times) increased the number of animals with a calm orientation-exploratory activity. Somato-vegetative manifestations of stress also dissipated in both groups.

The emotional reaction of anxiety and anxiety associated with the expectation of pain in a "dangerous" chamber was significantly enhanced when using additional provocation—bringing an unfamiliar object to the head of the animal. This was manifested as an increase in the number of rats with active (up to 40%) and passive (up to 55%) behavior and a decrease in the number of animals with calm behavior (down to 5%) (**Table 1B**). Respiratory symptoms, squeaking, frequency of defecation, and urination also increased. Both drugs (TP Abs to S100 and diazepam) reduced the severity of stress induced by expectation of pain. TP Abs to S100 reduced both the number of animals with a spontaneous active and passive reaction by 20%, while diazepam reduced the number of animals with active attempts to escape the chamber (by 35%) more than the number of animals with freezing (only by 10%). The same trend continued with additional negative provocation, which may be the result of the sedative activity of diazepam, which TP Abs to S100 do not have.

| Parameter | [A] Stress induced by anticipation of pain | | | [B] Stress induced by anticipation of pain with additional negative stimulation | | |
|---|---|---|---|---|---|---|
| | Control | Diazepam | TP Abs to S100 | Control | Diazepam | TP Abs to S100 |
| *Percent of animals with:* | | | | | | |
| Passive behavior (freezing) | 45 | 35 | **25*** | 55 | 45 | **15*** |
| Active behavior with attempts to get out of the chamber | 35 | 5* | **15*** | 40 | 5* | **20*** |
| Calm exploratory behavior | 20 | 60* | **60*** | 5 | 50* | **65*** |
| Freezing in response to provocation | *n/a* | *n/a* | *n/a* | 55 | 45 | **15*** |
| Aggression in response to provocation | *n/a* | *n/a* | *n/a* | 40 | 15 | **10*** |
| Hurried breathing | 55 | 35 | **25*** | 75 | 40 | **35*** |
| *Frequency (%) of:* | | | | | | |
| Squeaking | 25 | 5* | **5*** | 45 | 20* | **25*** |
| Fecal boluses | 50 | 25* | **25*** | 65 | 25* | **45** |
| Urinations | 35 | 25 | **25** | 60 | 25* | **25*** |

*Note: animals were intragastrically administered distilled water (2.5 ml/kg, control), TP Abs to S100 (2.5 ml/kg), or diazepam (1 mg/kg) at a single dose 30 minutes prior to testing. n/a, not applicable; TP Abs to S100, technologically processed highly diluted antibodies to S100 protein.*
*$p < 0.05$ *versus corresponding control.*
*Bold entries were made to emphasize the results in TP Abs to S100 group.*

**Table 1.**
*TP Abs to S100 antistress activity in a model of a conditioned emotional reflex to unescapable electric pain.*

### 2.1.1.1.2 Effect on c-Fos protein expression

It is known that immediate-early response *c-fos* gene expression in the hypothalamic paraventricular nucleus is one of the primary biological markers of stress [62]. The effectiveness of stress-protective compounds can be assessed by their ability to suppress *c-fos* expression in the brain.

The study was conducted on male Wistar rats weighing 250–280 g [63], classified as active or passive (stress-resistant or predisposed to stress, respectively) in the open field (OF) test [64]. The OF test is widely used to study the behavior of rats [65]: animals are placed in the center of the OF arena and the horizontal and vertical activity, the number of entries into the center zone, as well as the number of acts of defecation and urination (emotionality) is recorded.

Rats were administered TP Abs to S100 or imipramine (antidepressant drug that modulates *c-fos* expression) and then subjected to 1-hour immobilization with simultaneous electrocutaneous irritation. Immunohistochemical detection of c-Fos protein in the parvocellular neurons of the paraventricular nucleus of the hypothalamus was performed in samples obtained 90 min after the procedure, at the peak of the protein expression [62].

In response to stress, c-Fos protein level significantly increased (vs. intact animals) in both active and passive animals (20–25 fold), and in the latter, this increase was more pronounced (**Figure 1**). TP Abs to S100 and imipramine demonstrated equally and pronounced antistress activity in passive animals: 1.2- and 1.5-fold decrease in the number of Fos-positive cells was observed, respectively.

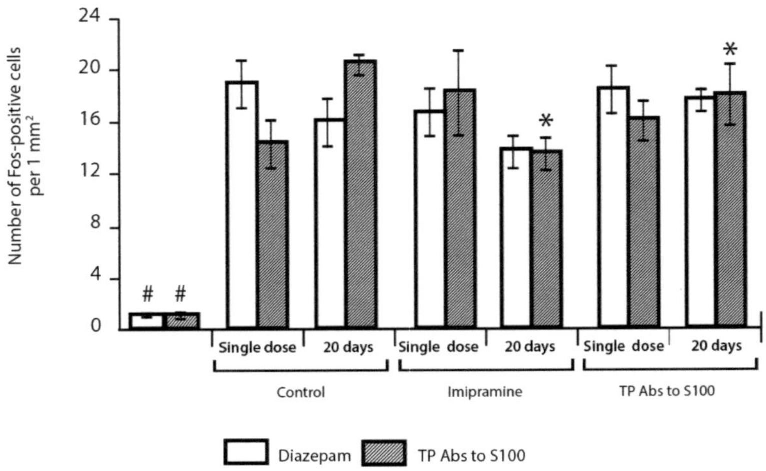


**Figure 1.**
*TP Abs to S100 effect on c-Fos protein expression (stress marker) in the rat hypothalamic paraventricular nucleus after 1-hour immobilization with simultaneous electrocutaneous irritation. Note: animals were intragastrically administered distilled water (2.5 ml/kg, control), TP Abs to S100 (2.5 ml/kg) or imipramine (12 mg/kg) at a single dose or for 20 days preceding stress exposure. Data are expressed as M ± SD.* $^{*}p < 0.05$ ($^{\#}p < 0.001$) *versus corresponding control. TP Abs to S100, technologically processed highly diluted antibodies to S100 protein.*

### *2.1.1.1.3 Effect on gastric ulcers after an immobilization stress*

Another important biological marker of stress is development of ulcers in the gastric mucosa. For example, it is known that immobilization stress is accompanied by severe gastric ulceration [66].

The study of antistress activity of TP Abs to S100 was carried out on male Wistar rats weighing 250–280 g, classified as active or passive in the OF test [67]. Animals were administered TP Abs to S100 at a dose of 2.5 ml/kg for 5 consecutive days or placebo. On the 6th day, half of the rats from each group were immobilized by fixing their paws on a special platform for 1 h, and then the number of animals with ulcers and total number of ulcers formed in the stomach was counted.

TP Abs to S100 decreased by 33.4% the number of animals with ulcers in the group of passive (but not active) rats, which complements the previously obtained results on the higher efficacy of the drug in passive, highly sensitive to stress animals.

TP Abs to S100 also reduced the total number of ulcers in both groups by more than 50%. Again, in control passive animals, there were 1.3 times more ulcers than in control active ones. However, after TP Abs to S100 administration, there was no such difference.

### *2.1.1.2 Anxiolytic activity of TP Abs to S100*

The studies were carried out on outbred white male rats weighing 230–250 g [31] using the most widely validated tests (the Vogel conflict test, the elevated plus maze test, and the OF test) [65]. The activity of TP Abs to S100 was compared to diazepam.

The conflict situation in the *Vogel test* was created by exposing animals to opposing behavioral tendencies: motivation to drink and fear, when every attempt to drink was punished by an electric shock. This lead to a significant reduction in water consumption. Drugs with anxiolytic properties alter behavior and cause an increase in drinking.

To study the activity of TP Abs to S100, depending on the individual reaction to stress, animals were grouped into highly (stress-resistant) and low active (predisposed to stress) in the forced swim test with water wheel (Nomura test), in which stress is modeled, and asthenia and depressive behavior are evaluated. Then, animals were treated with TP Abs to S100 or diazepam, and the Vogel conflict test was performed.

Anxiolytic effect of TP Abs to S100 was not inferior to that of diazepam: the number of punished water intakes in highly active groups increased by 27.4 and 28.7%, respectively (**Figure 2**). Meanwhile, in low-activity animals characterized by a predisposition to asthenia and depressive behavior [64], TP Abs to S100 efficacy was superior to diazepam (2.8 and 2 times vs. control, respectively). The data obtained indicate that in addition to the anxiolytic activity TP Abs to S100 have an antiasthenia activating effect, which distinguishes them from diazepam that induces both anxiolytic and sedative effects.

The *elevated plus maze test* is based on the fear of heights and open spaces: animals are placed on the central platform of the maze and the latent period before the first entry into the open arms, the number of full and incomplete entries and the duration of stay in them, as well as the number of head dips below the level of the open arms is recorded.

It was established that TP Abs to S100 and diazepam had a similar anxiolytic effect in this test: both drugs increased the number of entries into the open arms (1.9 and 2.3 times, respectively), the time spent in the open arms (5.4 and 7 times), as well as the number of head dips (5 and 9 times) versus control animals (**Table 2**).

In the *OF test*, the antianxiety activity of TP Abs to S100 and diazepam was demonstrated by the fact that rats began to go to the center of the field, which was not observed in the control group (**Table 3**). However, unlike diazepam, which reduced the horizontal activity of animals by 1.5 times, TP Abs to S100 did not change this parameter and, therefore, did not have a sedative effect.

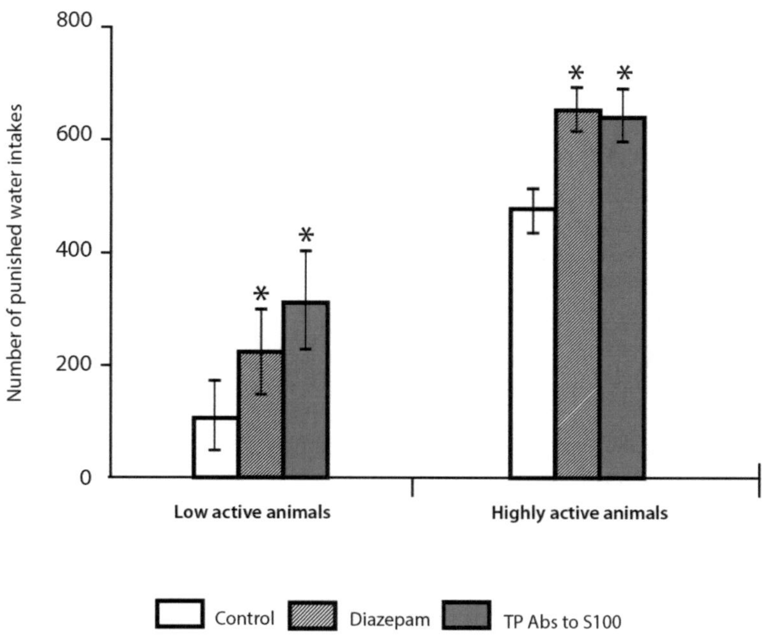


**Figure 2.**
*TP Abs to S100 demonstrate anxiolytic activity in the Vogel conflict test. Note: animals were intragastrically administered distilled water (2.5 ml/kg, control), TP Abs to S100 (2.5 ml/kg) or diazepam (2 mg/kg) at a single dose 30 minutes prior to testing. Data are expressed as M ± SD.* *$p < 0.05$ *versus corresponding control. TP Abs to S100, technologically processed highly diluted antibodies to S100 protein.*

| Parameter group | Number of entries into open arms | Number of entries into enclosed arms | Time spent in open arms, sec | Number of head dips |
|---|---|---|---|---|
| Control | 1.1 ± 0.55 | 2.8 ± 0.65 | 12.1 ± 8.15 | 0.5 ± 0.43 |
| Diazepam | 2.6 ± 0.80* | 1.5 ± 0.8 | 85.3 ± 38.5* | 4.5 ± 1.12* |
| **TP Abs to S100** | **2.1 ± 0.42*** | **2.3 ± 0.48** | **65.4±27.5*** | **2.4 ± 0.95*** |

*Note: animals were intragastrically administered distilled water (2.5 ml/kg, control), TP Abs to S100 (2.5 ml/kg), or diazepam (2 mg/kg) at a single dose 30 minutes prior to testing. Data are expressed as M ± SD. TP Abs to S100, technologically processed highly diluted antibodies to S100 protein.*
*$^{*}p < 0.05$ versus control.*
*Bold entries were made to emphasize the results in TP Abs to S100 group.*

**Table 2.**
*TP Abs to S100 anxiolytic activity in the elevated plus maze test.*

| Parameter group | Number of entries into the arena center | Horizontal activity | Vertical activity | Exploratory activity |
|---|---|---|---|---|
| Control | 0 ± 0 | 18.2 ± 2.4 | 8.2 ± 3.3 | 11.1 ± 3.1 |
| Diazepam | 1.8 ± 0.9* | 12.5 ± 1.8* | 6.2 ± 1.4 | 8.7 ± 1.5 |
| **TP Abs to S100** | **2.4 ± 0.7*** | **15.8 ± 2.1** | **5.8 ± 2.6** | **8.9 ± 1.6** |

*Note: animals were intragastrically administered distilled water (2.5 ml/kg, control), TP Abs to S100 (2.5 ml/kg), or diazepam (2 mg/kg) at a single dose 30 minutes prior to testing. Data are expressed as M ± SD. TP Abs to S100, technologically processed highly diluted antibodies to S100 protein.*
*$^{*}p < 0.05$ versus control.*
*Bold entries were made to emphasize the results in TP Abs to S100 group.*

**Table 3.**
*TP Abs to S100 anxiolytic activity in the open field test.*

#### *2.1.1.3 Antiaggressive activity of TP Abs to S100*

Anxiety disorders are often accompanied by covert or overt aggression. The antiaggressive activity of TP Abs to S100 was studied in the tests of motivated and unmotivated aggression on outbred adult white male rats weighing 200–250 g in comparison with diazepam [68].

In the *test of unmotivated aggression caused by inescapable shock*, the threshold of aggressive response of a pair of animals placed on a grid floor was determined by increasing the stimulating current. Animals manifested shock-elicited aggression when they assumed upright "boxing" posture and tried to bite and strike each other with front and hind paws.

TP Abs to S100 and diazepam after a single dose and course administration exerted antiaggressive activity: single TP Abs to S100 administration increased the threshold of aggressive response by 23.1%, and after a 4-day administration—by 31.3% compared with the control, while diazepam increased this threshold by 26.3 and 34.9%, respectively (**Figure 3**).

The *test of motivated aggression* is based on the study of the intensity of the aggressive reaction elicited in a pair of rats trying to escape electric shock. Rats were individually taught to avoid pain caused by electric irritation of the paws on a safe bench installed in the center of the chamber. Then, they were placed in pairs in the chamber, and their behavior was observed for 2 min. Control animals began to fight for a safety on the bench, which had a capacity to tightly fit both animals. The criterion for the effectiveness of substances with antiaggressive action in this test was the duration of joint avoidance of pain exposure.

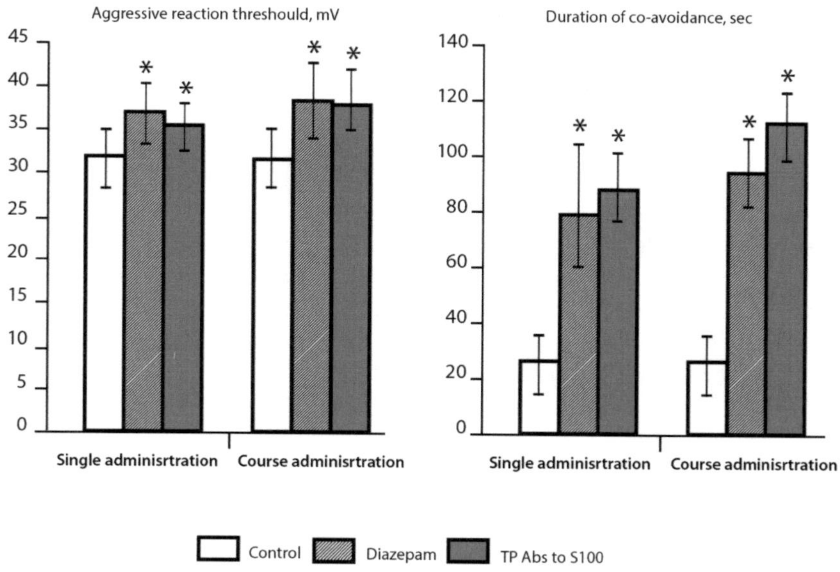


**Figure 3.**
*TP Abs to S100 and diazepam effects on rat's aggressive reaction parameters in the tests of motivated and unmotivated aggression. Note: animals were intragastrically administered distilled water (2.5 ml/kg, control), TP Abs to S100 (2.5 ml/kg) or diazepam (2 mg/kg) at a single dose or for 5 days (2 times per day) prior to testing. Data are expressed as M ± SD. *p < 0.05 versus corresponding control. TP Abs to S100, technologically processed highly diluted antibodies to S100 protein.*

TP Abs to S100 and diazepam had a pronounced antiaggressive effect, increasing the duration of joint avoidance: with a single dose, respectively, 3.4 and 3.1 times, and with a course—3.8 and 3.3 times (**Figure 3**).

#### 2.1.1.4 Other psychotropic and neurotropic activities of TP Abs to S100

Along with the above-described activities (stress-protective and anxiolytic), TP Abs to S100 were shown to exert:

- *antidepressant* effect in Porsolt's and Nomura's forced swimming tests [30, 31, 34];
- *antiamnestic* and *neuroprotective* effects in the models of ischemic and hemorrhagic stroke [35–39], multiple sclerosis [69], Alzheimer's disease [36], attention deficit hyperactivity disorder [37], and *in vitro* glucose and oxygen deprivation [70].

### 2.2 Mechanisms of action of TP Abs to S100

TP Abs to S100 belong to a novel class of drugs that are produced from various antibodies (drug substances) using a single technological platform. This technology allows to obtain active pharmaceutical ingredients that, while retaining antibody specificity (targeting), exert a modulating effect on the target and its biological activity [71–73]. As the endogenous target of TP Abs to S100 is the brain-specific protein S100 that can influence functional activity of GABA-, serotonin-, dopamine-, noradrenaline-, and glutamatergic systems and sigma$_1$ receptors [74–78], these CNS elements had been studied while screening TP Abs to S100 mechanisms of action (**Figure 7**). For this purpose, various *in vivo* and *in vitro* approaches have been used (including the *in vitro* assessment of receptor's functional activity providing the validated protocols existed).

### *2.2.1 GABA-ergic system involvement in TP Abs to S100 mechanisms of action*

#### *2.2.1.1 GABA-A-ergic system*

To assess the role of this system in the implementation of TP Abs to S100 anxiolytic effect, GABA-A receptors were selectively blocked, and the behavior of animals was evaluated in the Vogel conflict test [29].

The study was performed on outbred white male rats weighing 230–250 g. Before testing, animals were administered TP Abs to S100 or diazepam. For blockade of the GABA-A receptors and the chloride channel of the GABA-benzodiazepine receptor complex, bicuculline and picrotoxin, respectively, were administered simultaneously with the tested drugs.

With blockade of the GABA-A receptor, a 1.8-fold decrease in the anticonflict effect of TP Abs to S100 was observed, and a 2-fold decrease with diazepam; with blockade of the chlorine channel—1.6 and 2.4-fold decrease, respectively (**Figure 4**). The data obtained indicate the involvement of the abovementioned subunits of the GABA-benzodiazepine-chloride ionophore receptor complex in the implementation of the anxiolytic effect of TP Abs to S100.

#### *2.2.1.2 GABA-B-ergic system*

In this experiment, GABA-B receptors were selectively stimulated or blocked and anxiolytic or antidepressant effects of TP Abs to S100, diazepam and amitriptyline were evaluated in the Vogel conflict test and the Nomura test [40].

Outbred white male rats weighing 200–250 g were pretreated with baclofen, a selective agonist of GABA-B receptors, or phaclofen, an antagonist of GABA-B receptors. Then, the animals were administered test drugs, and their effect was evaluated.

In the Vogel conflict test, baclofen reduced the anxiolytic effect of TP Abs to S100 by 2.2-fold and did not affect the effect of diazepam. Phaclofen increased the anxiolytic effect of TP Abs to S100 by 1.4-fold (**Figure 5**). Moreover, as expected, none of the ligands influenced the effect of diazepam.

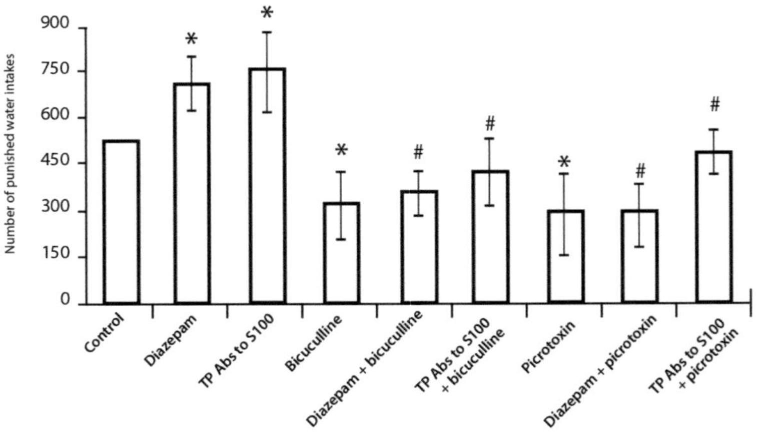


**Figure 4.**
*Influence of GABA-A-ergic agents on anxiolytic activity of TP Abs to S100 and diazepam in the Vogel conflict test. Note: animals were intragastrically administered distilled water (2.5 ml/kg, control), TP Abs to S100 (2.5 ml/kg) or diazepam (2 mg/kg) at a single dose alone or simultaneously with GABA-A receptor antagonist bicuculline (1 mg/kg) or GABA-benzodiazepine receptor complex chloride channel blocker picrotoxin (1 mg/kg) 30 minutes prior to testing. Data are expressed as M ± SD.* * $p < 0.05$ *versus control,* # $p < 0.05$ *versus TP Abs to S100 or diazepam. TP Abs to S100, technologically processed highly diluted antibodies to S100 protein.*

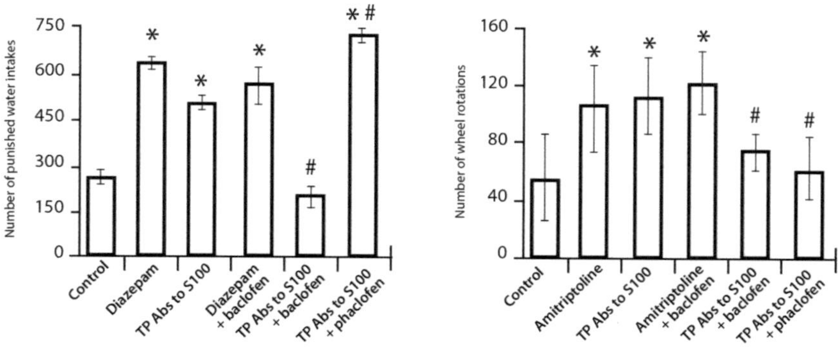


**Figure 5.**
*Influence of GABA-B-ergic agents on anxiolytic and antidepressant activity of TP Abs to S100, diazepam, and amitriptyline in the Vogel conflict test and the Nomura test. Note: animals were intragastrically administered distilled water (2.5 ml/kg, control), TP Abs to S100 (2.5 ml/kg), diazepam (2 mg/kg), or amitriptyline (10 mg/kg) at a single dose. GABA-B receptors agonist baclofen (1 mg/kg) or antagonist phaclofen (10 mg/kg) were intraperitoneally administered 40 min prior to testing and 10 min prior to the administration of the drugs. Data are expressed as M ± SD. * $p < 0.05$ versus control, # $p < 0.05$ versus TP Abs to S100. TP Abs to S100, technologically processed highly diluted antibodies to S100 protein.*

In the forced swim test, baclofen and phaclofen reduced the antidepressant effect of TP Abs to S100 by 1.5 and 2-fold, respectively, whereas these ligands did not affect the effectiveness of amitriptyline.

Thus, it was shown that the GABA-B-ergic system is involved in the realization of both the anxiolytic and antidepressant effects of TP Abs to S100.

In an *in vitro* study, the ability of TP Abs to S100 to influence binding of the standard radioligands to the corresponding GABA receptors and to change the effect of the standard GABA-$B_{1A/B2}$ receptor agonist (using functional analysis—measuring [$^{35}$S]GTPγS incorporation into G-proteins) was investigated [41]. The study was performed on the cell membranes of Chinese hamster cells (CHO) and human embryonic kidney cells (HEK293) that expressed human recombinant GABA-$B_{1A/B2}$ receptors.

In the presence of TP Abs to S100, a 25.8% decrease in standard ligand binding to GABA-$B_{1A/B2}$ receptor was observed, as well as 30.2% inhibition of the GABA-$B_{1A/B2}$ receptor's agonist-induced response was observed.

### *2.2.2 Serotoninergic system involvement in TP Abs to S100 mechanisms of action*

Similarly, this hypothesis was studied in experiments *in vivo* and *in vitro*.

For the *in vivo* experiments, ketanserin, a blocker of 5-$HT_2$/5-$HT_{1C}$ receptors involved in the development of both anxiety and depression, and the 5HT precursor, 5-hydroxytryptophan (5HTP), were used [79].

The anxiolytic effect of TP Abs to S100 was studied using the Vogel conflict test [30]. The antidepressant effect of the drugs was determined using the Nomura test [30]. Outbred white male rats weighing 200–250 g were pretreated with ketanserin or 5HTP, and before testing, they received a single dose of TP Abs to S100 or diazepam.

Ketanserin and 5HTP reduced both anxiolytic (2 and 1.3-fold, respectively) and antidepressant effects of TP Abs to S100 (2- and 1.6-fold, respectively) (**Figure 6**).

Thus, it was demonstrated that the 5HT system is involved in the realization of both the anxiolytic and antidepressant effects of TP Abs to S100.

In an *in vitro* study, the ability of TP Abs to S100 to influence binding of standard radiolabeled ligands to the corresponding 5HT receptors and the ability to change the magnitude of the effect on binding of standard ligands to their receptors

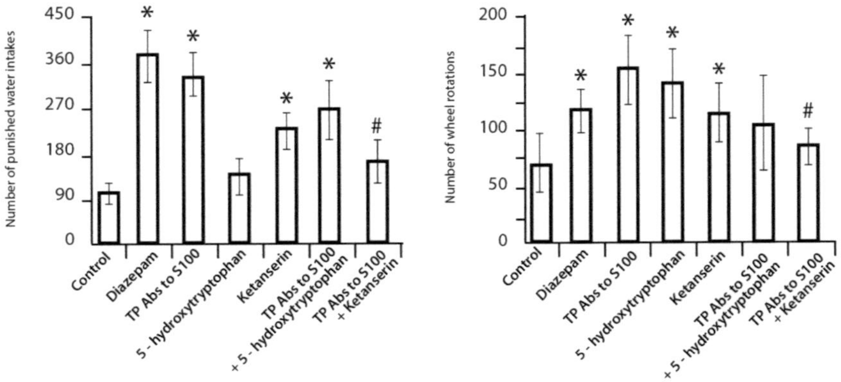


**Figure 6.**
*Influence of serotoninergic agents on anxiolytic and antidepressant activity of TP Abs to S100, diazepam, and amitriptyline in the Vogel conflict test and the Nomura test. Note: animals were intragastrically administered distilled water (2.5 ml/kg, control), TP Abs to S100 (2.5 ml/kg), diazepam (2 mg/kg), or amitriptyline (15 mg/kg) at a single dose. 5-HT2 receptors antagonist ketanserin (1 mg/kg) or the serotonin precursor 5-hydroxytryptophan (5-HTP, 50 mg/kg) were intraperitoneally administered 40 min prior to testing and 10 min prior to administration of the drugs. Data are expressed as M ± SD.* * $p < 0.05$ *versus control,* # $p < 0.05$ *versus TP Abs to S100. TP Abs to S100, technologically processed highly diluted antibodies to S100 protein.*

were tested. The latter was investigated using a functional analysis of the binding of $[^{35}S]GTP\gamma S$, calcium mobilization assay, and dielectric spectroscopy or by measuring the intracellular concentration of cAMP using HTRF (Homogenous Time Resolved Fluorescence) technology. The experiments were performed on CHO cells stably expressing human $5HT_{1A}$, $5HT_{1B}$, $5HT_{1D}$, $5HT_{1E}$, $5HT_{1F}$, $5HT_{2A}$, $5HT_{2B}$, $5HT_{2Cedited}$, $5HT_3$, $5HT_4$, $5HT_6$, or $5HT_7$ receptors [41].

TP Abs to S100 increased binding of the corresponding standard ligands to $5HT_{1A}$ (19.0%), $5HT_{1F}$ (42.0%), $5HT_{2B}$ (31.9%), $5HT_{2Cedited}$ (49.3%), and $5HT_3$ (20.7%) receptors. Moreover, the drug enhanced the effect of $5HT_{1A}$ receptor agonist by 27.8% and reduced the effect of $5HT_{1B}$ receptor agonist by 27.5%.

### *2.2.3 Dopaminergic system involvement in TP Abs to S100 mechanisms of action*

The *in vitro* experiment was carried out similar to the study of the effect of TP Abs to S100 on dopamine receptors [41].

The study was performed on CHO, HEK293, and pituitary rat tumor cells (GH4) stably expressing human $D_1$, $D_{2L}$, $D_{2S}$, $D_3$, $D_{4.4}$ or $D_5$ receptors.

TP Abs to S100 increased binding of the standard ligand to the human $D_3$ receptor by 26.3% and reduced the effect of an agonist of this type of receptor by 32.8%.

### *2.2.4 Glutamatergic system involvement in TP Abs to S100 mechanisms of action*

In this study that was performed *in vitro* using rat cerebral cortex cells, TP Abs to S100 significantly reduced binding of the standard radiolabeled ligand to the glycine site of NMDA receptors [80].

### *2.2.5 Sigma$_1$ receptors involvement in TP Abs to S100 mechanisms of action*

The study was carried out *in vitro* using MCF-7 or Jurkat cells [41].

TP Abs to S100 significantly (by 24.7–56.7%) reduced binding of the standard radiolabeled ligand to human sigma$_1$ receptors (**Figure 7**).

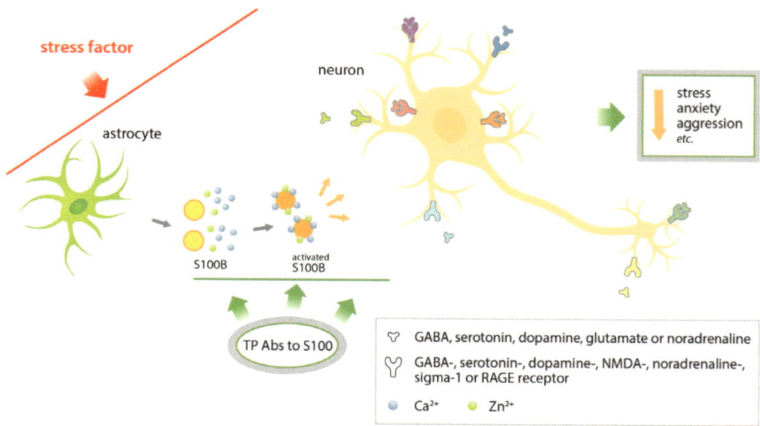


**Figure 7.**
*Schematic representation of TP Abs to S100 mechanisms of action. Note: TP Abs to S100 (technologically processed highly diluted antibodies to S100 protein) molecular target—brain-specific S100 protein. This protein is secreted mainly by astrocytes in the CNS and considered to be an important regulator of many intracellular and extracellular processes (e.g., protein phosphorylation, activity of various enzymes, the dynamics of cytoskeleton components, binding of transcription factors, calcium homeostasis, cell proliferation and differentiation, generation and transmission of nerve impulses, and synaptic transmission [81]). Moreover, S100 proteins interact with almost every neurotransmitter system (serotonin-, dopamine-, GABA-, glutamatergic, etc.) and sigma$_1$ receptors [74–78].* TP Abs to S100 *possess their pharmacological effects via modulating activity of brain-specific S100 protein and influencing functions of the major neurotransmitter systems as well as sigma$_1$ receptors.* In vivo *studies [29, 40] revealed 5-HT$_{2a}$, GABA$_A$, and GABA$_B$ receptor involvement in the drug psychotropic effects. Also, the drug was shown to normalize noradrenaline level [82].* In vitro *studies [41, 42] have shown that* TP Abs to S100 *increase standard radioligand binding to 5-HT$_{1F}$, 5-HT$_{2B}$, 5-HT$_{2Cedited}$, 5-HT$_3$, NMDA, and D$_3$ receptors. In addition, the drug inhibits binding of specific radioligands to GABAB$_{1A/B2}$ and sigma$_1$ receptors and exerts antagonism at GABAB$_{1A/B2}$, 5-HT$_{1B}$, and D$_3$ receptors and agonism at 5-HT$_{1A}$ receptor. The above listed* TP Abs to S100 *activities at the molecular level are involved in maintaining both emotional and physiological homeostasis, and thereby, the drug exerts its stress-protective, anxiolytic, antiamnestic, antidepressant, neuroprotective, and other activities.*

## 2.3 Safety investigation

### *2.3.1 Assessment of a possible sedative effect*

The study was performed on outbred white male rats weighing 230–250 g. Prior to testing (in OF test), animals were administered TP Abs to S100 or diazepam. The sedative effect was evaluated by a decrease in the horizontal activity of rats [7].

TP Abs to S100 did not decrease the motor activity of animals, while diazepam decreased this parameter by 1.5 times.

### *2.3.2 Assessment of a possible muscle relaxant effect*

This activity was investigated in the rotarod test on outbred white male rats weighing 230–250 g [33]. Before testing, animals were administered TP Abs to S100 or diazepam. Then, the time before falling off the rotating rod and the number of rats that fell off were recorded.

TP Abs to S100 did not affect the coordination of movements and did not have a muscle relaxant effect. In contrast, only 30% of rats from diazepam group were able to keep balance.

### *2.3.3 Toxicological studies of TP Abs to S100*

The drug safety investigation was performed in accordance with principles of Good Laboratory Practice. It included studies of the single and repeat dose toxicities, genotoxicity, reproductive and developmental toxicity, immunotoxicity, and local tolerance.

TP Abs to S100 exerted no toxic effects even at a dose significantly exceeding the human recommended daily dose. The drug was shown to be well tolerated and thereby considered to be a low-hazard substance.

## 3. Clinical efficacy and safety of TP Abs to S100 protein in the treatment of NDs

### 3.1 Treatment of AD, AjD, SD, and neurasthenia

To date, 453 patients with AD, AjD, and neurasthenia took part in double-blind randomized controlled CTs ($n$ = 2), and open-label comparative randomized CTs (n = 4) conducted in the Russian Federation and Kazakhstan according to International Conference on Harmonisation Good Clinical Practice and Declaration of Helsinki [55, 57–60, 83]. Two studies were registered and approved by the regulatory agency (Ministry of Health of the Russian Federation) [55, 57].

#### *3.1.1 Placebo-controlled studies*

##### *3.1.1.1 CT in patients with AD and neurological diseases*

A double-blind placebo-controlled CT of TP Abs to S100 in the treatment of AD in patients with neurological diseases [Parkinson's disease (PD) (G.20) and chronic cerebrovascular diseases (CCD)—cerebral atherosclerosis (I67.2), hypertensive encephalopathy (I67.4), unspecified sequelae of cerebral infarction (I69.3)] was conducted in 2010 ([55], unpublished data). Sixty-two patients of both sexes aged 18–75 years were enrolled and randomized in two groups to receive TP Abs to S100 ($n$ = 32) 10 tablets/day or placebo 10 tablets/day. Data from all 62 patients were included in the analysis, so that intention-to-treat and per-protocol sets were equal. The use of any antidepressants, antipsychotics, or antianxiety medications was prohibited in CT. The therapy of concurrent somatic and neurological diseases was permitted.

The study duration was 4 weeks with a 4-week follow-up period. Inclusion criteria were: manifested AD, the Hospital Anxiety and Depression Scale-Anxiety (HADS-A) score $\geq 11$, signed informed consent form (ICF). The percentage of patients with a $\geq$50% decrease in the severity of anxiety according to the Hamilton Anxiety Rating Scale (HAM-A) after 4 weeks of treatment and 4-week follow-up was set as a primary efficacy endpoint. Other efficacy endpoints were: mean decrease in HAM-A, HADS-A, and State-Trait Anxiety Inventory (STAI) scores after 4 weeks of treatment and 4-week follow-up. Safety was assessed based on the results of laboratory tests (blood and urine analysis) and adverse events reports. Mann-Whitney U test, Wilcoxon signed-rank test, Student $t$-test, and Fisher's exact test were used for analysis.

The mean age of patients enrolled was $59.5 \pm 2.0$ years in the TP Abs to S100 group and $60.0 \pm 1.9$ years in the placebo group. The mean duration of neurological disease was $6.13 \pm 1.2$ years in the TP Abs to S100 group and $6.55 \pm 0.89$ years in the placebo group. No differences in demographic and clinical characteristics of patients were found (**Table 4**).

The percentage of patients with a $\geq$50% decrease in HAM-A total score was 41.3% in the TP Abs to S100 group and 6.7% in the placebo group ($p < 0.05$ compared to placebo) after 4 weeks of therapy (**Table 4**). After 4 weeks of therapy, the total HAM-A score significantly decreased in the TP Abs to S100 group [a 1.8-fold decrease ($-45.63 \pm 2.61\%$) from baseline in the TP Abs to S100 group

| | TP Abs to S100 | | | Placebo | | |
|---|---|---|---|---|---|---|
| | **Total ($n$ = 32)** | **Patients with PD ($n$ = 16)** | **Patients with CCD ($n$ = 16)** | **Total ($n$ = 30)** | **Patients with PD ($n$ = 15)** | **Patients with CCD ($n$ = 15)** |
| *Demographic and clinical characteristics* | | | | | | |
| Age, years | 59.5 ± 2.0 | 61.4 ± 3.0 | 57.9 ± 2.5 | 60.0 ± 1.9 | 61.1 ± 2.9 | 58.9 ± 2.6 |
| Duration of neurological disease, years | 6.13 ± 1.22 | 6.13 ± 1.15 | 5.94 ± 2.03 | 6.55 ± 0.89 | 8.0 ± 1.48 | 5.29 ± 2.56 |
| *Baseline data* | | | | | | |
| HADS-A, score | 14.75 ± 0.46 | 15 ± 0.68 | 14.24 ± 0.63 | 15.7 ± 0.41 | 16.93 ± 0.34 | 14.47 ± 0.59 |
| STAI, trait anxiety, score | 62.28 ± 0.97 | 62.69 ± 1.76 | 60.82 ± 0.88 | 59.5 ± 1.25 | 61.53 ± 1.82 | 57.47 ± 1.61 |
| STAI, state anxiety, score | 60.09 ± 1.05 | 59.31 ± 1.71 | 59.82 ± 1.24 | 60.8 ± 1.07 | 63 ± 1.06 | 58.6 ± 1.7 |
| HAM-A, score | 27.28 ± 0.66 | 26.38 ± 0.82 | 28.19 ± 1.01 | 26.37 ± 0.6 | 27.13 ± 0.65 | 25.6 ± 0.9 |
| *After 4 weeks of treatment* | | | | | | |
| HADS-A, score | 7.74 ± 0.53 | 8.8 ± 0.97 | 6.75 ± 0.39 | 12.93 ± 0.8 | 16.0 ± 0.53 | 9.87 ± 1.0 |
| STAI, trait anxiety, score | 50.58 ± 1.25 | 53.2 ± 2.27 | 48.13 ± 0.82 | 55.93 ± 1.55 | 61.07 ± 1.55 | 50.8 ± 1.95 |
| STAI, state anxiety, score | 43.48 ± 1.06 | 46.4 ± 1.57 | 40.75 ± 1.07 | 54.0 ± 1.58 | 58.6 ± 1.59 | 49.4 ± 2.19 |
| HAM-A, score | 14.74 ± 0.74 | 16.4 ± 1.21 | 13.19 ± 0.7 | 22.83 ± 1.05 | 26.07 ± 1.05 | 19.6 ± 1.41 |
| After 4 weeks of follow-up | | | | | | |
| HADS-A, score | 7.61 ± 0.49 | 8.8 ± 0.74 | 6.5 ± 0.52 | 13.1 ± 0.69 | 15.6 ± 0.36 | 10.6 ± 0.97 |
| STAI, trait anxiety, score | 49.45 ± 1.04 | 51.0 ± 1.91 | 48.0 ± 0.84 | 56.47 ± 1.33 | 60.6 ± 1.43 | 52.33 ± 1.69 |
| STAI, state anxiety, score | 43.65 ± 0.85 | 46.67 ± 1.13 | 40.81 ± 0.78 | 56.67 ± 1.27 | 60.47 ± 1.19 | 60.47 ± 1.19 52.87 ± 1.8 |
| HAM-A, score | 14.13 ± 0.68 | 15 ± 1.01 | 13.31 ± 0.9 | 24.03 ± 0.89 | 26.78 ± 0.64 | 21.2 ± 1.31 |

*Note: Data are expressed as M ± SD. HAM-A, Hamilton Anxiety Rating scale; HADS-A, Hospital Anxiety and Depression Scale-Anxiety; STAI, State-Trait Anxiety Inventory; CCD, chronic cerebrovascular disease; PD, Parkinson's disease; TP Abs to S100, technologically processed highly diluted antibodies to S100 protein.*

**Table 4.**
*Demographic and clinical characteristics, baseline, and post-treatment data on patients in double-blind placebo controlled CT of TP Abs to S100.*

versus a 1.1-fold (or −13.09 ± 3.3%) decrease in the placebo group; Student's $t$-test $p < 0.05$]. The result of therapy persisted during the follow-up period in the TP Abs to S100 group. The anxiety level additionally decreased by 3% (−48.19 ± 2.1% from baseline in total) by the end of the follow-up period ($p < 0.05$ compared to placebo). The percentage of patients with a ≥50% decrease in HAM-A total score additionally increased by 3.3% after 4 weeks of follow-up ($p < 0.05$ compared to placebo) (**Figure 8**).

A significant decrease in the severity of anxiety was shown in patients receiving TP Abs to S100 according to HADS-A after 4 weeks of therapy and 4 weeks of follow-up ($p < 0.05$ compared to the placebo group). There was a 1.4-fold decrease

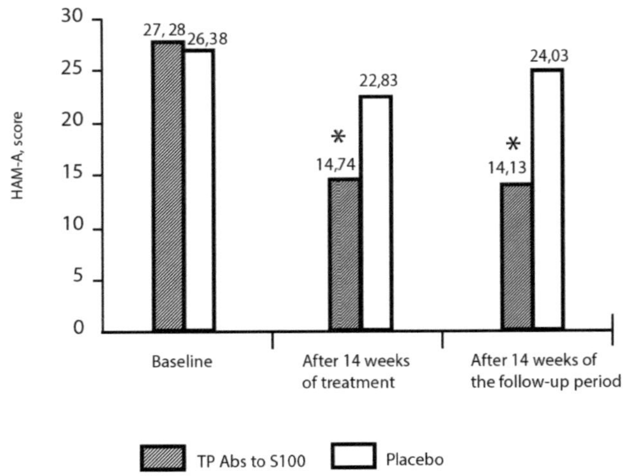


**Figure 8.**
*Dynamics of the severity of anxiety in TP Abs to S100 and placebo groups. *p < 0.05 versus placebo (Student's t-test). HAM-A, Hamilton Anxiety Rating scale; TP Abs to S100, technologically processed highly diluted antibodies to S100 protein.*

($60.09 \pm 1.05$ vs. $43.65 \pm 0.85$) in state anxiety according to STAI in the TP Abs to S100 group after 4 weeks of therapy and result of therapy persisted during the follow-up period. The efficacy rate in reduction of the anxiety was higher in CCD patients than in PD patients according to STAI.

Data from 62 patients were included in the safety analysis. There were two AEs (pyrosis and burping) in one patient received TP Abs to S100 and one AE (pyrosis) in one patient in the placebo group. There was no significant difference in the frequency of AEs between groups. Neither TP Abs to S100 nor placebo influenced results of blood or urine tests in patients. All AEs were of medium severity and had no definite relationship with the study drug. No serious AEs were registered.

TP Abs to S100 were shown to be an effective drug for the treatment of AD in adult patients with concurrent neurological diseases.

### 3.1.1.2 Clinical trials in patients with SD

An international multicenter double-blind randomized placebo-controlled study in 390 patients of both sexes aged 18–45 years with SD (mostly), AjD, or neurasthenia and ≥11 HADS-A points was conducted in 2017–2019 in the Russian Federation and Kazakhstan [57]. There were four treatment groups receiving TP Abs to S100 or placebo in two dosage regimens: 4 or 8 tablets/day. Preliminary (yet unpublished) data on primary efficacy endpoint showed the decrease in the mean HAM-A score by 11.25 points in TP Abs to S100 group (4 tablets/day) and by 11.91 points in TP Abs to S100 8 tablets/day groups observed after 12 weeks of treatment (vs. 9.71 points in merged placebo group; ANCOVA: $p_{TP}$ Abs to S100 4 tablets per day/placebo = 0.0055, $p_{TP}$ Abs to S100 8 tablets per day /placebo $< 0.0001$). A detailed analysis of the results is currently being prepared for a publication. Complete information on the study design is available at clinicaltrials.gov NCT 03036293 [57].

### 3.1.2 Comparison of the TP Abs to S100 efficacy and safety with benzodiazepines

To evaluate the advantages and limitations of novel medication, especially in the treatment of mental disorders, it is necessary to compare its efficacy and safety not only with placebo but also with the "golden standard" treatment [84].

Benzodiazepines are usually chosen as such a standard in CTs in patients with NDs and, in particular, ADs. Therefore, four CTs with the use of bromdihydrochlorphenylbenzodiazepine, diazepam, clonazepam, and tofisopam as the control therapy were conducted [58–60].

#### *3.1.2.1 Open-label comparative randomized CT of TP Abs to S100 and bromdihydrochlorphenylbenzodiazepine*

Outpatients aged 18–65 years ($n$ = 59) with a diagnosis of GAD (F41.1), AjD (F43.2), or neurasthenia (F48.0) who signed ICF participated in this open-label randomized CT [58]. One group of patients ($n$ = 32) received TP Abs to S100 4 tablets/day, and the other ($n$ = 27) was administered bromdihydrochlorphenylbenzodiazepine 1.5 mg/day for 28 days. Exclusion criteria were other mental diseases, severe somatic diseases, pregnancy, or lactation period. Any medications that could influence the emotional state of participants were prohibited for use for 1 week prior to the initiation of CT and during the study.

Efficacy was evaluated based on the results of the HAM-A test and Clinical Global Impression-Improvement scale (CGI-I) after 7, 14, and 28 days of treatment. The frequency of AEs and any deviations from the reference ranges in blood and urine tests was used for safety assessment. The Kruskal-Wallis test, ANOVA, and Mann-Whitney U-test were used for statistical analysis.

The mean age of patients was 34.8 ± 3.6 years in TP Abs to S100 and 36.3 ± 4.6 years in bromdihydrochlorphenylbenzodiazepine group. The mean duration of disease was 0.8 ± 0.6 years and 0.9 ± 0.5 years in TP Abs to S100 and bromdihydrochlorphenylbenzodiazepine groups, respectively (**Table 5**). No significant differences between groups in any demographic and clinical characteristics were found.

After 7 days of treatment, the severity of anxiety was reduced by 41% (from 18.2 ± 3.91 to 10.73 ± 5.02) in the TP Abs to S100 group and by 56.2% (from 21.24 ± 3.25 to 9.29 ± 4.24) in the comparison group according to HAM-A scale. No significant differences between groups were found after the first week of treatment ($p$ = 0.41), and TP Abs to S100 were shown to be as effective as bromdihydrochlorphenylbenzodiazepine in the short-term period. After 14 and 28 days the anxiolytic effect in the group, receiving benzodiazepine drug was superior to that in the TP Abs to S100 group ($p < 0.05$ between groups). In accordance with CGI-I results, the level of improvement was found to be similar in both groups ($p$ = 0.004) on the 7th and 14th days, but later, bromdihydrochlorphenylbenzodiazepine led to a significant decrease in the severity of illness after 28 days of treatment ($p > 0.05$ between groups).

The frequency of AEs was higher in the benzodiazepine group. There were several cases of severe daytime sleepiness, disturbance of accommodation, and muscle weakness in patients that received bromdihydrochlorphenylbenzodiazepine. Some patients in the study group reported mild sleepiness. No severe AEs were registered in the TP Abs to S100 group. Neither TP Abs to S100 nor benzodiazepine administration affected results of blood or urine tests in patients.

Thus, TP Abs to S100 were as effective as the control medication only in the short-term period according to HAM-A but caused no severe AEs in patients with GAD, AjD, and neurasthenia comparing to benzodiazepine.

#### *3.1.2.2 Open-label comparative randomized CT of TP Abs to S100 and diazepam*

Diazepam is the most frequent standard drug used in CTs of anxiolytic agents [85]. This open-label randomized CT was conducted under the regulation of the

| | TP Abs to S100 | Bromdihydrochlorphenylbenzodiazepine | $p$ |
|---|---|---|---|
| *Demographic and clinical characteristics* | | | |
| Age, years | 34.8 ± 3.6 | 36.3 ± 4.6 | >0.05 |
| Disease duration, years | 0.8 ± 0.6 | 0.9 ± 0.5 | >0.05 |
| *Baseline data* | | | |
| HAM-A, score | 18.2 ± 3.91 | 21.24 ± 3.25 | 0.41 |
| *After 7 days of treatment* | | | |
| HAM-A, score | 10.73 ± 5.02 | 9.29 ± 4.24 | 0.46 |
| CGI-I, score | 3.41 ± 1.1 | 3.05 ± 0.97 | 0.28 |
| *After 14 days of treatment* | | | |
| HAM-A, score | 11.14 ± 5.49 | 6.62 ± 2.80 | 0.003 |
| CGI-I, score | 3.14 ± 1.13 | 2.33 ± 1.39 | 0.004 |
| *After 28 days of treatment* | | | |
| HAM-A, score | 9.59 ± 6.08 | 5.62 ± 2.18 | 0.000023 |
| CGI-I, score | 2.86 ± 1.58 | 2.33 ± 1.06 | 0.21 |

*Note: Data are expressed as M ± SD. HAM-A, Hamilton Anxiety Rating scale; CGI-I, Clinical Global Impression-Improvement scale; TP Abs to S100, technologically processed highly diluted antibodies to S100 protein.*

**Table 5.**
*Demographic and clinical characteristics, baseline, and post-treatment data of patients in comparative CT of TP Abs to S100 and bromdihydrochlorphenylbenzodiazepine.*

Ministry of Health of the Russian Federation [unpublished data]. Outpatients aged 18–65 years with GAD (F41.1), AjD (F43.2), neurasthenia (F48.0) (total $n$ = 272), and mixed anxiety and depressive disorder (mADD) (F41.2) signed ICF and then were randomized to receive TP Abs to S100 ($n$ = 142) 6 tablets/day or diazepam ($n$ = 130) 15 mg/day for 28 days. All medications influencing the emotional state were prohibited for use 1 week prior to CT initiation and during the study. Diagnosis of any other psychiatric disorder, pregnancy, lactation period, substance abuse, and severe somatic diseases were set as the exclusion criteria. Efficacy was measured using the HAM-A scale and STAI. Safety was assessed based on the AE reports and results of blood and urine tests.

The mean age of patients was 40.4 ± 1.13 in TP Abs to S100 group and 39.6 ± 1.06 in the diazepam group. The mean duration of NDs was 31.9 ± 4.1 and 29.2 ± 3.23 months in the TP Abs to S100 and diazepam groups, respectively. In the TP Abs to S100 group, 27.5% of patients had GAD, 31.3%—neurasthenia, 24.4%—AjD, and 17%—mADD. Among patients administered diazepam 31.6% had GAD, 37%—neurasthenia, 17.5%—AjD, and 14.8%—mADD. Mean HAM-A score was 27.1 ± 0.5 in the TP Abs to S100 group and 28.1 ± 0.46 in the diazepam group ($p$ = 0.3). No differences in baseline characteristics were observed.

The total HAM-A score decreased to 22.0 ± 0.5 in TP Abs to S100 group at the end of the first week of therapy ($p < 0.001$ compared to baseline). There was a 57.2% decrease in total HAM-A score in the TP Abs to S100 group after 28 days of treatment (vs. 63% in the diazepam group, $p$ = 0.02) (**Figure 9**).

The percentage of patients with a ≥50% decrease in HAM-A total score was 72.6% in the TP Abs to S100 group (vs. 65.8% in the diazepam group) after 28 days of treatment. There were 12.8% of patients in TP Abs to S100 group with anxiety remission (less than 7 HAM-A scores) (vs. 22.1% in diazepam group). There were no significant differences between the TP Abs to S100 and diazepam groups on 7th

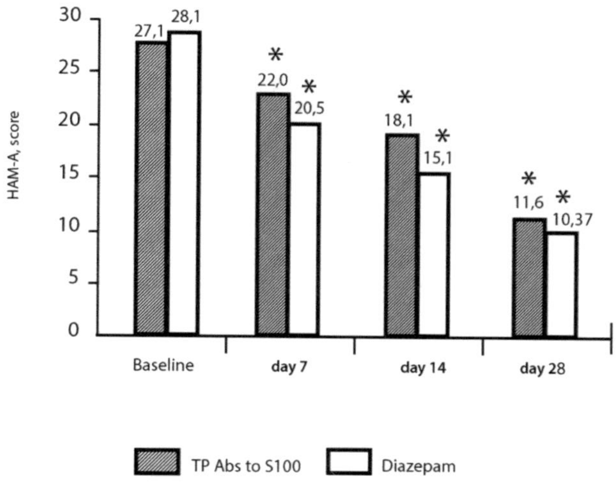


**Figure 9.**
*Dynamics of the severity of anxiety in the TP Abs to S100 and diazepam groups.* * p < 0.05 *versus baseline. HAM-A, Hamilton Anxiety Rating Scale; TP Abs to S100, technologically processed highly diluted antibodies to S100 protein.*

and 28th days of treatment according to the HAM-A section "anxiety mood" ($p$ = 0.2 and $p$ = 0.1 between groups). Treatment with diazepam was more effective only at the 14th day of treatment [48.0 ± 0.62 (diazepam) vs. 50.0 ± 0.52 (TP Abs to S100), $p$ = 0.02 comparing to the TP Abs to S100 group] according to STAI (state anxiety). The influence of TP Abs to S100 and diazepam on state anxiety was equal on the 7th and 28th days of therapy ($p$ = 0.2 between groups). Diazepam and TP As to S100 were of equal efficacy in reducing the trait anxiety after 14 days [49.7 ± 0.60 (TP Abs to S100) vs. 51.0 ± 0.55 (diazepam); $p$ = 0.1 between groups].

Only eight (5.6%) patients in the TP Abs to S100 group reported AEs (sleepiness, dizziness, dry mouth, pyrosis, bloating, excessive sweating, decreased libido, and tachycardia) of mild and moderate severity. In contrast, in the diazepam group, 51 (39.2%) patients had AEs (most frequent—daytime sleepiness, muscle relaxation, orthostatic hypotension) ($p < 0.01$).

To summarize the data, we consider TP Abs to S100 less effective than diazepam, though TP Abs to S100 were well tolerated by patients with GAD, AjD, neurasthenia, or mADD and exerted significantly less AEs in contrast to diazepam.

### *3.1.2.3 Open-label comparative randomized CT of TP Abs to S100 and clonazepam*

In this open-label CT, 60 patients with AjD ($n$ = 35) or SD ($n$ = 25) and cardiovascular diseases (CVDs) (coronary heart disease (CHD), arterial hypertension (AH) grades II–III, postmyocarditis cardiosclerosis, dyshormonal myocardial dystrophy with cardiac arrhythmias, ventricular and supraventricular extrasystoles, atrial fibrillation, and heart defects) were randomly prescribed to receive TP Abs to S100 6 tablets/day ($n$ = 30) or clonazepam 0.5–1 mg/day ($n$ = 20) as an anxiolytic treatment in addition to standard therapy of CVD for 28 days after signing an ICF [59]. The control group ($n$ = 10) was not administered any antianxiety medication. No drugs influencing the mental status of participants were allowed 1 week prior to CT and after the onset of CT. The reduction of HAM-A score was set as an efficacy endpoint. Safety was assessed based on the number of reported AEs, changes in electrocardiogram (in TP Abs to S100 group), and results of blood and urine tests.

At the baseline mean, HAM-A score was 20.75 ± 8.3 in the TP Abs to S100 group, 22.3 ± 8.1 in the clonazepam group, and 14.7 ± 5.6 in control. After 28 days of treatment, the mean HAM-A score was reduced by 30.1% in patients that received TP Abs to S100 (to 14.5 ± 5.6; $p < 0.01$ vs. baseline), by 30.04% in the clonazepam group (to 15.6 ± 6.2; $p < 0.01$ vs. baseline) and 24.5% in the control group (to 11.1 ± 4.1; $p > 0.05$ vs. baseline). Patients in the TP Abs to S100 group reported no AEs and no changes were found on electrocardiogram or blood and urine tests. On the contrary, the extrasystoles in two participants with dyshormonal myocardial dystrophy that received TP Abs to S100 became less frequent (from 3122 to 2040) after 14 days of treatment. Patients in the clonazepam group ($n$ = 5) noted a slowdown in mental and motor reactions, a feeling of tiredness, and daytime sleepiness.

Thus, TP Abs to S100 appeared to be slightly less effective than clonazepam but at the same time exerted less AEs that are important for patients with not only the AjD alone but also for those with CVD.

#### *3.1.2.4 Open-label comparative randomized CT of TP Abs to S100 and tofisopam*

Patients ($n$ = 51) with GAD or mADD and CVD (CHD or AH grades II–III) signed ICF and then were randomized into two groups. The first group ($n$ = 31) received TP Abs to S100 4 tablets/day, the second ($n$ = 20)—tofisopam 100 mg/day for 4 weeks in addition to standard CVD therapy [60]. After 4 weeks of treatment, patients were followed up for the next 4 weeks. Patients that previously received antianxiety or antidepressant medications, diagnosed with other mental diseases, having a history of substance abuse or lactose intolerance were not included in CT. The changes in HAM-A score after 2 and 4 weeks of treatment and after 4-week follow-up were set as efficacy endpoints. Safety was evaluated by analysis of AEs.

The mean age of patients in the TP Abs to S100 group was 49.3 ± 7.0 years, and the mean duration of CVD was 8.2 ± 4.5 years. In the tofisopam group, the mean age was 54 ± 5.2, and the duration of CVD was 7.6 ± 2.9 years. No differences in baseline characteristics were registered. During the treatment, anxiety was reduced by 63% after 1 week, by 73.1% after 2 weeks, and by 78.5% after 4 weeks in the TP Abs to S100 group according to HAM-A. There was a decrease in HAM-A scores by 62.5% after 1 week, by 75% after 2 weeks, and by 78.5% after 4 weeks in the tofisopam group. A positive effect of TP Abs to S100 on anxiety state was maintained for 4 weeks during follow-up, while there was a tendency for an increase in HAM-A score in the tofisopam group. The addition of TP Abs to S100 to standard CVD therapy helped to decrease the mean systolic blood pressure (SBP) by 25% (from 161.5 ± 18.5 mmHg to 122 ± 5.0 mmHg) after 4 weeks of treatment, whereas only 15.9% decrease in mean SBP was shown in the tofisopam group. No serious AEs were registered in both groups. In the TP Abs to S100 and tofisopam groups, 3.2 and 10% of patients, respectively, discontinued the treatment for personal reasons.

Thus, TP Abs to S100 were shown to be as effective as tofisopam. The compliance in the TP Abs to S100 group was slightly higher than that in the tofisopam group. The addition of TP Abs to S100 to standard CVD treatment led to a more prominent decrease in the mean SBP than the addition of tofisopam. TP Abs to S100 achieved more prolonged action on anxiety state than tofisopam.

### 3.2 Treatment of anxiety, accompanying somatic diseases

The use of anxiolytic treatment in the patients with chronic somatic diseases is challenging [86]. Many side effects of benzodiazepines such as drowsiness, sleepiness, cognitive impairment, dizziness, and addiction can be crucial for these patients [87]. Polypharmacy is also an unwanted phenomenon. The negative interaction of antianxiety medications with standard therapy of somatic diseases is frequently observed [88]. For instance, the use of SSRI in combination with nonsteroidal anti-inflammatory drugs increases the risk of gastrointestinal tract bleeding [89]. Some authors described the association between high risk of myocardial infarction and the use of benzodiazepines and antidepressants [90]. So, the search for a possible role of TP Abs to S100 in treatment of patients with the somatic disease is relevant.

#### *3.2.1 Cardiovascular diseases*

Around 40% of patients with CVD experience anxiety that can have a negative impact on the risk of adverse cardiovascular events [91, 92]. Thus, it is important to reduce anxiety symptoms in CVD patients.

Two CTs that compared TP Abs to S100 with clonazepam and tofisopam in patients with CVD were described above [59, 60]. The results showed equal efficacy of TP Abs to S100 and tofisopam in CVD patients.

In another open-label randomized comparative CT by Nikol'skaya et al., TP Abs to S100 were used in combination with the standard treatment of patients with AH grades II–III and anxiety ($n$ = 60, 23 women, 37 men; mean age—61.4 ± 6.9, mean AH duration—10.6 ± 4.1 years) [93]. All patients received diuretics, β blockers, and angiotensin-converting-enzyme inhibitors (ACE inhibitors). Randomly chosen participants ($n$ = 30) were additionally prescribed TP Abs to S100 6 tablets/day for 4 weeks. At the baseline, there were 40% of patients with severe anxiety and 60% with the anxiety of moderate severity in the TP Abs to S100 group according to the Taylor Manifest Anxiety Scale (TMAS) modified by Nemchinov. Sixty percent of patients with severe anxiety and 56.6% with the anxiety of moderate severity made up the control group were receiving no antianxiety therapy.

The 1.3-fold reduction of severity of anxiety (from 23.76 ± 2.81 to 18.83 ± 2.75 TMAS points) after 2 weeks of therapy was shown in the TP Abs to S100 group ($p < 0.0001$ vs. baseline and the control group). There was a 24.28% decrease in SBP from 181.7 ± 10.8 to 140.0 ± 8.3 ($p < 0.0001$ vs. baseline and control) after 4 weeks of therapy in the TP Abs to S100 group. There was a 17.7% decrease in diastolic blood pressure from 102.3 ± 4.3 to 85.0 ± 5.7 in the study drug group after 4 weeks of therapy ($p < 0.0001$ vs. baseline and the control group). No negative interactions with standard therapy were registered for TP Abs to S100.

Matyushin et al. demonstrated the efficacy and safety of TP Abs to S100 in an open-label randomized comparative CT in patients ($n$ = 60) with anxiety measured with HAM-A and CHD, AH grades II–III, angina pectoris I–III functional classes by Canadian Cardiovascular Society Classification, heart rhythm disturbances (extrasystole, paroxysmal supraventricular tachyarrhythmias) receiving standard CVD therapy (β blockers, amiodarone, sotalol, lappaconitine hydrobromide, diethylaminopropionylethoxycarbonylaminophenothiazine, etc.) [94]. The study drug group ($n$ = 30) received TP Abs to S100 6 tablets/day, and the control group ($n$ = 30) was administered only CVD treatment for 8 weeks. The mean age of patients in TP Abs to S100 and control groups was 64.4 ± 8.6 and 63.1 ± 8.5, respectively.

The addition of TP Abs to S100 to the standard therapy in patients with angina pectoris I–III functional classes helped to decrease the severity of anxiety (50.4% decrease vs. 32.3% decrease in the TP Abs to S100 group vs. the control group; $p < 0.05$) and caused cardiac rhythm normalization [80% patients with more than 75% decrease in the frequency of daily episodes of rhythm disturbances in the study group ($p < 0.05$ vs. control)]. There were 60% of patients with a decrease in angina pectoris functional class in the study drug group (vs. 33.3% in control; $p < 0.05$ between groups). No AEs and negative drug interactions were registered.

An open-label placebo-controlled study in 85 patients with acute coronary syndrome and anxiety (diagnosed with HADS-A) showed significant improvement in the quality of life assessed with the Short Form-36 in the TP Abs to S100 group after 6 month of therapy [95]. The 1.7-fold decrease in HADS-A score (from 12.1 [9;17] to 7.1 [6;8]) was observed in patients receiving TP Abs to S100 in combination with standard therapy after 6 months ($p = 0.00008$ vs. baseline). No reduction of anxiety according to HADS-A was found in the placebo group after 6 months ($p = 0.07$ vs. baseline). No negative interaction with standard therapy (acetylsalicylic acid, clopidogrel, enoxaparin, statins, ACE inhibitors, β blockers, nitrates, calcium agonists) was registered.

Thus, TP Abs to S100 is an effective anxiolytic medication that helps to reduce the severity of anxiety as well as to avoid drug interaction, polypharmacy and increase the quality of life. According to some CTs mentioned above, TP Abs to S100 increase the efficacy of standard treatment in patients with AH, angina pectoris, and some heart rhythm disturbances due to their antianxiety action. Due to reduction in severity of anxiety, the improvement of compliance in CVD patients is possible, though this consideration requires further investigation.

#### 3.2.2 Gastrointestinal diseases

Anxiety is common in 20% of patients with gastrointestinal (GI) problems [96] and in 27% of patients with gastritis in particular [97]. Some publications revealed an association between mood disorders and the risk of carcinogenesis in patients with GI diseases [98, 99]. The necessity for antianxiety therapy in these patients is justified.

An open-label comparative study by Tsukanov et al. in patients with anxiety (diagnosed with HAM-A) complicating ulcerative gastritis associated with *Helicobacter pylori* and duodenal ulcers was conducted [100]. One hundred and two participants received standard helicobacter eradication therapy (clarithromycin, amoxicillin, omeprazole, algeldrate—magnesium hydroxide combination drug), and 49 of them were prescribed TP Abs to S100 6 tablets/day for 20 days. Mean age of participants was $41.8 \pm 2.4$ in the TP Abs to S100 group ($n = 49$) and $42.3 \pm 2.8$ in the control group ($n = 53$). The dynamics of HAM-A scale scores was evaluated.

Anxiety was significantly reduced in the TP Abs to S100 group after 20 days of treatment. The mean HAM-A score decreased by 55.2% from $23.43 \pm 1.8$ to $10.5 \pm 0.98$ (vs. 28% in the control group; $p < 0.001$ vs. baseline; $p < 0.001$ vs. control group). No serious AEs were registered in both groups.

According to another open-label noncomparative CT by Karpin et al. in patients with chronic gastritis and duodenal ulcers, the addition of TP Abs to S100 to standard treatment leads to a prominent reduction in GI symptoms (pain, intestinal dyspepsia, appetite changes) ($p = 0.003$ vs. baseline for pain and dyspepsia, $p = 0.045$ for appetite changes) [101].

So, the treatment of patients with GI diseases with TP Abs to S100 helps to reduce anxiety and indirectly decrease the severity of somatic symptoms via its anxiolytic action.

## 4. Conclusions

In this review, the data obtained from experimental and clinical studies of TP Abs to S100 efficacy, safety, and mechanisms of action are summarized.

In nonclinical trials, TP Abs to S100 were shown to exert stress-protective, anxiolytic, antidepressant, antiamnestic, and neuroprotective activities. All these effects were manifested at the same level as the activity of comparator drugs. At the same time, toxicological studies have shown a high safety level of TP Abs to S100: there was no any toxic activity of drug reviled even when it was administered to laboratory animals at the maximal dose for 6 consecutive months (every day).

The mechanisms of action studies confirmed the hypothesis that TP Abs to S100 biological effects are realized via recruiting of GABA-, serotonin-, dopamine-, noradrenaline-, and glutamatergic systems, as well as via $sigma_1$ receptors.

Clinical efficacy and safety of TP Abs to S100 were demonstrated in multicenter double-blind randomized placebo-controlled trials and in open-label randomized comparative trials. In all conducted placebo-comparative studies or studies with nonmedicated control group, the main symptom of most NDs—the anxiety—was significantly reduced in TP Abs to S100 action. It should be stressed that in these CTs, the equal efficacy of TP Abs to S100, tofisopam, and bromdihydrochlorphenylbenzodiazepine (in the short-term use) with a notably higher tolerance level was demonstrated. Meanwhile, TP Abs to S100 increased the efficacy of standard treatment of somatic diseases (due to its anxiolytic activity), and there was a lower number of AEs and lack of drug interactions observed in the TP Abs to S100 group.

Thus, the discussed drug—TP Abs to S100—has been extensively studied and demonstrated favorable efficacy and safety profile. The presented evidence justifies TP Abs to S100 to be a promising treatment option for patients with NDs.

## Acknowledgements

We thank Dr. Kovalchuk A.L. for valuable comments on the paper and language editing.

## Conflict of interest

All authors are the employees of OOO NPF Materia Medica Holding pharmaceutical company. The substance TP ABS to S100 is produced and marketed by OOO NPF Materia Medica Holding.

## Abbreviations

| | |
|---|---|
| ACE | angiotensin-converting-enzyme |
| AD | anxiety disorder |
| AE | adverse event |
| AH | arterial hypertension |
| AjD | adjustment disorder |
| CCD | chronic cerebrovascular disease |
| CHD | coronary heart disease |
| CGI-I | global impression-improvement scale |
| GI | gastrointestinal |
| CNS | central nervous system |
| CT | clinical trial |
| CVD | cardiovascular diseases |
| DSM | Diagnostic and Statistical Manual of Mental Disorders |
| HADS-A | Hospital Anxiety and Depression Scale-Anxiety |

| | |
|---|---|
| HAM-A | Hamilton Anxiety Rating Scale |
| HPAA | hypothalamic-pituitary-adrenal axis |
| HTP | hydroxytryptophan |
| GABA | γ-aminobutyric acid |
| GAD | generalized anxiety disorder |
| ICD | International Disease Classification |
| ICF | informed consent form |
| mADD | mixed anxiety and depressive disorder |
| ND | neurotic disorder |
| NMDA | N-methyl-D-aspartate |
| OCD | obsessive-compulsive disorder |
| OF | open field test |
| PD | Parkinson's disease |
| SBP | systolic blood pressure |
| SD | somatoform disorder |
| SSRI | selective serotonin reuptake inhibitors |
| STAI | State-Trait Anxiety Inventory |
| TCA | tricyclic antidepressants |
| TMAS | Taylor Manifest Anxiety Scale |

## Author details

Kristina Konstantinovna Khacheva*, Gulnara Rinatovna Khakimova, Alexey Borisovich Glazunov and Victoria Vyacheslavovna Fateeva
OOO NPF Materia Medica Holding, Moscow, Russia

*Address all correspondence to: hachevakk@materiamedica.ru

## References

[1] Holubova M, Prasko J, Ociskova M, Kantor K, et al. Quality of life, self-stigma, and coping strategies in patients with neurotic spectrum disorders: A cross-sectional study. Psychology Research and Behavior Management. 2019;**12**:81. DOI: 10.2147/PRBM.S179838

[2] Ni C, Ma L, Wang B, Hua Y, et al. Screening and correlates of neurotic disorders among general medical outpatients in Xi'an China. Perspectives in Psychiatric Care. 2015;**51**(2):128-135. DOI: 10.1111/ppc.12074

[3] Diagnostic and Statistical Manual of Mental Disorders (DSM) V [Internet]. Available from: https://dsm.psychiatryonline.org/doi/full/10.1176/appi.books.9780890425596.dsm08 [Accessed: 05 March 2020]

[4] International Disease Classification (ICD-10) [Internet]. Available from: https://icd.who.int/browse10/2019/en. [Accessed: 05 March 2020]

[5] O'Donnell ML, Agathos JA, Metcalf O, et al. Adjustment disorder: Current developments and future directions. International Journal of Environmental Research and Public Health. 2019;**16**(14):2537. DOI: 10.3390/ijerph16142537

[6] Baxter AJ, Scott KM, Vos T, Whiteford HA. Global prevalence of anxiety disorders: A systematic review and meta-regression. Psychological Medicine. 2013;**43**(5):897-910

[7] Weiland A, Blankenstein AH, Van Saase JL, Van der Molen HT, Jacobs ME, Abels DC, et al. Training medical specialists to communicate better with patients with medically unexplained physical symptoms (MUPS). A randomized, controlled trial. PLoS One. 2015;**10**(9):e0138342. DOI: 10.1371/journal.pone.0138342

[8] Haller H, Cramer H, Lauche R, Dobos G. Somatoform disorders and medically unexplained symptoms in primary care. Deutsches Ärzteblatt International. 2015;**112**(16):279-287. DOI: 10.3238/arztebl.2015.0279

[9] Versace A, Graur S, Greenberg T, et al. Reduced focal fiber collinearity in the cingulum bundle in adults with obsessive-compulsive disorder. Neuropsychopharmacology. 2019;**44**(7):1182-1188. DOI: 10.1038/s41386-019-0353-4

[10] Sar V. Epidemiology of dissociative disorders: An overview. Epidemiology Research International. 2011;**2011**:1-8. DOI: 10.1155/2011/404538

[11] Bandelow B, Michaelis S. Epidemiology of anxiety disorders in the 21st century. Dialogues in Clinical Neuroscience. 2015;**17**(3):327

[12] Grover S, Aneja J, Sharma A, et al. Do the various categories of somatoform disorders differ from each other in symptom profile and psychological correlates. International Journal of Social Psychiatry. 2015;**61**(2):148-156. DOI: 10.1177/0020764014537238

[13] Essau CA. Course and outcome of somatoform disorders in non-referred adolescents. Psychosomatics. 2007;**48**(6):502-509. DOI: 10.1176/appi.psy.48.6.502

[14] Michopoulos V, Powers A, Gillespie CF, et al. Inflammation in fear- and anxiety-based disorders: PTSD, GAD, and beyond. Neuropsychopharmacology. 2017;**42**(1):254-270. DOI: 10.1038/npp.2016.146

[15] de la Mora MP, Gallegos-Cari A, Arizmendi-García Y, et al. Role of dopamine receptor mechanisms in the amygdaloid modulation of fear and anxiety: Structural and functional

analysis. Progress in Neurobiology. 2010;**90**(2):198-216. DOI: 10.1016/j.pneurobio.2009.10.010

[16] Fryers T, Melzer D, Jenkins R, et al. The distribution of the common mental disorders: Social inequalities in Europe. Clinical Practice and Epidemiology in Mental Health. 2005;**1**(1):14. DOI: 10.1186/1745-0179-1-14

[17] Andlin-Sobocki P, Wittchen HU. Cost of anxiety disorders in Europe. European Journal of Neurology. 2005; **12**(1):39-44. DOI: 10.1111/j.1468-1331.2005.01196.x

[18] Gustavsson A, Svensson M, Jacobi F. Cost of disorders of the brain in Europe 2010. European Neuropsychopharmacology. 2011;**21**: 718-779. DOI: 10.1016/j.euroneuro.2011.08.008

[19] Trautmann S, Rehm J, Wittchen HU. The economic costs of mental disorders. EMBO Reports. 2016; **17**(9):1245-1249. DOI: 10.15252/embr.201642951

[20] Wang SY. Survey of help-seeking behavior of patients with mental disorders. Sichuan Mental Health. 2002; **15**:16 [in Chinese]

[21] Piontek K, Shedden-Mora MC, Gladigau M, Kuby A, Löwe B. Diagnosis of somatoform disorders in primary care: Diagnostic agreement, predictors, and comparisons with depression and anxiety. BMC Psychiatry. 2018;**18**(1): 361. DOI: 10.1186/s12888-018-1940-3

[22] Baldwin DS, Anderson IM, Nutt DJ, Allgulander C, et al. Evidence-based pharmacological treatment of anxiety disorders, post-traumatic stress disorder and obsessive-compulsive disorder: A revision of the 2005 guidelines from the British Association for Psychopharmacology. Journal of Psychopharmacology. 2014;**28**(5): 403-439. DOI: 10.1177/0269881114525674

[23] Grassi G, Pallanti S. Current and up-and-coming pharmacotherapy for obsessive-compulsive disorder in adults. Expert Opinion on Pharmacotherapy. 2018;**19**(14):1541-1550. DOI: 10.1080/14656566.2018.1528230

[24] Kleinstaeuber M, Witthoeft M, Steffanowski A, van Marwijk H, Hiller W, Lambert MJ. Pharmacological interventions for somatoform disorders in adults. Cochrane Database of Systematic Reviews. 2014;**11**:1465-1858. DOI: 10.1002/14651858.CD010628.pub2

[25] Donato R, Cannon BR, Sorci G, et al. Functions of S100 proteins. Current Molecular Medicine. 2013;**13**(1):24-57. DOI: 10.2174/156652413 804486214

[26] Parfenov VA, Ostroumova OD, Ostroumova TM, Kochetkov AI, Fateeva VV, Khacheva KK, et al. Vascular cognitive impairment: Pathophysiological mechanisms, insights into structural basis, and perspectives in specific treatments. Neuropsychiatric Disease and Treatment. 2019;**15**:1381-1402. DOI: 10.2147/NDT.S197032

[27] Larentsova LI, Grinin VM, Fokina TY, et al. Eksperimental'no-klinicheskoe izuchenie tenotena (antitela k mozgospetsificheskomu belku S-100) i vozmozhnosti ego primeneniya v kachestve sredstva premedikatsii na ambulatornom stomatologicheskom prieme. Rossiyskaya Stomatologiya. 2008;**1**: 48-51 [in Russian]

[28] Castagne V, Lemaire M, Kheyfets I, Dugina JL, Sergeeva SA, Epstein OI. Antibodies to S100 proteins have anxiolytic-like activity at ultra-low doses in the adult rat. Journal of Pharmacy and Pharmacology. 2008;**60**(3):309-316. DOI: 10.1211/jpp.60.3.0005

[29] Voronina TA, Molodavkin GM, Sergeeva SA, Epsteyn OI. GAMK-ergicheskaya sistema v realizatsii

anksioliticheskogo deystviya "Proprotena": Eksperimental'noe issledovanie. Byulleten' eksperimental'noy biologii i meditsiny. 2003;**1**:37-39 [in Russian]

[30] Heyfets IA, Dugina YL, Voronina TA, Molodavkin GM, Martyushev-Poklad AV, Sergeeva SA. Uchastie serotoninergicheskoy sistemy v mekhanizme deystviya antitel k belku S-100 v sverhmalyh dozah. Byulleten' eksperimental'noy biologii i meditsiny. 2007;**143**(5):535-537 [in Russian]

[31] Voronina TA, Sergeeva SA, Martyushev-Poklad AV, Dugina JL, Epstein OI. Antibodies to S-100 protein in anxiety-depressive disorders in experimental and clinical conditions. In: Animal Models in Biological Psychiatry. New York: Nova Science Publishers; 2006. pp. 137-152 [in Russian]

[32] Heyfets IA, Voronina TA, Dugina YL, Molodavkin GM, Sergeeva SA. Zavisimost' anksioliticheskoy aktivnosti ot usloviy provedeniya testa konfliktnoy situatsii po VOGEL na primere tenotena i diazepama. Byulleten' eksperimental'noy biologii i meditsiny. 2011;**3**:311-314 [in Russian]

[33] Voronina TA, Molodavkin GM, Sergeeva SA, Epstein OI. Anksioliticheskiy effekt "Proprotena" v usloviyah nakazuemogo i nenakazuemogo povedeniya. Byulleten' eksperimental'noy biologii i meditsiny. 2003;**1**:31-33 [in Russian]

[34] Epstein OI, Molodavkin GM, Voronina TA, Sergeeva SA. Antidepressivnye svoystva proprotena i amitriptilina: Sravnitel'noe eksperimental'noe issledovanie. Byulleten' eksperimental'noy biologii i meditsiny. 2003;**145**(6):34-36 [in Russian]

[35] Voronina TA, Borodavkina MV, Heyfets IA, et al. Eksperimental'noe izuchenie nootropnoy i antiamnesticheskoy aktivnosti deystviya tenotena v teste uslovnogo refleksa passivnogo izbeganiya u krys. In: Vtoroy natsional'nyy kongress po sotsial'noy psihiatrii «Sotsial'nye preobrazovaniya i psihicheskoe zdorov'e»; Moskva. 2006. p. 171 [in Russian]

[36] Voronina TA, Belopol'skaya MV, Heyfets IA, Dugina YL, Sergeeva SA, Epstein OI. Deystvie sverhmalyh doz antitel k S-100 pri narushenii kognitivnyh funktsiy, emotsional'nogo i nevrologicheskogo statusov v usloviyah eksperimental'noy modeli bolezni Al'tsgeymera. Byulleten' eksperimental'noy biologii i meditsiny. 2009;**148**(8):174-176 [in Russian]

[37] Voronina TA, Molodavkin GM, Borodavkina MV, Heyfets IA, Dugina YL, Sergeeva SA. Nootropnyy i antiamnesticheskiy effekty tenotena detskogo u nepolovozrelyh krysyat. Byulleten' eksperimental'noy biologii i meditsiny. 2009;**148**(8):164-166 [in Russian]

[38] Romanova GA, Voronina TA, Sergeeva SA, Barskov IV, Dugina YL, Epstein OI. Issledovanie protivoishemicheskogo, neyroprotektornogo deystviy proprotena. Sibirskiy vestnik psihiatrii i narkologii. 2003;**1**(27):123-125 [in Russian]

[39] Voronina TA, Heyfets IA, Dugina YL, Sergeeva SA, Epstein OI. Izuchenie effektov preparata sverhmalyh doz antitel k S-100 v usloviyah eksperimental'noy modeli gemorragicheskogo insul'ta. Byulleten' eksperimental'noy biologii i meditsiny. 2009;**148**(8):170-173 [in Russian]

[40] Heyfets IA, Molodavkin GM, Voronina TA, Dugina YUL, Sergeeva SA, Epstein OI. Uchastie GAMK-V-sistemy v mekhanizme deystviya antitel k belku S-100 v sverhmalyh dozah. Byulleten' eksperimental'noy biologii i meditsiny. 2008;**145**(5):552-554 [in Russian]

[41] Gorbunov EA, Ertuzun IA, Kachaeva EV, Tarasov SA, Epstein OI. In vitro screening of major neurotransmitter systems possibly involved in the mechanism of action of antibodies to S100 protein in released-active form. Neuropsychiatric Disease and Treatment. 2015;**11**:2837-2846. DOI: 10.2147/NDT.S92456

[42] Ertuzun IA. Mekhanizmy anksioliticheskogo i antidepressatnogo deystviya Tenotena (eksperimental'noe issledovanie). Avtoreferat dissertatsii na soiskanie uchenoy stepeni kandidata meditsinskih nauk. 2012;**23** [in Russian]

[43] Matsumoto RR. σ receptors: Historical perspective and background. In: Su TP, Matsumoto RR, Bowen WD, editors. Sigma Receptors. Boston: Springer; 2007. pp. 1-23. DOI: 10.1007/978-0-387-36514-5_1

[44] Nguyen L, Lucke-Wold BP, Mookerjee S, Kaushal N, Matsumoto RR. Sigma-1 receptors and neurodegenerative diseases: Towards a hypothesis of sigma-1 receptors as amplifiers of neurodegeneration and neuroprotection. In: Sigma Receptors: Their Role in Disease and as Therapeutic Targets. Springer; 2017. pp. 133-152. DOI: 10.1007/978-3-319-50174-1_10

[45] Mohler H. GABAA receptors in central nervous system disease: Anxiety, epilepsy, and insomnia. Journal of Receptor and Signal Transduction Research. 2006;**26**(5–6):731-740. DOI: 10.1080/10799890600920035

[46] Atack JR. The benzodiazepine binding site of GABA(A) receptors as a target for the development of novel anxiolytics. Expert Opinion on Investigational Drugs. 2005;**14**(5): 601-618. DOI: 10.1517/13543784.14.5.601

[47] Nakagawa Y, Ishima T, Ishibashi Y, Tsuji M, Takashima T. Involvement of GABAB receptor systems in action of antidepressants. II: Baclofen attenuates the effect of desipramine whereas muscimol has no effect in learned helplessness paradigm in rats. Brain Research. 1996;**728**(2):225-230. DOI: 10.1016/0006-8993(96)00413-1

[48] Nakagawa Y, Ishima T, Ishibashi Y, Tsuji M, Takashima T. Involvement of GABAB receptor systems in experimental depression: Baclofen but not bicuculline exacerbates helplessness in rats. Brain Research. 1996;**741**(1–2): 240-245. DOI: 10.1016/0006-8993(95)01273-7

[49] Pytliak M, Vargová V, Mechírová V, Felšöci M. Serotonin receptors—From molecular biology to clinical applications. Physiological Research. 2011;**60**(1):15-25. DOI: 10.33549/physiolres.931903

[50] Karcz-Kubicha M, Jessa M, Nazar M, Plaznik A, Hartmann S, Parsons CG, et al. Anxiolytic activity of glycine-B antagonists and partial agonists—No relation to intrinsic activity in the patch clamp. Neuropharmacology. 1997;**36**(10): 1355-1367. DOI: 10.1016/S0028-3908(97)00130-5

[51] Zarrabian S, Nasehi M, Farrahizadeh M, Zarrindast M-R. The role of CA3 GABA(B) receptors on anxiolytic-like behaviors and avoidance memory deficit induced by D-AP5 with respect to Ca(2+) ions. Progress in Neuro-Psychopharmacology & Biological Psychiatry. 2017;**79**(Pt B): 515-524. DOI: 10.1016/j.pnpbp.2017.08.007

[52] Kotlinska J, Liljequist S. A characterization of anxiolytic-like actions induced by the novel NMDA/glycine site antagonist, L-701,324. Psychopharmacology. 1998;**135**(2): 175-181. DOI: 10.1007/s002130050499

[53] Przegaliński E, Tatarczyńska E, Chojnacka-Wójcik E. Anxiolytic- and antidepressant-like effects of an

antagonist at glycineB receptors. Polish Journal of Pharmacology. 1998;**50**(4–5): 349-354

[54] Moraga-Amaro R, Gonzalez H, Pacheco R, Stehberg J. Dopamine receptor D3 deficiency results in chronic depression and anxiety. Behavioural Brain Research. 2014;**274**:186-193. DOI: 10.1016/j.bbr.2014.07.055

[55] Domashenko MA, Bolotova TA, Ershova MV, Illarioshkin SN, Dugina YL. Tenoten v lechenii trevogi u patsientov s hronicheskimi tserebrovaskulyarnymi zabolevaniyami i bolezn'yu Parkinsona. In: VI mezhdunarodnaya konferentsiya «Klinicheskie issledovaniya lekarstvennyh sredstv»; 12 October 2007; Moscow. 2007. pp. 48-49 [in Russian]

[56] Khacheva KK, Glazunov AB, Kamchatnov PR. The efficacy and safety of the most prescribed drugs with anxiolytic effect in the Russian federation. Lechebnoye Delo. DOI: 10.24411/2071-5315-2019-12153

[57] Clinical trials.gov NCT03036293 [Internet]. Available from: https://clinicaltrials.gov/ct2/show/NCT03036293?cond=NCT03036293&draw=2&rank=1 [Accessed: 05 March 2020]

[58] Shamrey VK, Kurpatov VI, Habarov IY, Shabanov PD. Klinicheskoe primenenie Tenotena v kachestve anksioliticheskogo i antiastenicheskogo sredstva. Psihofarmakologiya i biologicheskaya narkologiya. 2006;**6** (1-2):1212-1219 [in Russian]

[59] Romasenko LV, Nedostup AV, Artyuhova MG, Parhomenko IM. Primenenie preparata Tenoten pri lechenii nevroticheskih rasstroystv u patsientov s zabolevaniyami serdechno-sosudistoy sistemy. Rossiyskiy psihiatricheskiy zhurnal. 2007;**2**(1): 81-84 [in Russian]

[60] Vanchakova NP, Popov AP. Trevozhnye rasstroystva u patsientov s gipertonicheskoy bolezn'yu i ishemicheskoy bolezn'yu serdtsa i opyt ih korrektsii Tenotenom. Poliklinika. 2007;**2**:56-60 [in Russian]

[61] Vorob'eva OV. Stress–indutsirovannye psihovegetativnye reaktsii. Russkiy meditsinskiy zhurnal. 2005;**13**(12):798 [in Russian]

[62] Meyza KZ, Boguszewski PM, Nikolaev E, Zagrodzka J. The effect of age on the dynamics and the level of c-Fos activation in response to acute restraint in Lewis rats. Behavioural Brain Research. 2007;**180**(2):183-189. DOI: 10.1016/j.bbr.2007.03.007

[63] Umryuhin PE, Heyfets IA, Sergeeva SA, Epstein OI, Sudakov KV. Deystvie subnanomolyarnyh kontsentratsiy antitel k belku s-100 na stressindutsirovannuyu ekspressiyu rannego gena s–fos v paraventrikulyarnyh yadrah gipotalamusa u krys. In: Funktsional'nye sistemy organizma v norme pri patologii Sbornik nauchnyh trudov. Minsk: Citeseer; 2008. pp. 348-353 [in Russian]

[64] Koplik EV, Salieva RM, Gorbunova AV. Test «otkrytogo polya» kak prognosticheskiy kriteriy ustoychivosti krys linii Vistar k emotsional'nomu stressu. Zhurnal vysshey nervnoy deyatel'nosti im IP Pavlova. 1995;**45**(4):775-781 [in Russian]

[65] Griebel G, Holmes A. 50 years of hurdles and hope in anxiolytic drug discovery. Nature Reviews Drug Discovery. 2013;**12**(9):667-687. DOI: 10.1038/nrd4075

[66] Khaleva A. Obestatin protective role againest stress gastric ulcer in rat. Medical Journal Cairo University. 2016; **84**(3):56-58

[67] Umryuhin AE, Epstein OI, Chekmareva NY, et al. Tenoten kak

antistressornyy faktor. Trudy nauchnogo soveta po eksperimental'noy i prikladnoy fiziologii «Sistemnaya samoregulyatsiya funktsiy organizma». 2011;**16**:226-238 [in Russian]

[68] Voronina TA, Heyfets IA, Molodavkin GM, et al. Antiagressivnaya aktivnost' antitel k belku S-100 v sverhmalyh dozah. Byulleten' eksperimental'noy biologii i meditsiny. 2009;**148**(8):167-169 [in Russian]

[69] Ganina KK, Dugina YL, Zhavbert KS, Ertuzun IA, Epstein OI, Abdurasulova IN. Reliz-aktivnye antitela k belku S100 sposobny korrektirovat' techenie jeksperimental'nogo allergicheskogo jencefalomielita. Zhurnal nevrologii i psihiatrii im. SS Korsakova. 2015;**115**(6):78-82. DOI: 10.17116/jnevro20151156178-82 [in Russian]

[70] Pankova TM, Starostina MV, Shtark MB, Epstein OI. Neyroprotektornoe deystvie sverhmalyh doz antitel k belku S100 v kul'ture neyroblastomy pri deprivatsii kisloroda i glyukozy. Byulleten' eksperimental'noy biologii i meditsiny. Izdatel'stvo Rossiyskoy akademii meditsinskih nauk. 2007;**144**(9): 260-263 [in Russian]

[71] Epstein OI. Sverhmalye dozy (istoriya odnogo issledovaniya). Moskva: Izdatel'stvo RAMN; 2008. p. 336

[72] Epstein OI, Beregovoy NA, Sorokina NS, Starostina MV, Shtark MB. Vliyanie razlichnyh razvedeniy potentsirovannyh antitel k mozgospetsificheskomu belku S-100 na dinamiku posttetanicheskoy potentsiatsii v perezhivayuschih srezah gippokampa. Byulleten' eksperimental'noy biologii i meditsiny. 2002;**127**(3):317-320 [in Russian]

[73] Epstein OI. The spatial homeostasis hypothesis. Symmetry (Basel). Multidisciplinary Digital Publishing Institute. 2018;**10**(4):103. DOI: 10.3390/sym10040103

[74] Tramontina F, Tramontina AC, Souza DF, Leite MC, Gottfried C, Souza DO, et al. Glutamate uptake is stimulated by extracellular S100B in hippocampal astrocytes. Cellular and Molecular Neurobiology. 2006;**26**(1): 81-86. DOI: 10.1007/s10571-006-9099-8

[75] Liu Y, Buck DC, Neve KA. Novel interaction of the dopamine D2 receptor and the $Ca^{2+}$ binding protein S100B: Role in D2 receptor function. Molecular Pharmacology. 2008;**74**(2):371-378. DOI: 10.1124/mol.108.044925

[76] Palacios G, Muro A, Verdu E, Pumarola M, Vela JM. Immunohistochemical localization of the sigma1 receptor in Schwann cells of rat sciatic nerve. Brain Research. 2004; **1007**(1–2):65-70. DOI: 10.1016/j.brainres.2004.02.013

[77] Azmitia EC, Dolan K, Whitaker-Azmitia PM. S-100B but not NGF, EGF, insulin or calmodulin is a CNS serotonergic growth factor. Brain Research. 1990;**516**(2):354-356. DOI: 10.1016/0006-8993(90)90942-5

[78] Hyden H, Lange PW, Larsson S. S100-glia regulation of GABA transport across the nerve cell membrane. Journal of the Neurological Sciences. 1980;**45** (2–3):303-316. DOI: 10.1016/0022-510X(80)90173-2

[79] Eison MS. Serotonin: A common neurobiologic substrate in anxiety and depression. Journal of Clinical Psychopharmacology. 1990;**10**(3):26-30

[80] Bespalov AU, Zvartau EE. Neyropsihofarmakologiya antagonistov NMDA-retseptorov. Nevskiy dialekt: Sankt-Peterburg; 2000. p. 297 [in Russian]

[81] Donato R, Shimomura O, Musicki B, Kishi Y. S100: A multigenic family of

calcium-modulated proteins of the EF-hand type with intracellular and extracellular functional roles Cause of spectral variation in the luminescence of semisynthetic aequorins Semi-synthetic aequorins with improved sensitivity. International Journal of Biochemistry & Cell Biology. 2001;**33**(7):637-668. DOI: 10.1016/S1357-2725(01)00046-2

[82] Titkova AM, Epstein OI. Vliyanie potentsirovannyh antitel k mozgospetsificheskomu belku S-100 na sistemu biogennyh monoaminov i intensivnost' perekisnogo okisleniya lipidov u krys v usloviyah alkogolizatsii. Proproten-100 Sbornik Statey. 2002: 95-99 [in Russian]

[83] ICH Good Clinical Practice [Internet]. Available from: https://ichgc p.net/ [Accessed: 05 March 2020]

[84] Hertzman M, Adler L. Clinical Trials in Psychopharmacology: A Better Brain. Chichester: John Wiley & Sons; 2010. p. 403

[85] Costa M, Kirchner H, Klotz U, Kraker J, Patierno R, Werner G. Essential and Non-Essential Metals Metabolites with Antibiotic Activity Pharmacology of Benzodiazepines Interferon Gamma Research. Vol. 1. Berlin: Springer Science & Business Media; 2012. 204 p. DOI: 10.1007/978-3-642-69872-9

[86] Arbanas G, Arbanas D, Dujam K. Adverse effects of benzodiazepines in psychiatric outpatients. Psychiatria Danubina. 2009;**21**(1):103-107

[87] Baldwin DS, Aitchison K, Bateson A, et al. Benzodiazepines: Risks and benefits. A reconsideration. Journal of Psychopharmacology. 2013;**27**(11): 967-971. DOI: 10.1177/026988111 3503509

[88] Low Y, Setia S, Lima G. Drug–drug interactions involving antidepressants: Focus on desvenlafaxine. Neuropsychiatric Disease and Treatment. 2018;**14**:567. DOI: 10.2147/ NDT.S157708

[89] de Abajo FJ, Garcia-Rodriguez LA. Risk of upper gastrointestinal tract bleeding associated with selective serotonin reuptake inhibitors and venlafaxine therapy: Interaction with nonsteroidal anti-inflammatory drugs and effect of acid-suppressing agents. Archives of General Psychiatry. 2008; **65**:795-803. DOI: 10.1001/ archpsyc.65.7.795

[90] Balon R, Rafanelli C, Sonino N. Benzodiazepines: A valuable tool in the management of cardiovascular conditions. Psychotherapy and Psychosomatics. 2018;**87**(6):327-330. DOI: 10.1159/000493015

[91] Ouakinin SRS. Anxiety as a risk factor for cardiovascular diseases. Frontiers in Psychiatry. 2016;**7**:25. DOI: 10.3389/fpsyt.2016.00025

[92] Małyszczak K, Rymaszewska J. Depression and anxiety in cardiovascular disease. Kardiologia Polska (Polish Heart Journal). 2016; **74**(7):603-609. DOI: 10.5603/KP. a2016.0063

[93] Nikol'skaya IN, Guseva IA, Bliznevskaya EV, Tret'yakova TV. Rol' trevozhnyh rasstroystv pri gipertonicheskoy bolezni i vozmozhnosti ih korrektsii. Lechaschiy vrach. 2007;**3**:89-91 [in Russian]

[94] Matyushin GV, Yurin VV, Golovenkin SE, Savchenko EA, Kuskaev AP. Opyt primeneniya anksioliticheskogo sredstva v terapii bol'nyh s ekstrasistoliey i paroksizmal'nymi nadzheludochkovymi tahiaritmiyami. Lechaschiy vrach. 2009; **2**:76-78 [in Russian]

[95] Poponina TM, Gunderina KI, Poponina YS, Soldatenko MV, Markov VA. Vozmozhnosti

uluchsheniya kachestva zhizni patsientov s ostrym koronarnym sindromom. Sibirskiy meditsinskiy zhurnal. 2015;**30**(4):19-23 [in Russian]

[96] Mussell M, Kroenke K, Spitzer RL, Williams JB, Herzog W, Löwe B. Gastrointestinal symptoms in primary care: Prevalence and association with depression and anxiety. Journal of Psychosomatic Research. 2008;**64**(6): 605-612. DOI: 10.1016/j.jpsychores.2008.02.019

[97] Goodwin RD, Cowles RA, Galea S, Jacobi F. Gastritis and mental disorders. Journal of Psychiatric Research. 2016; **47**(1):128-132. DOI: 10.1016/j.jpsychires.2012.09.016

[98] Hou N, Zhang X, Zhao L, et al. A novel chronic stress-induced shift in the Th1 to Th2 response promotes colon cancer growth. Biochemical and Biophysical Research Communications. 2013;**439**:471-476. DOI: 10.1016/j.bbrc.2013.08.101

[99] Lee SP, Sung IK, Kim JH, et al. The effect of emotional stress and depression on the prevalence of digestive diseases. Journal of Neurogastroenterology and Motility. 2015;**21**(2):273. DOI: 10.5056/jnm14116

[100] Tsukanov VV, Kupershteyn EY, Sharypova VN. Effektivnost' primeneniya protivotrevozhnogo preparata Tenoten v sostave kompleksnoy terapii u patsientov s Helicobacter Pylori – assotsiirovannoy yazvennoy bolezn'yu dvenadtsatiperstnoy kishki. Poliklinika. 2008;**2**:52-53 [in Russian]

[101] Karpin VA, Burmasova AV, Voronova EI. Vliyanie Tenotena na neyrovegetativnyy status i konsolidatsiyu remissii u bol'nyh hronicheskim gastroduodenitom i yazvennoy bolezn'yu dvenadtsatiperstnoy kishki. Poliklinika. 2010;**1**:78-83 [in Russian]

Chapter 11

# The Role of Personal and Immune Variables in the Development of Co-Morbid Affective and Related Psychopathological Syndromes in Partial Epilepsies in Relation to Handedness

*Vladimir V. Kalinin, Kirill Y. Subbotin, Natalia G. Yermakova, Anna A. Zemlyanaya and Lyudmila V. Sokolova*

## Abstract

The current study was performed in order to find the influence of premorbid personality traits and immune variables on psychopathological constructs including affective and related syndromes in patients with epilepsy separately for right-handers and left-handers. Ninety two patients with epilepsy have been included into the study. There were 85 right-handers and 7 left-handers. Assessment of psychopathological status of patients has been performed by using of Symptom Check List –90 (SCL-90) and the Hamilton rating scales for Depression and Anxiety. The Munich Personality test (MPT) was used for the assessment of personality trait. The amounts of different lymphocytes clusters were calculated. The multiple stepwise regression analysis was used to find the relationships between personality, immunity variables and affective and related psychopathological syndromes separately for right-handers and left-handers.In the right-handers significant relationships between the Neuroticism level (MPT) and value of HAM-D, Depression construct (SCL-90), Anxiety (SCL-90), Obsessions (SCL-90) and Phobia construct (SCL-90) have been obtained. In the left-handers stochastically significant correlations between Regulatory Index (CD4/CD8) with Depression construct (SCL-90) and Obsession construct (SCL-90) were revealed. Premorbid personality traits determine the affective, anxiety, obsessive and phobia syndromes strictly in right-handed patients with epilepsy, while immunity variables (CD4/CD) quite the contrary predispose to affective and obsessive syndromes strictly in left-handed patients.

**Keywords:** epilepsy, cerebral lateralization, handedness, immunity variables, personality constructs, depression, anxiety, obsessions, phobia

## 1. Introduction

Psychiatric co-morbidity in form affective and anxiety disorders are commonest among patients with epilepsy. The frequency of these disorders achieves 40–80% and 11–16% respectively [1, 2]. Principally, that these disorders cause additional issues in life of patients with epilepsy and make worse the social and clinical prognosis.

Several probable mechanisms explaining the development of concomitant psychopathological disorders in patients with epilepsy have been proposed during the last several decades. Thus, some authors regard the temporal lobe epilepsy especially with the left hemisphere focus and concomitant function reduction of frontal lobes (hypofrontality) and focal seizures with impaired awareness (FSIA) as the main risk factors for the development of co-morbid psychopathology and especially depression [3–11].

Nevertheless, such pure neurobiological approach may hardly be regarded as perfect since it can't explain the specific nature of different psychopathological disorders in epilepsy and shouldn't be regarded as universal one. In other words, why in some cases depression and anxiety, while in other cases psychosis or obsessive–compulsive disorder can origin is not properly understood.

In one our previous article we have shown that origin of depression or anxiety in temporal lobe epilepsy depends not only on focus localization but focus lateralization too. Thus, depression development has been observed mostly in patients with the right focus, while the anxiety in case of left focus [12].

In another study the interaction between depression and anxiety in dependence on focus lateralization in temporal lobe epilepsy has been studied [13]. Obtained results have shown that depression and anxiety had stronger and more close correlation in patients with the right focus compared with the left-sided focus. It implies the more solid and less differentiated syndrome in case of right-sided focus activity and more differentiated and looser association between depression and anxiety in case of left-focus activity [13].

Suggestion can be made, that some other pathogenetic mechanisms may take part in the origin of psychopathology in epilepsy, and premorbid personality constructs and immune mechanisms may be responsible for such role, since the psychoneuroimmunological interrelationship at present is regarded as principal factor in the pathogenesis of depressions, anxiety and psychoses. Nevertheless, the exact specific mechanisms which could explain the involvement of immunity in the pathogenesis of psychopathology are absent [14–17].

The certain role of immunity mechanisms in the pathogenesis of partial forms of epilepsy has been confirmed in our previous studies [18, 19]. Thus, the combination of immunity variables with focus lateralization, gender and handedness had influence on the frequency of focal sensory seizures (FSS) in epilepsy. Principally, that most high frequencies of FSS were observed in patients with low CD4/CD8 ratio with left temporal focus, female gender and left-handedness. Quite the contrary, the maximal frequency of FSS was observed in the patients with left frontal focus and high B-lymphocyte level. The left-handed patients with low CD8 and high CD4/CD8 ratio were characterized by more severe seizures. Similarly, severe seizures were also observed in left-handers with frontal left focus and high T-lymphocyte level. The stochastically significant correlation between CD4 cell level and length of remission has been also observed [18].

In the other article [19] the interaction between alexithymia score and immunity variables has been studied. The obtained results have shown that between alexithymia score and regulatory index CD4/CD8 the positive correlation exists. It implies that patients with epilepsy and alexithymic traits are characterized by higher immunity tension compared with non-alexithymic patients.

Obviously, the role of immunity variables in the genesis of co-morbid psychopathological symptoms and syndromes has not been properly studied yet. It concerns also the role of premorbid personality in relation to motor asymmetry in patients with epilepsy.

Here must be stressed, that motor asymmetry itself isn't important for the development of psychopathology and immunity functions but underlying cerebral structure and functions that determine the handedness can influence on psychopathological structure and immunity mechanisms in epilepsy.

In this context the data obtained by Knecht et al. [20], should be mentioned. In order to illustrate the relationship between the handedness and language dominance the authors have shown that the incidence of right hemisphere language dominance increases linearly with degree of left-handedness from 4% in strong right-handers to 27% in strong left-handers [20].

Obviously, the structural and functional cerebral organization in the right- and the left-handers is different, and by that may differently determine their psychopathology [21–23].

On the other hand, according to the model proposed by Geschwind and Behan, [21] and Geschwind and Galaburda [22, 23] between handedness and immune mechanisms the close relationships exist. The authors stressed the fact that frequency of auto-immune disorders in the left-handers is higher than in the right-handers. Taking into account these data the suggestion can be made that anomalous cerebral organization (lateralization) correlates with higher immunity tension that, in turn, can determine the specific psychopathology distinct from psychopathological symptoms of right-hander persons.

The role of cerebral lateralization in the development of some psychopathological syndromes and intelligence deficiency in patients with epilepsy has been revealed earlier in our previous works, although the state of immunity mechanisms in this context has not been studied properly yet [24, 25].

## 2. Objective

The current pilot study has been designed and performed in order to find the possible influence of cellular immune and premorbid personality constructs on co-morbid affective, obsessive and anxiety psychopathology in relation to handedness in patients with partial forms of epilepsy.

## 3. Material and methods

For the current study ninety and two patients with epilepsy have been selected and included into research design. There were 38 men and 54 women. Among them were 40 patients with diagnosis of symptomatic epilepsy and 52 - with diagnosis of cryptogenic epilepsy. The temporal-lobe epilepsy was diagnosed in 36 patients, the frontal-lobe epilepsy – in 16 patients and temporal-frontal epilepsy – in 40 patients.

The mean age of patients was 32,13 + −9,78 and varied from 18,0 to 74,0 years. The duration of epilepsy was 15,16 + −9,69 with range from 0 to 35 years. Neither age of patients, nor duration of epilepsy revealed stochastically significant discrepancies between left-hander and right-hander groups of patients (27,57 + −5,22 vs. 32,52 + −10,00; $p = 0,06$) and (16,86 + −8,76 vs. 15,00 + −9,81; $p = 0,61$) respectively.

All patients were scanned through MRT. No any visible pathology (hippocampal sclerosis or limbic pathologies) could be found in the left-hander and right-hander groups.

The visual EEG-method was used in order to detect the focus laterality, while data on ictal semiotics have not been taken into account. The left-sided foci were detected in 32 patients, the right-sided foci – in 30 patients, and bilateral foci – in 30 patients.

The new operational classification of seizure types by the International League Against Epilepsy has been used in the current study [26].

The assessment of seizures severity in accordance with National Hospital Seizure Severity Scale (NHS3) has been performed [27]. Principally, that statistically significant discrepancy between left-handers and right-handers for NHS3 score has not been observed (16,71 + −12,78 vs. 13,15 + −8,67; p = 0,495).

All patients were receiving antiepileptic drugs (AED) before and after inclusion into the study and any change of AED has not been designed and permitted. The antiepileptic drugs included mostly valproates, carbamazepine and lamotrigine in recommended standard doses. The left-hander and right-hander patients received the similar therapy.

Assessment of psychopathological status of patients has been performed by using of Symptom Check List −90 (SCL-90). This questionnaire represents a self-rated scale that has 9 psychiatric symptom groups, consisting of 90 items with a range of five degrees severity (0,1,2,3,4). The evaluated psychiatric constructs include somatization, obsessive–compulsive symptoms, interpersonal sensitivity, depression, anxiety, hostility, phobic anxiety, paranoid ideations, and psychoticism [28, 29]. This scale is widely used in psychiatry and its validity has been proved in many studies, including our trials [24, 30].

Along with SCL-90 for the assessment of affective and anxiety constructs the Hamilton rating scale for Depression [31] and Hamilton rating scale for Anxiety [32] have been used.

For assessment of the premorbid personality features the Munich Personality Test (MPT) has been used [33]. The MPT represents a self-rating questionnaire and includes 51 questions depicting the different personality traits. The patients have filled in all rating scales themselves, and after that the obtained raw data have been transformed into six constructs in line with specific structure of scales. These constructs include Extraversion, Neuroticism, Rigidity, Frustration Tolerance, Tendencies to Isolation and Esoteric Tendency. The last two constructs form Schizoidia scale [33]. The other two control scales of MPT (Orientation towards Social Norms and Motivation) were not included in the final analysis [33].

The choice of MPT was dictated by fact that this test was widely used in different psychiatric disorders and has proved its efficacy [33].

Along with MPT the Toronto Alexithymia Scale (TAS-26) [34] was explored for assessment of alexithymia. This scale consists of 26 items, and each item can be scored in points from 1 to 5. The global alexithymia score in TAS-26 may be expressed from 26 to 130 points. All patients whose global TAS-26 score exceeds 74 points were regarded as alexithymic persons.

For the assessment of handedness Annett's scale was used [35]. Persons, with global score on that scale lower than – 5 points were regarded as left-handers, while persons with global score exceeded +5 points - as right-handers. Among all studied patients 85 persons were considered as right-handers (Mean + – Std. Dev.: + 21,9 + −2,7) in Annett's score and 7 persons as left-handers (Mean + – Std. Dev: −9,9 + −12,9).

The so-called pathological left-handedness has not been observed in our studied group. All patients were scanned through MRT and any visible pathology (hippocampal sclerosis or limbic pathologies) has not been observed in the left-hander group.

The blood samples were taken in every patient after he or she had been admitted to hospital. The analyses have been performed on cytofluorimeter FC 500 (Beckman Coulter).

The amounts of different lymphocytes clusters were calculated. Among them the number of T-lymphocytes (CD3+), T-helpers (CD3 + CD4+), T-cytotoxic (CD3 + CD8+), T-NK (CD3 + CD16 + CD56+), B-lymphocytes (CD3 + CD19+), Natural Killers (CD3-CD16 + CD + 56) and regulatory index (CD4/CD8 ratio) were analyzed.

## 4. Statistical analysis

The multiple regression analysis has been used in order to find any possible relationships between neurobiological and immunity variables on the one hand and SCL-90 constructs on the other hand separately within left-handers group and right-handers group [36, 37].

That method is usually used in order to find a probable dependence of one variable on several independent variables [36, 37].

Comparison of means of neurobiological, Immunological and psychopathological variables between right-handers and left-handers has also been done using Student's test.

## 5. Results

The main obtained results are shown in **Tables 1-3**. In **Table 1** the comparison of means of immunological and personality variables between right-handers and

| Variable | Left-handers | Right-handers | Significance |
|---|---|---|---|
| Extraversion (MPT) | 15,57 + −4,54 | 14,59 + −4,59 | n.s. |
| Neuroticism (MPT) | 15,43 + −4,08 | 13,41 + −5,89 | n.s. |
| Frustration Tolerance (MPT) | 8,00 + −4,12 | 9,37 + −4,20 | n.s. |
| Rigidity (MPT) | 13,29 + −5,02 | 13,04 + −4,80 | n.s. |
| Isolation Tendency (MPT) | 4,14 + −1,57 | 5,71 + −2,80 | n.s. |
| Tendencies (MPT) | 1,71 + −1,25 | 3,71 + −2,87 | n.s. |
| Schizoidia (MPT) | 5,86 + −1,35 | 9,39 + −4,74 | n.s. |
| **Alexithymia (TAS-26)** | **58,43 + -9,27** | **67,94 + -9,26** | **p = 0,013** |
| T-lymphocytes | 77,63 + −5,19 | 73,97 + −6,60 | n.s. |
| T-helpers CD3 + CD4 | 46,59 + −8,94 | 46,59 + −6,71 | n.s. |
| T-cytotoxic (CD3 + CD8+) | 28,87 + −7,51 | 25,62 + −6,22 | n.s. |
| T-NK (CD3 + CD16 + CD56+) | 9,29 + −5,91 | 6,01 + −4,16 | n.s. |
| B-lymphocytes (CD3 + CD19+) | 10,24 + −3,02 | 12,62 + −4,97 | n.s. |
| Natural Killers (CD3-CD16 + CD + 56) | 9,81 + −3,20 | 11,69 + −5,69 | n.s. |
| Regulatory index (CD4/CD8) ratio | 1,79 + −0,79 | 1,97 + −0,65 | n.s. |

*Note: statistically significant discrepancies are marked in boldface.*

**Table 1.**
*Comparison of mean values of Munich Personality Test constructs, and immune variables in groups of left-handers and right-handers.*

| Variable | Left-handed patients (N = 7) | Right-handed patients (N = 59) | Significance |
|---|---|---|---|
| HAM-D | 3,86 + −3,08 | 8,08 + −7,65 | N.S. |
| HAM-A | 4,29 + −3,45 | 8,0 + −7,26 | N.S. |
| Depression (SCL-90) | 6,14 + −5,55 | 9,47 + −8,68 | N.S. |
| Anxiety (SCL-90) | 5,00 + −2,65 | 5,59 + −6,01 | N.S. |
| Obsession (SCL-90) | 6,14 + −4,45 | 8,34 + −6,47 | N.S. |
| Phobia (SCL-90) | 1,43 + −2,07 | 3,45 + −3,98 | N.S. |

**Table 2.**
*Comparison of psychopathological variables in patients with left-handedness and right-handedness.*

| Group | *B* Neuroticism | *B* Frustration tolerance | *B* Alexithymia | *B* CD4/CD8 ratio | R2 |
|---|---|---|---|---|---|
| HAM-A RH | — | **0,298** | — | — | **0,089** |
| HAM-A LH | — | — | — | — | — |
| HAM-D RH | **0,326** | — | — | — | **0,106** |
| HAM-D LH | — | — | — | — | — |
| Depression (SCL-90) RH | **0,751** | — | — | — | **0,250** |
| Depression (SCL-90) LH | — | — | — | **0,834** | **0,695** |
| Anxiety (SCL-90) RH | **0,401** | **-0,334** | **0,257** | — | **0,292** |
| Anxiety (SCL-90) LH | — | — | — | — | — |
| Obsession (SCL-90) RH | **0,432** | — | — | — | **0,186** |
| Obsession (SCL-90) LH | — | — | — | **0,780** | **0,608** |
| Phobia (SCL-90) RH | **0.317** | — | — | — | **0,101** |
| Phobia (SCL-90) LH | — | — | — | — | — |

*All statistically significant regression coefficients are marked in boldface.*

**Table 3.**
*Multiple forward stepwise regression analysis (values of beta coefficients) for different psychopathological constructs as dependent variable in right-handers and left-handers.*

left-handers has been done. As can be seen the left-handers were characterized by less alexithymia score compared with right-handers (58,43 + −9,27 vs. 67,94 + −9,26, p = 0,013) The other personality constructs didn't show any differences.

Data on comparison of psychopathological data (SCL-90 constructs) and HAM-D and HAM-A are included in **Table 2**. Once again neither one difference has been obtained.

**Table 3** include the results of multiple regression analysis between premorbid personality constructs, immunity variables and HAM-D, HAM-A and SCL-90 constructs separately for group of the right-handers and the left-handers.

As can be seen in the group of right-handers stochastically significant correlations exist between Neuroticism level (MPT) and expression of HAM-D (b = 0,326), Depression SCL-90 (b = −0,751), Anxiety SCL-90 (b = 0,401), Obsession SCL-90 (b = 0,432) and Phobia SCL-90 (b = 0,317). It implies that the high level of Neuroticism predisposes to high expression of all mentioned psychopathological syndromes, although the role of this relationship should not be exaggerated due the small size of correlation and the final level of explained total variance (R2) was within 0.101–0,357 range.

In addition, in the right-hander group the level of Anxiety (SCL-90) was dependent on Frustration tolerance (b = −0,334), Alexithymia score (b = 0,257), and the final value of explained variance here achieved 0,292. In other words, the high Alexithymia level predisposes to Anxiety, while the high level of Frustration tolerance reduces the risk of Anxiety development.

Quite the contrary, in the group of left-handers have been revealed much more statistically significant correlations of high values despite the small size of left-handers group.

Thus, the regulatory index (CD4/CD8 ratio) correlates positively with Obsessions SCL-90 (b = 0.780) and Depression SCL-90 (b = 0,834). The final value of explained variance here achieved 0,695 for Depression and 0,608 for Obsession SCL-90. It implies that high immunity tension relates to high expression of mentioned variables and determines the affective psychopathological syndrome with co-morbid obsessions in left-handers with epilepsy.

## 6. Discussion

The current study is characterized by the unequal size of compared groups and too small left-handers group, that may be regarded as shortcoming and may be criticized. Here must be stressed that frequency of left-handedness in a general population usually reaches near 8–11% [38–41] and our findings are in full accordance with these data.

In one of our previous work has been shown that left-handers with epilepsy are characterized by much more frequencies of focal seizures (FS) and focal sensory seizures (FSS). In other words, the cerebral organization of left-handed patients with epilepsy predisposes to development of more frequent FS and FSS. Nevertheless, no any statistically significant correlations between mentioned seizure types and SCL-90 constructs have been revealed. It implies, that these seizure types *per se* don't determine the psychopathology constructs and affective and anxiety syndromes particularly. The exact mechanisms of such phenomenon remain unknown [42].

On the other hand, focal seizures with impaired awareness (FSIA) and focal to bilateral tonic–clonic seizures (FBTCS) had no significant discrepancies between right-handers and left-handers, but both significantly correlated with SCL-90 constructs. In implies that only these seizures can determine the psychopathology in left-handed patients. Although the FSIA and FBTCS frequencies have no significant discrepancies between left-handers and right-handers [42].

The obtained results in the current study have shown that only Alexithymia construct has discrepancy between right- and left-handers (67,94 + −9,26 versus 58,43 + −9,27, p = 0,013). The other personality constructs didn't show any discrepancy between right-handers and left-handers with epilepsy. It implies that right-handed patients are able to recognize respectively their affective incapability unlike left-handers.

Principally, that despite the small number of studied left-handers the statistically significant correlation between immunity variables and psychopathological constructs of SCL-90, have been observed.

Moreover, the values of observed correlations in the left-handers group reached 0,780 for Obsessions and 0,834 for Depression and explained respectively 0,608 and 0,695 of total variance. This implies the strong and practically functional connections between mentioned above variables.

The principal results of current study have shown that right-handers and left-handers with epilepsy have discrepancies in terms of interaction between premorbid personality traits and affective and related psychopathological variables on one hand, and between immunity variables and psychopathological constructs, on the other hand.

Thus, in right-handers the psychopathological syndromes are practically independent from immunity variables, while in the left-handers the strong positive correlations between immunity variables and psychopathological constructs exist.

In other words, the studied immune variables determine the psychopathological structure of co-morbid disorder strictly in left-handers.

Here must be stressed, that immunity variables were quite comparable in groups of left- and right-handers. It means that immunity tension as a whole doesn't depend on the handedness. In this context our data contradict the hypothesis of Geschwind, Behan [21], Geschwind, Galaburda [22, 23] about higher risk of immune pathology, including auto-immune disorders in patients with left-handedness. Nevertheless, not all studies could confirm this hypothesis [43–45].

Thus, In the study by McKeever and Riche [43] the Laterality quotients from the Edinburgh Handedness Inventory were unrelated to immune disorders in both sexes. Based on received data the authors conclude, that the Geschwind-Behan-Galaburda model about linkage between left-handedness and immune pathology couldn't be confirmed [43–45].

Nevertheless, the strong linkage between immunity and psychopathology seems to be the prerogative of left-handedness, but not of right-handedness in epilepsy.

Thus, in left-handers the high regulatory index CD4/CD8 score resulted in the more severe syndromes of Obsession and Depression. In other words, in such cases the more severe conglomerate of affective, and obsessive syndromes can appear in comparison with right-handers.

## 7. Conclusion

The principal conclusion from the current study concerns the fact, that prediction of co-morbid psychopathological syndromes in patients with epilepsy is quite possible based upon immunity data strictly in patients with left-handedness, but not in right-handedness.

Quite the contrary, in the right-handed patients with epilepsy the prediction of comorbid affective disorders is possible based on the premorbid personality traits, but not on the immunological variables. It implies that stronger interaction between immunity and psychopathological mechanisms seems to be the prerogative of left-handed patients.

The exact mechanism of such discrepancies between right-handers and left-handers with epilepsy are not known and should be elucidated in the future studies.

## Conflict of interest

The authors have no conflict of interest to declare.

*DOI: http://dx.doi.org/10.5772/intechopen.95318*

## Author details

Vladimir V. Kalinin*, Kirill Y. Subbotin, Natalia G. Yermakova, Anna A. Zemlyanaya and Lyudmila V. Sokolova
Department of Brain Organic Disorders and Epilepsy, Moscow Research Institute of Psychiatry—The Branch of Serbsky's National Center of Psychiatry and Narcology of Ministry of Health of Russian Federation, Russia

*Address all correspondence to: doct.kalinin@mail.ru

## References

[1] Heuser I., Moller A.A. Depression. In: Moller A.A., Froscher W.(Hrsg) Psychische Storungen bei Epilepsie. Thieme, Stuttgart, 1992, S.37-44 (In German)

[2] Wetterling T., Lanfermann H. Organische psychische Storungen. Hirnorganische Psychosyndrome. Steinkopff, Darmstadt, 2002-574 SS. (In German).

[3] Mendez M.F., Cummings J.L., Benson D.F. Depression in epilepsy. Significance and phenomenology. Arch Neurology 1986; 43: 766-770.

[4] Mendez M.F., TaylorJ.L., Doss R.C., Salguero P. Depression in secondary epilepsy: relation to lesion laterality. J.Neurol. Neurosurg. Psychiatry. 1994; 57(2), p.232-233.

[5] Altshuler L.L., Devinsky O., Post R.M.,Theodore W. Depression, anxiety and temporal lobe epilepsy. Laterality of focus and symptoms. Archives of Neurology 1990; 47 (3):284-288.

[6] Blumer D. Postictal depression: significance for the neurobehavioral disorder of epilepsy. J. Epilepsy 1992;5: pp.214-219.

[7] Perini G.I., Tosin C., Carraro C., Bernasconi G., Canevini M.P., Canger R. et al. Interictal mood and personality disorders in temporal lobe epilepsy and juvenile myoclonic epilepsy. J Neurol Neurosurg Psychiatry 1996; 61 (6): 601 – 605.

[8] Schmitz B. Depressive disorders in epilepsy. In: Seizures, affective disorders and anticonvulsant drugs (Eds.M.Trimble, B. Schmitz) Clarius Press-2002 :19-34.

[9] Schmitz B. Depression and mania in patients with epilepsia. Epilepsia 2005; 46 (Suppl): 45 -49.

[10] Attarian H, Vahle V, Carter J, Hykes E, Gilliam F Relation between Depression and Intractability of Seizures Epilepsy & Behav 2003;4:298-301

[11] Kanner A. Depression in neurological disorders. Lundbeck Institute, Cambridge Medical Communication Ltd, 2005 – 161pp.

[12] Kalinin V.V., Polyanskiy D.A. Focus laterality and interictal psychiatric disorder in temporal lobe epilepsy // Seizure, 2009, v.18, №3 – p.176 -179.

[13] Kalinin V.V., Zheleznova E.V., Sokolova L.V., Zemlyanaya A.A., Subbotin K.Y. Focus laterality and interface between depression and anxiety in patients with temporal lobe epilepsy. In: Epileptology. The modern state of science (Ed. V. Kalinin), Intech, 2016: 145-155.

[14] Ader R. Psychosomatic and psychoimmunologic research. Psychosomatic Medicine, 1980, 42: 307-321.

[15] Birnbaum G. Introduction to immunology/ In: Antel J., Birnbaum G., Hartung H.P. (eds) Clinical neuroimmunology, Blackwell Science Ltd, London, 1998, p.1-12.

[16] Daruna J.H. Introduction to psychoneuroimmunology. Elsevier Academic Press, 2004 – 280 pp.

[17] Vedhara K., Irwin M. Human psychoneuroimmunology. Oxford University Press, 2005- 356 pp.

[18] Kalinin V.V., Subbotin K.Y., Yermakova N.G. The interrelationship between clinical and immunity variables in epilepsy// J.Epileptology, 2016, 24 (2), p.95-104.

[19] Kalinin V.V., Subbotin K.Y., YermakovaN.G.Alexithymia:relationships with neurobiological and immune variables in patients with epilepsy// Current developments in alexithymia. A cognitive and affective deficit/ Eds.R.J.Teixeira, B. Bermond, P.P.Moormann, Nova Publishers, 2018 – pp.121-130.

[20] Knecht S.,Dräger B, Deppe M, Bobe L, Lohmann H, Flöel A, et al. Handedness and hemispheric language dominance in healthy humans// Brain, 2000,123, p.2512-2518.

[21] Geschwind N., Behan P. Left-handedness: association with immune disease, Migraine, and developmental learning disorder. Proc. National Academy of Sciences, 1982, Vol.79: 5097 -5100.

[22] Geschwind N., Galaburda A. Cerebral Lateralization. Biological mechanisms, associations and pathology: I. a hypothesis and program for research. Arch Neurol, 1985, Vol.42 (6): 428-459.

[23] Geschwind N., Galaburda A. Cerebral Lateralization. Biological mechanisms, associations and pathology: II. a hypothesis and program for research. Arch Neurol, 1985, Vol.42 (6): 521-552.

[24] Kalinin V.V., Zemlyanaya A.A., KrylovO.E.,ZheleznovaE.V.Handedness, alexithymia, and focus laterality as risk factors for psychiatric comorbidity in patients with epilepsy //Epilepsy & Behavior, 2010, 17(3) – P.389-394.

[25] Kalinin V.V., Nazmetdinova D.M., Basamygin A.V. Handedness, cognitive processing and intelligence in patients with epilepsy// J.Epileptology, 2014, 22, p.26-32.

[26] Fisher R., Cross J.H., French J.A., Higurashi N., Hirsch E., Jansen F.E. et al. Operational classification of seizure types by the ILAE Commission for Classification and Terminology. Epilepsia,2017, Vol.58 (4): 522-530.

[27] O'Donoghue M.F., Duncan J.S., Sander J.W. The National Hospital Seizure Severity Scale: a further development of the Chalfont Seizure Severity Scale. Epilepsia, 1996, 37: 563- 571.

[28] Derogatis L.R., Lipman R., Covi L. SCL-90: an outpatient psychiatric rating scale: preliminary report. Psychopharmacol Bull, 1973; 9: 13-28.

[29] Derogatis L.R., Cleary P.A. Confirmation of the dimensional structure of SCL-90: a study of construct validation. J Clin Psychol 1977; 33: 981-989.

[30] Kalinin V.V., Zemlyanaya A. A., Zheleznova E.V., Sokolova L.V. Neurobiological and clinical predictors of remission and antiepileptic treatment efficacy in partial epilepsies// J.Epileptology, 2013, 21, p.23-33.

[31] Hamilton M. A rating scale for depression. J.Neurol.Neurosurg. Psychiatry. 1960, Vol.23: 56-62.

[32] Hamilton M. The assessment of anxiety states by rating. Br.J.Med. Psychol. 1959, Vol.32:50-55.

[33] Zerssen D. von, Pfister H., Koeller D-M. The Munich Personality Test (MPT): a short questionnaire for self-rating and relatives' rating of personality traits: Formal properties and clinical potential. Eur Arch Psychiatry Neurol Sci, 1988, 238: 73-93.

[34] Bagby R.M., Taylor G.J., Ryan D. Toronto Alexithymia Scale: Relationship with personality and psychopathology measures. Psychother Psychosom., 1986, Vol.45, P.207-215.

[35] Annett, M. A classification of hand preference by association analysis.

British Journal of Psychology, 1970, 61, 303-321.

[36] Feinstein A.R. Principles of medical statistics. Boca Raton, Chapman&Hall/ CRC, 2002- 701 P.

[37] Mathews D.E., Farewell V.T. Using and Understanding Medical Statistics, Basel, Karger, 2007- 322p.

[38] Hardyck C., Petrinovich L.F. Left-handedness. Psychol.Bull., 1977, 84: 385-404.

[39] Brackenbridge C.J. Secular variation in handedness over ninety years // Neuropsychologia, 1981, 19 (4)- pp.493-508.

[40] Raymond M., Pontier D., Doufour A.B., Moller A.P. Frequency-dependent maintenance of left-handedness in humans. Proc.Biol. Sci. 1996, Dec.22, 263(1377): 1627-1633.

[41] McManus I.C. The history and geography of human handedness // Language lateralization and psychosis/ Eds. I.E.C. Sommer, R.S. Kahn, Cambridge University Press, 2009 - pp. 37-57.

[42] Kalinin V.V., Zheleznova E.V., Subbotin K.Y., Yermakova N.G., Zemlyanaya A.A., Sokolova L.V. The influence of clinical and immune variables on psychopathological syndromes in partial epilepsies in relation to handedness// J. Epileptology, 2019, 27 (2), p.37-45.

[43] McKeever W.F., Riche D.A. Left-handedness and immune disorders. Cortex, 1990, 26: 33-40.

[44] Bryden P.J., McManus I.C., Bulman-Fleming M.B. Evaluating the empirical support for the Geschwind-Behan-Galaburda model of cerebral lateralization. Brain Cognition, 1994, 26: 103-167.

[45] Bryden P.J., Bruyn J., Fletcher P. Handedness and health: an examination of association between different handedness classification and health disorders. Laterality, 2005, 10:429-440.

Chapter 12

# Association of Personal Anxiety with Dopamine Receptor D4 (DRD4), DAT Genes Polymorphism

*Valery V. Gafarov, Elena A. Gromova, Vladimir N. Maksimov, Igor V. Gagulin and Almira V. Gafarova*


## Abstract

Modern studies in the world have attached high priority to the role of genetics in human psychosocial stress. People who have strong biochemical responses to stress are more inclined to develop acute and posttraumatic stress disorders. Why do such unusually strong biological reactions occur in certain people? Psychogenetics focuses on many aspects: personality traits that can affect human behavior directly. Their individual variability has been found to be a genetic trait. At present we already know a number of genes, certain allelic variants and genotypes associated with some neuropsychological characters. Among these are genes encoding intracellular and plasma protein neurotransmitter transporters and their receptors; to date, there are only several dozen genes. Of particular interest are dopaminergic system genes. However, information about the polymorphism of known genes associated with personality traits is quite limited and contradictory for open population. Under these circumstances, the chapter is devoted to the association of polymorphisms of candidate genes of the dopaminergic system with anxiety in the open population.


**Keywords:** DRD4 gene, DAT gene, anxiety, psychosocial factors, open population

## 1. Introduction

An individual's unique pattern of behaviors, feelings and thoughts is his or her personality expression, which is a strong predictor of the physical, mental and social aspects of current and future health across the lifespan [1]. The psychobiological model of personality Cloninger C.R. (1987) became the prerequisite for the genetic basis search of personality and temperament where temperament traits are correlated with certain biochemical systems in the brain. Cloninger C.R. identified four dimensions for temperament: 'harm avoidance', 'novelty seeking', 'reward dependence' and 'persistence'.

People with high grades on the 'novelty seeking' scale are impulsive, irritable, and tend to break rules blocking access to what they believe will bring satisfaction or allow them to shake themselves. On the other hand, there is conventionality, adherence to rules. Cloninger C.R. connected the 'novelty seeking' - with the dopamine system [2]. Dopamine is a neurotransmitter that provides neurochemical transmission in the nigrostriatal, mesolimbic, mesocortical and tuberoinfundibular dopaminergic systems in mammals. These brain structures play a vital part in the implementation of psychomotor, cognitive, neuroendocrine functions [3]. Relationship between 'novelty seeking' and dopamine system has been found: an association of temperament with genetic polymorphism encoding the fourth type dopamine receptor (DRD4) was established [4].

The dopamine D4 receptor gene is located on chromosome 11 (11p 15.5) [5]. The human D4 gene has the regions homologous to the regions of the human D1 and D2 genes and other G-proteins and contains 7 transmembrane domains [6]. Unlike the D2 gene containing 7 exons, the D4 gene contains 5 exons. The encoded polypeptide has a molecular weight of 41,000 Da and consists of 387 amino acids. Currently, four polymorphic regions have been identified in the dopamine D4 receptor gene. Three of these polymorphic alleles in humans are not widely distributed. The widespread polymorphism of variable numbers of tandem repeats 48 bp (VNTR) in exon 3 of the D4 gene is most important. The third exon of the dopamine D4 receptor gene contains alleles with a variable number (2–10) of imperfect DNA repeats 48 bp long encoding the region in the third cytoplasmic loop of a 16 amino acid with a general consensus PXAPXLPXXPXGXXCA [7]. A different number of amino acids in the cytoplasmic loop affects the conformation of transmembrane domains and changes the characteristics of ligand binding. Sequenced at least 19 monomers of nucleotide sequences of imperfect repeats in 48 bp and 25 variations of a polymorphic region containing from 2 to 10 repeats [6]. The study on the global frequency distribution of allelic variations of the D4 gene [8] showed that in the healthy population the most common is 4-repeat allete (D4.4) (global frequency in the world is 64.3%). The D4.4 allele is found in all populations with a frequency of 16–96%. The second most frequent variant was 7 repetitions (D4.7) (global frequency in the world 20.6%), which is quite frequent in the American population (average frequency 48.3%) and is rarely represented in populations of East and South Asia (average frequency 1.9%). 2-repeat allete (D4.2) is the third most frequent (global frequency in the world is 8.2%). More often this allele is found in populations of East and South Asia (average frequency 18.1%) and is almost absent in American and African populations (average frequency 2.9% and 1.7%, respectively). The universality of the polymorphism (three repeat-number alleles) indicates that this polymorphism arose before the global dispersion of modern humans [9].

Unused dopamine is moved back to the presynaptic neuron or oxidized by enzymes in the synaptic cleft. Protein dopamine transporter (DAT) provides a reuptake of the mediator in the synaptic cleft. The gene for the DAT1 protein (dopamine transporter) is localized to chromosome 5p15.3, consists of 64 thousand nucleotide pairs, contains 15 exons and 14 introns. Analysis of the 3′untranslated region revealed the presence of the polymorphic locus in it associated with a different number of repeats of 40-nucleotide sequence, repeated from 3 to 11 times [10].

VNTR allele frequencies of the DAT gene in representatives of different ethnic groups differ significantly. The 10-repeat allele has been indicated as the most represented one in all studied populations. Its frequency ranges from 60% (Italians) to 93% (Japanese). The frequency of the 9-repeat allele, which is the second most frequent allele, varies from 4.2% (Japanese) to 39% (Italians). The remaining alleles are present in all populations, but the frequency is less than 3%. The shortest variation with 3 repeats has been found with a low-frequency only in white Americans and African Americans [11].

As in the case of the D4 gene, the DAT gene polymorphism can be associated with some pathological conditions in the pathogenesis, which play the main role in disorders of dopamine metabolism. However, the results of the study on the association between DAT and the 'novelty seeking' are inconsistent so far [12].

Anxiety may be due to neurotransmitter disorders: impaired dopamine synthesis. Nevertheless, the search for a relationship between disturbing traits and the DRD2, DRD3, DRD4, DAT1 genes has yielded conflicting results at present [13].

There is a wide range of convincing clinical studies in laboratory animals that indicate a disorder in the dopaminergic system in depression [14]. López León et al. (2005) performed a meta-analysis of 12 studies of VNTR of the DRD4 gene polymorphism with depression. According to the results of the study, it turned out that the 'short' allele 2 is associated with depression [15].

Most people believe that a state of vital exhaustion arises from long-term psychosocial problems they are not able to solve [16]. As has been shown, dopamine is involved in certain responses to surrounding stressful events [17], and some dopamine reuptake inhibitors have an antidepressant effect [18]. It is still open to question whether the development of vital exhaustion, as a variant of minor depression, is due to certain changes in the dopaminergic system.

We note that at present, predominantly molecular genetics "leads" psychological research to find associations of personality traits, as well as affective disorders. Given these circumstances, the chapter is devoted to the association of candidate gene polymorphisms in dopaminergic system with psychosocial risk factors.

## 2. Materials and methods

The research of the association of candidate gene polymorphisms with psychosocial factors was carried out on the basis of a large-scale epidemiological study performed as part of the III screening of the WHO MONICA program (Multinational Monitoring of Trends and Determinants of Cardiovascular Disease) in 1994 [19]. We examined men 25–64 years of age, residents of a district in Novosibirsk. The representative sample was generated according to the requirements of the protocol of the MONICA program [19] on the basis of electoral lists using a random number table. 657 men were examined (average age 44.3 ± 0.4 years). The response was –82.1%.

## 3. Psychosocial testing

The Spielberger test was used to assess anxiety level. The result was interpreted as follows: up to 30 points – mild anxiety level; 34–45 points – moderate anxiety level, 46 and above – severe anxiety level [20]. To evaluate depression, we used the form of the depression scale - the MOPSY test (Depression Scale), consisting of 15 questions. For each question there are 2 answers given: 'agree', 'disagree'. The severity of depression was assessed as no depression (No D), moderate (Mod. D), major (Major D). To assess vital exhaustion, the MOPSY test [19], consisting of 14 statements, was used. For each question there are three answers given: 'yes', 'no', 'I don't know'. The level of vital exhaustion was regarded as: no vital exhaustion, vital exhaustion (average, high). Questionnaires were filled out by the participants. The methods were strictly standardized and complied with the requirements of the protocol of the MONICA project. Material processing performed in

Helsinki (Finland). Quality control was carried out in MONICA quality control centers: Dundee (Scotland), Prague (Czech Republic), Budapest (Hungary). The presented results were found to be satisfactory [19].

## 4. Molecular genetic analysis

Genotyping of the studied polymorphisms of the DRD4, DAT genes was performed in the Laboratory of Molecular Genetic Studies of Therapeutic Diseases Research Institute of Internal and Preventive Medicine - Branch of the Institute of Cytology and Genetics SB RAS, Novosibirsk, Russia. DNA preparation was conducted there as well. The phenol-chloroform extraction method was used [21, 22]. 5–6 volumes of buffer A (10 mM Tris–HCl, pH = 7.5; 10 mM NaCl; 3 mM MgCl2) were added to a blood sample (~ 10 ml) and hemodialysis was performed by grinding clots in a Potter homogenizer. The precipitates were obtained after centrifugation at 2500 g and washed twice with buffer A, then resuspended in 0.5 ml of buffer B (10 mM EDTA; 100 mM NaCl; 50 mM Tris–HCl, pH = 8.5). After adding SDS to 0.5% and proteinase K to 200 µg / ml, the mixture was incubated for 2 hours at 65° C, or overnight at 37° C. Deproteinization was carried out sequentially with water-saturated phenol, a mixture of phenol-chloroform (1: 1) and chloroform. DNA was precipitated by the addition of NH4Ac to 2.5 M and 2.5 V ethanol. The precipitate obtained by centrifugation in an Eppendorf microcentrifuge for 10 minutes was washed with 70% ethanol and dissolved DNA in water to a concentration of 0.5 µg / µl.

## 5. Genotyping of VNTR DRD4 gene polymorphism

Genotyping was performed according to a modified technique of Nanko et al. [23]. A DNA fragment of the DRD4 gene (GenBank identification number L12398) containing a DNA region with a variable size of 96–384 bp was amplified using primers: 5′-AGGTG-GCACG-TCGCG-CCAAG-CTGCA-3 ‘straight, pos. 668–692; 5’-TCTGC-GGTGG-AGTCT-GGGGT-GGGAG-3 ‘reverse, pos. 1129–1105. The amplification reaction mixture contained 0.5–1 µg of genomic DNA, direct and reverse primers at a concentration of 0.4 µM each, dNTP at a concentration of 0.1 mm each, 1.5 mm MgCl2, 10% dimethyl sulfoxide (DMSO), 0.01% by volume Tween-20, 20 mm (NH4) SO4, 75 mM TrisHCl (pH 9.0) and 1.25 units of Taq polymerase. The total volume of the mixture was 25 µl. PCR was performed using a Mastercycler gradient (Eppendorf Scientific Inc., USA). The amplification conditions were as follows: 95°C for 4 min, then 35 cycles: 95°C for 1 min, 65°C for 1 min, 72°C for 1 min. PCR products were analyzed using polyacrylamide gel electrophoresis (4%), in a buffer containing 90 mM Tris-borate (pH 8.0) and 2 mM EDTA, followed by staining with ethidium bromide. DNA markers of 100 bp were used as a molecular weight marker. (Sibenzyme, Russia).

## 6. Genotyping of VNTR DAT gene polymorphism

For genotyping, we used a modified method of Mitchell et al. [24]. The DNA fragment of the DAT gene (identification number in GenBank M95167), containing a DNA region with a variable size of 240–480 bp, was amplified using primers: 5′-TGTGG-TGTAG- GGAAC-GGCCT-GAG-3 ‘straight, pos. 2718–2740; 5’-CTTCC-TGGAG-GTCAC-GGCTC-AAGG-3 ‘reverse, pos. 3201–3178. The reaction mixture with a volume of 25 μl contained 0.5–1 μg of genomic DNA, forward and reverse primers at a concentration of 0.4 μM each, dNTP at a concentration of 0.4 mm each, 2 mm MgCl2, 0.01% by volume Tween-20, 98 mm beta mercaptoethanol, 67 mm Tris HCl (pH 8.8) and 1.25 units of Taq polymerase. Each of the 35 amplification cycles consisted of denaturation (95°C, 0.5 min), annealing (66°C, 5 min) and synthesis (72°C, 1.5 min). PCR products were analyzed using polyacrylamide gel electrophoresis (4%), followed by staining with ethidium bromide. DNA markers of 100 bp were used as a molecular weight marker. (Sibenzyme, Russia).

Statistical analysis was performed using the SPSS-19 software package [25]. The distribution of attributes and their numerical characteristics were analyzed. The analysis of simple relationships between variables (contingency tables) was carried out. Using the method of constructing contingency tables, we conducted the hypothesis of factors A and B independence or the homogeneity of factor B with respect to the levels of factor A. The reliability of the factor independence was evaluated using $\chi^2$criterion [26].

## 7. Results

In the open population among men aged 25–64 years, the frequency of 4/4 homozygous genotype of the D4 subtype of the dopamine receptor (DRD4) was 57.9%, 2/2 genotype was found to be less frequent - 6.1%, 2/4 genotype - 12, 5% and 3/4 genotype - 5.6%; even less frequent: 4/6 genotype - 4.2%, 2/6 genotype, 4/7 and 6/6 genotypes were found in the identical proportions of 2.1%. The frequency distribution of alleles showed that the 4 allele predominates - 70.7%, the 2 allele was found at 14%, the 6 allele was at 6%. The other alleles make up 0.8% - 5.4% (**Table 1**).

The distribution of carriers of VNTR genotypes of DRD4 gene polymorphism by anxiety level is presented in **Table 1**. Associative analysis revealed that carriers of the DRD4 genotype 4/4 are much more likely to be found in the group with moderate anxiety (59.8%) and mild anxiety (66.7%) than in the group with severe anxiety (54.8%). Carriers of the 2/4 genotype were much more frequent in the group with moderate anxiety (14.5%) than with severe anxiety where the level was 9.6% ($\chi 2 = 69.569$ $\upsilon = 36$ $p = 0.001$). On the contrary, carriers of the 4/6 genotype were more frequently found in the group with a severe level of anxiety - 7.8%, versus with a moderate level of anxiety - 2%. Moreover, the occurrence of carriers of the 4/6 genotype in the group with severe anxiety was more frequent than in the group with moderate anxiety, in comparison with carriers of all other genotypes OR = 4.2 (95% CI 1.4–12.1); ($\chi 2 = 8.521$ $\upsilon = 1$ $p < 0.01$), 2/2 genotype ($\chi 2 = 7.326$ $\upsilon = 1$ $p = 0.007$), 2/4 genotype ($\chi 2 = 9.825$ $\upsilon = 1$ $p = 0.002$), 4/4 genotype ($\chi 2 = 8.543$ $\upsilon = 1$ $p = 0.003$). The similar situation can be seen in groups of anxiety and carriage of alleles 2, 3, 4 and 6. Carriers of alleles 2 and 4 prevailed in the group with moderate anxiety - 15.6% and 72.1%, respectively, whereas, in the group with severe anxiety they were represented - 11.7% and 68.7%, respectively ($\chi 2 = 15.980$ $\upsilon = 12$ $p > 0.05$). Carriers of allele 3 in the group with severe anxiety were found in 7.5%, and with moderate anxiety –3.9%, with severe anxiety found in them 2 times (95% CI 1–3.6) more often than carriers of all other alleles ($\chi 2 = 5240$ $\upsilon = 1$ $p = 0{,}022$), carriers of allele 2 ($\chi 2 = 7122$ $\upsilon = 1$ $p < 0{,}01$) and allele 4 OR = 2 (95% CI 1–3,7); ($\chi 2 = 5.284$ $\upsilon = 1$ $p < 0.05$). Similarly, carriers of the allele 6 in the group with severe anxiety were found in 7.8%, and in the group with moderate anxiety - 4.7%, and the frequency of severe levels of anxiety was higher than in the carriers of all other alleles OR = 1, 7 (95% CI 0.9–3; $\chi 2 = 3.5$ $\upsilon = 1$, $p < 0.05$), carriers of allele 2 ($\chi 2 = 5.499$ $\upsilon = 1$ $p < 0.01$), carriers of allele 4 ($\chi 2 = 3689$ $\upsilon = 1$ $p < 0{,}05$).

| Genotype | Population | | Anxiety | | | | | | Depression | | | | Vital exhaustion | | | | | |
|---|---|---|---|---|---|---|---|---|---|---|---|---|---|---|---|---|---|---|
| | | | Mild | | Moderate | | Severe | | No D | | Depression | | None | | Moderate | | Severe | |
| | n | % | n | % | n | % | n | % | n | % | n | % | n | % | n | % | n | % |
| 2/2 | 26 | 6.1 | 0 | 0 | 18 | 7 | 8 | 4.8 | 19 | 6.4 | 7 | 5.4 | 8 | 6.3 | 17 | 7.7 | 1 | 1.3 |
| 2/3 | 1 | 0.2 | 0 | 0 | 0 | 0 | 1 | 0.6 | 1 | 0.3 | 0 | 0 | 0 | 0 | 1 | 0.5 | 0 | 0 |
| 2/4 | 53 | 12.5 | 0 | 0 | 37 | 14.5 | 16 | 9.6 | 43 | 14.5* | 10 | 7.8 | 20 | 15.6 | 23 | 10.4 | 10 | 13.2 |
| 2/5 | 2 | 0.5 | 0 | 0 | 1 | 0.4 | 1 | 0.6 | 0 | 0 | 2 | 1.6 | 1 | 0.8 | 1 | 0.5 | 0 | 0 |
| 2/6 | 10 | 2.4 | 0 | 0 | 5 | 2 | 5 | 3 | 6 | 2.0 | 4 | 3.1 | 4 | 3.1 | 6 | 2.7 | 0 | 0 |
| 2/7 | 1 | 0.2 | 0 | 0 | 1 | 0.4 | 0 | 0 | 1 | 0.3 | 0 | 0 | 1 | 0.8 | 0 | 0 | 0 | 0 |
| 3/3 | 8 | 1.9 | 0 | 0 | 3 | 1.2 | 5 | 3.0 | 6 | 2.0 | 2 | 1.6 | 1 | 0.8 | 4 | 1.8 | 3 | 3.9 |
| 3/4 | 24 | 5.6 | 0 | 0 | 12 | 4.7 | 12 | 7.2 | 16 | 5.4 | 8 | 6.2 | 8 | 6.3 | 9 | 4.1 | 7 | 9.2 |
| 3/6 | 3 | 0.7 | 1 | 33.3 | 1 | 0.4 | 1 | 0.6 | 1 | 0.3 | 2 | 1.6 | 1 | 0.8 | 1 | 0.5 | 1 | 1.3 |
| 3/7 | 2 | 0.5 | 0 | 0 | 1 | 0.4 | 1 | 0.6 | 2 | 0.7 | 0 | 0 | 0 | 0 | 2 | 0.9 | 0 | 0 |
| 4/4 | 246 | 57.9 | 2 | 66.7 | 153 | 59.8*** | 91 | 54.8 | 179 | 60.5 | 67 | 51.9 | 69 | 53.9 | 133 | 60.2 | 44 | 57.9 |
| 4/5 | 4 | 0.9 | 0 | 0 | 4 | 1.6 | 0 | 0 | 3 | 1.0 | 1 | 0.8 | 1 | 0.8 | 1 | 0.5 | 2 | 2.6 |
| 4/6 | 18 | 4.2 | 0 | 0 | 5 | 2 | 13 | 7.8** | 6 | 2.0 | 12 | 9.3** | 7 | 5.5 | 8 | 3.6 | 3 | 3.9 |
| 4/7 | 9 | 2.1 | 0 | 0 | 5 | 2 | 4 | 2.4 | 5 | 1.7 | 4 | 3.1 | 2 | 1.6 | 6 | 2.7 | 1 | 1.3 |
| 4/8 | 1 | 0.2 | 0 | 0 | 0 | 0 | 1 | 0.6 | 0 | 0 | 1 | 0.8 | 0 | 0 | 0 | 0 | 1 | 1.3 |
| 5/5 | 3 | 0.7 | 0 | 0 | 0 | 0 | 1 | 0.6 | 2 | 0.7 | 1 | 0.8 | 1 | 0.8 | 2 | 0.9 | 0 | 0 |
| 5/6 | 2 | 0.5 | 0 | 0 | 1 | 0.4 | 1 | 0.6 | 1 | 0.3 | 1 | 0.8 | 1 | 0.8 | 0 | 0 | 1 | 1.3 |
| 6/6 | 9 | 2.1 | 0 | 0 | 6 | 2.3 | 3 | 1.8 | 4 | 0.3 | 5 | 3.9 | 3 | 2.3 | 6 | 2.7 | 0 | 0 |
| 7/7 | 3 | 0.7 | 0 | 0 | 2 | 0.8 | 1 | 0.6 | 1 | 1.4 | 2 | 1.6 | 0 | 0 | 1 | 0.5 | 2 | 2.6 |
| | | | $\chi^2 = 69.569$ υ = 36 p = 0.001 | | | | | | $\chi^2 = 32.811$ υ = 18 p = 0.018 | | | | $\chi^2 = 39.186$ υ = 36 p = 0.329 | | | | | |

| Allele | Population | | Anxiety | | | | | | Depression | | | | Vital exhaustion | | | | | |
|---|---|---|---|---|---|---|---|---|---|---|---|---|---|---|---|---|---|---|
| | | | Mild | | Moderate | | Severe | | No D | | Depression | | None | | Moderate | | Severe | |
| | n | % | n | % | n | % | n | % | n | % | n | % | n | % | n | % | n | % |
| 2 | 26 | 6.1 | 0 | 0 | 80 | 15.6 | 39 | 11.7 | 89 | 15 | 30 | 11.6 | 42 | 16.4 | 65 | 14.7 | 12 | 7.9 |
| 3 | 9 | 2.1 | 1 | 16.7 | 20 | 3.9 | 25 | 7.5 | 32 | 5.4 | 14 | 5.4 | 11 | 4.3 | 21 | 4.8 | 14 | 9.2 |
| 4 | 323 | 76.0 | 4 | 66.7 | 369 | 72.1 | 228 | 68.7 | 431 | 72.8 | 170 | 65.9 | 176 | 68.8 | 313 | 70.8 | 112 | 73.7 |
| 5 | 9 | 2.1 | 0 | 0 | 8 | 1.6 | 6 | 1.8 | 8 | 1.4 | 6 | 2.3 | 5 | 2 | 6 | 1.4 | 3 | 2 |
| 6 | 42 | 9.9 | 1 | 16.7 | 24 | 4.7 | 26 | 7.8 | 22 | 3.7 | 29 | 11.2 | 19 | 7.4 | 27 | 6.1 | 5 | 3.3 |
| 7 | 15 | 3.5 | 0 | 0 | 11 | 2.1 | 7 | 2.1 | 10 | 1.7 | 8 | 3.1 | 3 | 1.2 | 10 | 2.3 | 5 | 3.3 |
| 8 | 1 | 0.2 | 0 | 0 | 0 | 0 | 1 | 0.3 | 0 | 0 | 1 | 0.4 | 0 | 0 | 0 | 0 | 1 | 0.7 |
| | | | $\chi^2$ = 15.980 υ = 12 p = 0.192 | | | | | | $\chi^2$ = 24.678 υ = 6 p = 0.00001 | | | | $\chi^2$ = 20.495 υ = 12 p = 0.058 | | | | | |

*$^*p < 0.05$, $^{**}p < 0.01$, $^{***}p < 0.001$.*

**Table 1.**
*Frequencies of VNTR genotypes and alleles of DRD4 gene polymorphism in a population and their association with psychosocial factors.*

The distribution of carriers of VNTR genotypes of DRD4 gene polymorphism by depression level is shown in **Table 1**. Carriers of the DRD4 genotype 4/4 and 2/4 were most frequently found in the group where there was no depression (60.5% and 14.5%, respectively) than in the group with depression (51.9% and 7.8%, respectively) ($\chi 2 = 32.811$ $\upsilon = 18$ $p < 0.05$). In contrast, carriers of the 4/6 genotype were more likely to be found in the group with depression (9.3%) than in the group without depression (2%), and compared with carriers of all other genotypes, OR = 4.9 (95% CI 1.8–13.5); ($\chi 2 = 11.725$ $\upsilon = 1$ $p < 0.001$), carriers of the 2/2 genotype ($\chi 2 = 6.848$ $\upsilon = 1$ $p < 0.01$), 2/4 genotype ($\chi 2 = 14.356$ $\upsilon = 1$ $p < 0.0001$), 3/4 genotype ($\chi 2 = 4582$ $\upsilon = 1$ $p < 0{,}05$) and 4/4 genotype ($\chi 2 = 12{,}436$ $\upsilon = 1$ $p = 0{,}00001$). Carriers of 6/6 homozygous genotype were also more frequently found in the group with depression (3.9%) than without depression (0.3), compared with carriers of the 2/4 genotype (without depression –14.5%, with depression –7, 8%) ($\chi 2 = 5645$ $\upsilon = 1$ $p = 0{,}017$). The similar situation can be seen in the groups with and without depression in the carriage of long and short alleles of the DRD4 gene (**Table 1**). Carriers of allele 2 and 4 are more frequent in the group without depression (15% and 72.8%, respectively) than in the group with depression (11.6% and 65.9%, respectively) ($\chi 2 = 24.678$ $\upsilon = 6$ $p < 0.00001$). Carriers of the long allele 6, on the contrary, are more frequently found in the group with depression (11.2%) than in the group without depression (3.7%), and compared with carriers of all other alleles, OR = 3.2 (95% CI 1 8–5.8); ($\chi 2 = 18.036$ $\upsilon = 1$ $p < 0.0001$), carriers of allele 2 ($\chi 2 = 15.784$ $\upsilon = 1$ $p < 0.0001$), allele 3 ($\chi 2 = 6.845$ $\upsilon = 1$ $p < 0.01$) and allele 4 ($\chi 2 = 18.103$ $\upsilon = 1$ $p < 0.0001$). DRD4 genotype 4/4, the most widely represented in the male population, was most frequently found in the group with a moderate level of vital exhaustion (60.2%). Carriers of the second most common genotype in the population: 2/4 genotype were more often found in the group where there was no vital exhaustion (15.6%). Carriers of the 3/3 and 3/4 genotype were more frequently found in the group with a severe level of vital exhaustion (3.9% and 9.2%, respectively) than in the group with moderate vital exhaustion (1.8% and 4, 1%, respectively). Carriers of the 4/5 and 7/7 genotype are more likely to be found in the group with a severe level of vital exhaustion (2.6%, respectively) than in other groups. Carriers of the 2/6 genotype (3.1%) and 4/6 genotype (5.5%) were more frequently found in the group with no vital exhaustion. Carriers of the 4/7 genotype (2.7%) and 6/6 genotype (2.7%) were most often found in the group with moderate vital exhaustion ($\chi 2 = 39.186$ $\upsilon = 36$ $p > 0.05$). Carriers of the 2/2 genotype were more likely to be found in the group with a moderate level of vital exhaustion (7.7%) than in the group with a severe level of vital exhaustion (1.3%) in comparison with: representatives of all other DRD4 genotypes ($\chi 2 = 4.039$ $\upsilon = 1$ $p < 0.05$), carriers of the 2/4 genotype ($\chi 2 =4.217$ $\upsilon = 1$ $p < 0.05$); 3/3 genotype ($\chi 2 = 5.218$ $\upsilon = 1$ $p < 0.05$); 3/4 genotype ($\chi 2 = 6.868$ $\upsilon = 1$ $p < 0.01$); 3/6 genotype ($\chi 2 = 3951$ $\upsilon = 1$ $p < 0{,}05$); 4/5 genotype ($\chi 2 = 7.843$ $\upsilon = 1$ $p < 0.01$); 7/7 genotype ($\chi 2 = 7.843$ $\upsilon = 1$ $p < 0.01$). Furthermore, carriers of the 2/2 genotype were more frequently found in the group with no vital exhaustion (6.3%) than in the group with severe vital exhaustion, compared with carriers of the DRD4 genotype 3/3 ($\chi 2 = 5306$ $\upsilon = 1$ $p < 0.05$).

The distribution of the other carriers of the DRD4 genotype does not exceed 1.3% (**Table 1**). The different picture can be seen in men with vital exhaustion in the carriage of long and short alleles of the DRD4 gene. Carriers of the DRD4 gene allele 2 are more frequently represented in the male group without vital exhaustion (16.4%) than in the group with a severe level of vital exhaustion (7.9%), moreover, in comparison with: carriers of all other DRD4 gene alleles ($\chi 2 = 6.017$ $\upsilon = 1$ $p < 0.01$); carriers of allele 3 ($\chi 2 = 8.830$ $\upsilon = 1$ $p < 0.01$); carriers of allele 4 ($\chi 2 = 5.466$ $\upsilon = 1$ $p < 0.01$); allele 7 ($\chi 2 = 5680$ $\upsilon = 1$ $p < 0{,}01$). Also, carriers of allele 2 were more often found in the group with a moderate level of vital exhaustion (14.7%) than in the group with a severe level (7.9%) as compared with carriers of all other alleles ($\chi 2 = 4.651$ df = 1 $p = 0.031$); carriers of allele 3 ($\chi 2 = 8.047$ df = 1 $p = 0.005$); allele 4 ($\chi 2 = 4.064$ df = 1 $p = 0.044$). Carriers of the allele 3 are more frequently represented in the group with severe vital exhaustion (9.2%) than in the group where there was no vital exhaustion (4.3%) compared with carriers of all other alleles of the DRD4 gene OR = 2.26 (95% CI 0.9–5.1); ($\chi 2 = 4.003$ $\upsilon = 1$ $p < 0.05$); carriers of the allele 6 OR = 4.83 (95% CI 1.3–17); ($\chi 2 = 6.379$ $\upsilon = 1$ $p < 0.01$). Carriers of the allele 3 were also more often found in the group with moderate vital exhaustion (4.8%) than in the group with severe vital exhaustion (9.2%), compared with the carriers of all other alleles OR = 2 (95% CI1–4.1); ($\chi 2 = 4.056$ $\upsilon = 1$ $p < 0.05$); carriers of the allele 6 OR = 3.6 (95% CI 1.1–11.5); ($\chi 2 = 4.889$ $\upsilon = 1$ $p < 0.05$). Carriers of allele 7 were more frequently found in the group with severe vital exhaustion (3.3%) than in the group where there is no vital exhaustion (1.2%), compared with carriers of allele 6, which are more often represented in the group of men without vital exhaustion (7.4%) ($\chi 2 = 4.848$ $\upsilon = 1$ $p < 0.05$). Carriers of the allele 4 of the DRD4 gene are represented at approximately the same frequency in all groups with and without vital exhaustion (68.8%, 70.8%, and 73.7%, respectively). Carrier of all other alleles of the DRD4 gene does not exceed 2% and is presented in **Table 1**. ($\chi 2 = 20.495$ $\upsilon = 12$ $p < 0.05$).

We determined that the 10/10 homozygous genotype is found more frequently (54.8%), and the heterozygous 9/10 genotype is more rare - 36.6% in the frequency distribution of the VNTR genotypes of DAT gene polymorphism in the population among of men aged 25–64 years. 9/9 genotype was observed in 3.7%. The prevalence of the other genotypes was from 1.7% and lower. The similar situation in the population and in the carriage of alleles is 9–22% and 10–74.2%, which were more common than carriers of all other alleles (**Table 2**).

The distribution of carriers of VNTR genotypes of DAT gene polymorphism by the level of anxiety is presented in **Table 2**. Men, carriers of the 10/10 genotype in the group with moderate anxiety were found in 58.4%, and in the group with a severe level of anxiety - 50.6%, carriers of the heterozygous genotype 9/10 were respectively in the group with the moderate level of anxiety - 35% and in the group with a severe level of anxiety - 38.8% ($\chi 2 = 51.105$ $\upsilon = 16$ $p < 0.0001$). Carriers of the 9/9 genotype were found much more frequently in the group with a severe level of anxiety (6.3%) than in the group with a moderate level of anxiety (1.6%), moreover, in comparison with representatives of all other genotypes, OR = 3.9 (95% CI 1.2–12.9); ($\chi 2 = 6.098$ $\upsilon = 1$ $p < 0.01$), carriers of the 9/10 genotype OR = 3.4 (95% CI 1–11.1); ($\chi 2 = 4.424$ $\upsilon = 1$, $p < 0.05$), and carriers of the 10/10 genotype OR = 4.3 (95% CI 1.3–14.4); ($\chi 2 = 6.863$ $\upsilon = 1$, $p < 0.01$).

The distribution of carriers of VNTR genotypes of DAT gene polymorphism by the level of anxiety is presented in **Table 2**. Men, carriers of the 10/10 genotype in the group with moderate anxiety, were found in 58.4%, and in the group with severe anxiety - 50.6%, carriers of the heterozygous 9/10 genotype were respectively in the group with moderate anxiety - 35% and in the group with severe anxiety - 38.8% ($\chi 2 = 51.105$ $\upsilon = 16$ $p < 0.0001$). Carriers of the 9/9 genotype were found much more frequently in the group with a severe level of anxiety (6.3%) than in the group with a moderate level of anxiety (1.6%), moreover, in comparison with representatives of all other genotypes, OR = 3.9 (95% CI 1.2–12.9); ($\chi 2 = 6.098$ $\upsilon = 1$ $p < 0.01$), carriers of the 9/10 genotype OR = 3.4 (95% CI 1–11.1); ($\chi 2 = 4.424$ $\upsilon = 1$, $p < 0.05$), and carriers of the 10/10 genotype OR = 4.3 (95% CI 1.3–14.4); ($\chi 2 = 6.863$ $\upsilon = 1$, $p < 0.01$).

The distribution of carriers of VNTR genotypes of DAT gene polymorphism by depression level is presented in **Table 2**. Carriers of the 10/10 and 9/10 genotypes were found approximately equally in the group with depression (57.7%, 37.9%, respectively) and in the group without depression (56% and 36.1%, respectively)

| Genotype | Population | | Anxiety | | | | | | Depression | | | | Vital exhaustion | | | | | |
|---|---|---|---|---|---|---|---|---|---|---|---|---|---|---|---|---|---|---|
| | | | Mild | | Moderate | | Severe | | No D | | Depression | | None | | Moderate | | Severe | |
| | n | % | n | % | n | % | n | % | n | % | n | % | n | % | n | % | n | % |
| 8/8 | 4 | 1 | 0 | 0 | 2 | 0.8 | 2 | 1.3 | 4 | 1.4 | 0 | 0 | 2 | 1.6 | 2 | 0.9 | 0 | 0 |
| 9/9 | 15 | 3.7 | 1 | 25* | 4 | 1.6 | 10 | 6.3 | 6 | 2.1 | 9 | 7.8 | 0 | 0 | 5 | 2.3 | 10 | 15.2*** |
| 6/10 | 3 | 0.7 | 1 | 25 | 0 | 0 | 2 | 1.3 | 3 | 1.0 | 0 | 0 | 1 | 0.8 | 1 | 0.5 | 1 | 1.5 |
| 8/10 | 1 | 0.2 | 0 | 0 | 1 | 0.4 | 0 | 0 | 1 | 0.3 | 0 | 0 | 1 | 0.8 | 0 | 0 | 0 | 0 |
| 9/10 | 149 | 36.6 | 2 | 50*** | 85 | 35** | 62 | 38.8* | 105 | 36.1 | 44 | 37.9 | 49 | 38.3 | 79 | 37.1 | 21 | 31.8 |
| 10/10 | 223 | 54.8 | 0 | 0 | 142 | 58.4** | 81 | 50.6 | 163 | 56 | 60 | 51.7 | 73* | 57 | 118 | 55.4 | 32 | 48.5 |
| 10/11 | 4 | 1.0 | 0 | 0 | 3 | 1.2 | 1 | 0.6 | 4 | 1.4 | 0 | 0 | 1 | 0.8 | 3 | 1.4 | 0 | 0 |
| 10/12 | 1 | 0.2 | 0 | 0 | 1 | 0.4 | 0 | 0 | 1 | 0.3 | 0 | 0 | 1 | 0.8 | 0 | 0 | 0 | 0 |
| 11/11 | 7 | 1.7 | 0 | 0 | 5 | 2.1 | 2 | 1.3 | 4 | 1.4 | 3 | 2.6 | 0 | 0 | 5 | 2.3 | 2 | 3.0 |
| | | | $\chi^2 = 51.105$ υ = 16 p = 0.0001 | | | | | | $\chi^2 = 13.549$ υ = 8 p = 0.094 | | | | $\chi^2 = 41.076$ υ = 16 p = 0.001 | | | | | |
| **Allele** | **Population** | | **Anxiety** | | | | | | **Depression** | | | | **Vital exhaustion** | | | | | |
| | | | Mild | | Moderate | | Severe | | No D | | Depression | | None | | Moderate | | Severe | |
| | n | % | n | % | n | % | n | % | n | % | n | % | n | % | n | % | n | % |
| 6 | 3 | 0.4 | 1 | 12.5* | 0 | 0 | 2 | 0.6 | 3 | 0.5 | 0 | 0 | 1 | 0.4 | 1 | 0.2 | 1 | 0.8 |
| 8 | 9 | 1.1 | 0 | 0 | 5 | 1.0 | 4 | 1.3 | 9 | 1.5 | 0 | 0 | 5 | 2 | 4 | 0.9 | 0 | 0 |
| 9 | 179 | 22 | 4 | 50*** | 93 | 19.1** | 82 | 25.6* | 117 | 20.1 | 62 | 26.7 | 49 | 19.1 | 89 | 20.9 | 41 | 31.1** |
| 10 | 604 | 74.2 | 3 | 37.5** | 374 | 77*** | 227 | 70.9 | 440 | 75.6 | 164 | 70.7 | 199 | 77.7 | 319 | 74.9 | 86 | 65.2 |
| 11 | 18 | 2.2 | 0 | 0 | 13 | 2.7 | 5 | 1.6 | 12 | 2.1 | 6 | 2.6 | 1 | 0.4* | 13 | 3.1 | 4 | 3 |
| 12 | 1 | 0.1 | 0 | 0 | 1 | 0.2 | 0 | 0 | 1 | 0.2 | 0 | 0 | 1 | 0.4 | 0 | 0 | 0 | 0 |
| | | | $\chi^2 = 45.402$ υ = 10 p = 0.0001 | | | | | | $\chi^2 = 9.235$ υ = 5 p = 0.1 | | | | $\chi^2 = 19.792$ υ = 10 p = 0.031 | | | | | |

*$^{*}p < 0.05$, $^{**}p < 0.01$, $^{***}p < 0.001$.*

**Table 2.**
*Frequencies of VNTR genotypes and alleles of DAT gene polymorphism in a population and their association with psychosocial factors.*

($\chi 2 = 13.549$ $\upsilon = 8$ $p > 0.05$). Carriers of the 9/9 genotype were more common in the group with depression (7.8%) than in the group without depression (2.1%), moreover, in comparison with representatives of all other genotypes, OR = 3.9 (95% CI 1.3–11.4); ($\chi 2 = 7.583$ $\upsilon = 1$ $p < 0.001$) and carriers of the 10/10 genotype OR = 4 (95% CI 1.3–11.9); ($\chi 2 = 7.477$ $\upsilon = 1$, $p = 0.006$). The ratio of the frequency of alleles 9 and 10 among men in groups with depression and without depression is similar to the distribution of these genotypes ($\chi 2 = 9.235$ $\upsilon = 5$ $p < 0.05$) (**Table 2**). Carriers of allele 9 and allele 10 were found in the group with depression (26.7% and 70.7%, respectively) and in the group without depression (20.1% and 75.6%, respectively). Moreover, carriers of allele 9 were more frequently found in the group with depression than without it, in comparison with carriers of all other alleles OR = 1.4 (95% CI 1–2); ($\chi 2 = 4.390$ $\upsilon = 1$, $p < 0.05$).

The distribution of carriers of VNTR genotypes of DAT gene polymorphism by level of vital exhaustion is presented in **Table 2**. Carriers of the DAT gene 9/10 and 10/10 genotypes were more common in the group where there was no vital exhaustion (38.3% and 57%, respectively); either in a group with a moderate level of vital exhaustion (37.1% and 55.4%, respectively); and in the group with a severe level, they were less common (31.8% and 48.5%, respectively) ($\chi 2 = 41.076$ $\upsilon = 16$ $p < 0.001$). Men, carriers of the DAT gene 9/9 genotype, were significantly more likely to be found in the group with a severe level of vital exhaustion (15.2%) than in the group with a moderate level of vital exhaustion (2.3%) in comparison with carriers of other genotypes OR = 7.4 (95% CI 2.4–22.6); ($\chi 2 = 16.238$ $\upsilon = 1$ $p < 0.0001$), carriers of the 9/10 genotype OR = 7.5 (95% CI 2.3–24.3); ($\chi 2 = 13.815$ $\upsilon = 1$ $p < 0.0001$), carriers of the 10/10 genotype OR = 7.3 (95% CI 2.3–23.11); ($\chi 2 = 14.769$ $df = 1$ $p = 0.0001$). The ratio of the frequencies of alleles 9 and 10 of the DAT gene in men in different groups of vital exhaustion is similar to the distribution of these genotypes ($\chi 2 = 19.792$ $\upsilon = 10$ $p < 0.05$). Carriers of allele 9 were more frequently found in the group with a severe level of vital exhaustion (31.1%) than in the group with a moderate level (20.9%), in comparison with carriers of all alleles of the DAT gene OR = 1.7 (95% CI 1, 1–2.6); ($\chi 2 = 5.831$ $\upsilon = 1$ $p < 0.01$), carriers of the allele 10 OR = 1.7 (95% CI 1.1–2.6); ($\chi 2 = 5.772$ $\upsilon = 1$ $p < 0.01$) and than in the group where there was no vital exhaustion (19.1%) in comparison with carriers of all alleles of the gene DAT OR = 1.9 (95% CI 1.1–3); ($\chi 2 = 6.946$ $\upsilon = 1$ $p < 0.01$), carriers of the 10 allele of the OR gene = 1.9 (95% CI 1.1–3.1); ($\chi 2 = 7.224$ $\upsilon = 1$ $p < 0.01$). In contrast, carriers of the 10 allele of the DAT gene, compared with carriers of all other alleles of the DAT gene, were more likely to have a moderate level of vital exhaustion (74.9%) ($\chi 2 = 4.795$ $\upsilon = 1$ $p < 0.05$) or there was no vital exhaustion (77,7%) ($\chi 2 = 7.072$ $\upsilon = 1$ $p < 0.01$), than a high level of vital exhaustion was observed (62.2%) (**Table 2**).

## 8. Discussion

In this study, we made an attempt to analyze the relationship between the DRD4 and DAT genes, since dopamine is involved in many cognitive and motivational processes; dopaminergic neurons are located in several parts in the midbrain; and dopaminergic axons extend to several regions of the striatum, hippocampus, tonsil, thalamus and cortex, and psychosocial factors, because the coordinated work of mediators and brain modulators underlies the emotional state and behavior of animals and humans [27].

The most frequent VNTR polymorphism of the DRD4 gene in the male population was the 4/4 homozygous genotype (57.9%), which is generally characteristic of Caucasoid populations. In second place we can see carriers of genotypes with short allele 2 of the DRD4 gene from 6 to 12% in frequency of occurrence in our population. This allele is more characteristic of Central Asian populations [28]. The frequency of carriage of longer alleles 6 and higher of the DRD4 gene did not exceed 6% among the participants. In the world the variant with 7 repetitions of DRD4 (20.6%) is more frequently found, and more often we can see this genotype in the US population [28].

In this study, male carriers of the 4/6 genotype of the DRD4 gene were more likely to be found in the group with a severe level of anxiety and depression. We have established a certain trend among men with different levels of vital exhaustion: with an increase in the number of tandem turns of the VNTR of the DRD4 gene polymorphism, the level of vital exhaustion increased. Carriers of the DRD4 allele 6 were more common among men with depression. Severe levels of vital exhaustion were more common among carriers of the allele 7. According to modern concepts of dopamine biosynthesis, it is known to take part in the so-called adaptation process.

Lack of dopamine results in depletion of the nervous system, and its increased level causes bipolar disorders [4, 27]. It has been shown that in people with the long form of the DRD4 gene (the number of repeats is six or more), the affinity of dopamine for the receptor is reduced and the number of receptors is reduced. These individuals are less sensitive to dopamine. So, they need more stimulation than people with a short form of the gene to get the same reaction [29]. Probably this is the reason for the high frequency of occurrence of genotypes with long allele of the DRD4 gene in men with anxiety, depression, and vital exhaustion.

As in the case of the DRD4 gene, VNTR polymorphic variants of the DAT gene can be associated with some pathological conditions in the pathogenesis, which play the main role in dopamine metabolism disorders [30]. In the studied population, the homozygous 10/10 genotype of the DAT gene prevailed - more than 50%, less often the 9/10 genotype was found slightly more than 36%, and finally, the third place was occupied by the 9/9 genotype - 3.7%. The incidence of the other genotypes was below 1.7%. According to literature data, the most represented was the allele with 10 repeats (60% - 93%) in all studied populations. The frequency of the allele with 9 repeats, which is the second most common, varies from 4.2–39%. The other alleles are present in all populations with a frequency of less than 3% [31]. Carriers of VNTR polymorphism of the 9/9 genotype of the DAT gene were more common among men with a severe level of anxiety, depression, and vital exhaustion. Similarly, carriage of allele 9 increased the chance of falling into the groups mentioned above.

Although studies on the association between anxiety, depression, life exhaustion, and VNTR polymorphism in the dopamine transporter gene are not available in the world literature, it may be associated with some pathological conditions in a number of cases; in the pathogenesis of which disorders in the dopaminergic system of the brain play the main role. It is known that individuals having a short version of the DAT gene in the genome, often develop post-traumatic stress disorder [32], which to some extent explains the results.

In summary, we should note that the genetic features found in the open male population may be responsible for the pathophysiological changes in the functioning and compensatory abilities of the dopaminergic system and are a background predisposing to the development of psychological and social risk factors for cardiovascular diseases (arterial hypertension, myocardial infarction, stroke).

## 9. Summary

In the population among men aged 25–64 years, the 4/4 homozygous genotype of the dopamine receptor 4-subtype DRD4 gene (57.9%) is the most represented.

2/2 genotype - 6.1%, 2/4 genotype - 12.5%, and 3/4 genotype - 5.6% are less frequently found; and more rarely - 4/6 genotype (4.2%), 2/6 genotype, 4/7 genotypes and 6/6 genotype were present in equal proportions of 2.1%.The frequency distribution of alleles showed that the 4 allele predominates - 70.7%, the 2 allele was found at 14%, the 6 allele was at 6%. The other alleles make up 0.8% - 5.4%.

We have found that the 10/10 homozygous genotype is more common (54.8%), and the heterozygous 9/10 genotype is more rare (36.6%) with the frequency distribution of the VNTR genotypes of the DAT gene polymorphism. The 9/9 genotype was observed in 3.7%. The prevalence of the other genotypes was from 1.7% and lower. The frequency distribution of alleles showed that the alleles were 9–22%, 10–74.2%, which were more common than carriers of all other alleles. The 4/6 genotype of the DRD4 gene is strongly associated with mild anxiety, depression. The 7 allele of the DRD4 gene is strongly associated with a severe level of vital exhaustion. The 9/9 genotype of the DAT gene is strongly associated with severe anxiety, depression, and vital exhaustion.

## Acknowledgements

The research was carried out under the state assignment within the framework of budget theme No. AAAA-A17-117112850280-2.

## Author details

Valery V. Gafarov[1,2], Elena A. Gromova[1,2]*, Vladimir N. Maksimov[3], Igor V. Gagulin[1,2] and Almira V. Gafarova[1,2]

1 Laboratory of Psychological and Sociological Issues of Internal Diseases, Institute of Internal and Preventive Medicine - Branch of Institute of Cytology and Genetics SB RAS, Novosibirsk, Russia

2 Collaborative Laboratory of Cardiovascular Diseases Epidemiology, Novosibirsk, Russia

3 Laboratory of Molecular Genetic Investigation of Internal Diseases, Institute of Internal and Preventive Medicine - Branch of Institute of Cytology and Genetics SB RAS, Novosibirsk, Russia

*Address all correspondence to: elena.a.gromova@gmail.com

## References


[1] Zohar AH, Zwir I, Wang J, Cloninger CR, Anokhin AP. The development of temperament and character during adolescence: the processes and phases of change. Dev Psychopathol. 2019;31:601-17.

[2] Cloninger CR. A systematic method for clinical description and classification of personality variants: A proposal. Arch. Gen. Psychiatry. 1987; 44: 573-588.

[3] Belkaid M, Krichmar JL. Modeling uncertainty-seeking behavior mediated by cholinergic influence on dopamine. Neural Networks. 2020. V.125, P.10-18 https://doi.org/10.1016/j.neunet.2020.01.032

[4] Silva PA, Trigo S, Marques CI, Cardoso GC, Soares MaC. Experimental evidence for a role of dopamine in avian personality traits. Journal of Experimental Biology. 2020. V. 223, jeb216499. doi:10.1242/jeb.216499

[5] Gelernter J., Kennedy J.L., Van Tol H.H.M.et al. The D4 dopamine receptor (DRD4) maps to distal 11p close to HRAS. Genomics.1992; 13: 208-210.

[6] Lichter J.B., Barr C.L., Kennedy G.L. et al. A hypervariable segment in the human dopamine receptor (DRD4) gene. Hum. Mol. Genet. 1993; 2: 767-773.

[7] Van Tol H.H.M., Bunzow J.R., Guan H.C. et al. Cloning of the gene for a human dopamine D4 receptor with high affinity for the antipsychotic clozapine. Nature, 1991; 350: 610-614.

[8] Chang F.M., Kidd J.R., Livak K.J. et al. The world-wide distribution of allele frecuencies at the human dopamine D4 receptor locus. Hum. Genet. 1996; 98: 91-101.

[9] Bonvicini C, Faraone SV, Scassellati C. *DRD4* 48 bp multiallelic variants as age-population-specific biomarkers in attention-deficit/hyperactivity disorder. Transl Psychiatry. 2020;10: 70.doi: 10.1038/s41398-020-0755-4

[10] Vanderberg D.G., Persico M., Hawkins A.L. et al. Human dopamine transporter gene (DAT1) maps to chromosome 5p15.3 and displays a VNTR. Genomics.1992; 14: 1104-1106.

[11] Gelenter J., Kranzler H.R., Satel S.L. et al.Genetic association between dopamine transporter protein alleles and cocaine-induced paranoia/ J. Gelenter. Neuropsychopharmacology. 1994; 11: 195-200.

[12] Kazantseva AV, Gaysina DA, Malykh SB, Khusnutdinova EK. Role of Dopamine Transporter Gene (DAT1) Polymorphisms in Personality Traits Russian Journal of Genetics, 2009; 45(8):974-980.

[13] Avila G, Picazo O, Chuc-Meza E, García-Ramirez M Reduction of dopaminergic transmission in the globus pallidus increases anxiety-like behavior without altering motor activity. Behavioural Brain Research. 2020; 386:112589 https://doi.org/10.1016/j.bbr.2020.112589

[14] Gururajan A, Cryan J, Dinan TG.Chapter 26 - Molecular biomarkers in depression: Toward personalized psychiatric treatment. Personalized Psychiatry 2020; 319-338https://doi.org/10.1016/B978-0-12-813176-3.00026-2

[15] López León S., Sayed-Tabatabaei F.A., Croes E.A. et al. The dopamine D4 receptor gene 48-base-pair-repeat polymorphism and mood disorders: a

meta-analysis. *Biol. Psychiatry.* 2005; 57: 999-1003.

[16] Szekely A, Balota D. A. , Duchek J. M., Nemoda Z. , Vereczkei A., Sasvari-Szekely M.Genetic factors of reaction time performance: DRD4 7-repeat allele associated with slower responses. Genes, Brain and Behavior. 2011; 10 (2):129-136 https://doi.org/10.1111/j.1601-183X.2010.00645.x

[17] Douma EH, Kloet ER. Stress-induced plasticity and functioning of ventral tegmental dopamine neurons Neuroscience & Biobehavioral Reviews. 2020; 108: 48-77 https://doi.org/10.1016/j.neubiorev.2019.10.015

[18] Sharma H, Santra S, Dutta A. Triple reuptake inhibitors as potential next-generation antidepressants: a new hope? Future Med Chem. 2015; 7(17): 2385-2405. doi: 10.4155/fmc.15.134

[19] MONICA Monograph and Multimedia Sourcebook. Helsinki. 2003; 237 p.

[20] Spielberger, C. D. (2012, February). State-trait anxiety inventory for adults.. Retrieved from http://www.mindgarden.com/products/staisad.htm.

[21] Cantor CR, Smith CL, Mattew MK. Pulsed-field gel electrophoresis of very large DNA molecules. Annu Rev Biophys Biophys Chem. 1988;17:287-304. doi: 10.1146/annurev.bb.17.060188.001443.

[22] Maniatis T, Fritsch EF. and Sambrook J. Molecular Cloning: A Laboratory Manual, X + 545 S., 61 Abb., 28 Tab. Cold Spring Harbor, N. Y. 1982. Cold Spring Harbor Laboratory. Journal of Basic Microbiology. 1984; V 24(1):32-32 https://doi.org/10.1002/jobm.19840240107.

[23] Nanko S., Hattori M., Ikeda K. et al. Dopamone D4 receptor polymorphism and schizophrenia // Lancet. 1993. V. 341. P. 689-690.

[24] Mitchell R.J., Howlett S., Earl L. et al. Distribution of the 3' VNTR polymorphism in the human dopamine transporter gene in world populations // Human Biology. 2000. V. 72. No. 2. P. 295-304.

[25] Buhl A, Zofel P SPSS: The art of information processing. Analysis of statistical data and recovery of hidden patterns. SPb.:JSC «DiaSoft».2015; p.608.

[26] Pandis N. The chi-square test. Am J Orthod Dentofacial Orthop. 2016;150(5):898-899. doi: 10.1016/j.ajodo.2016.08.009.

[27] De Young CG. The neuromodulator of exploration: A unifying theory of the role of dopaminein personality. Frontiers in Human Neuroscience.2013; 7(762): 1-26

[28] Korsten P., Korsten J.C., Mueller P., Hermannstädter C.et al. Association between DRD4 gene polymorphism and personality variation in great tits: a test across four wild populations. Mol Ecol. 2010; 19: 832-843.

[29] Matthews L.J., Butler P.M. Novelty-seeking DRD4 polymorphisms are associated with human migration distance out-of-Africa after controlling for neutral population gene structure. Am J Phys Anthropol. 2011; 145: 382-389.

[30] Maul S, Giegling I, Fabbri C, Corponi F, Serretti A, Rujescu D. Genetics of Resilience: Implications From Genome-Wide Association Studies and Candidate Genes of the Stress Response System in Posttraumatic Stress Disorder and Depression Am J Med Genet B Neuropsychiatr Genet. 2020 Mar;183(2):77-94. doi: 10.1002/ajmg.b.32763.

[31] Salatino-Oliveira A, Rohde LA., Hutz MH. The dopamine transporter role in psychiatric phenotypes Am J Med Genet. 2018; 177B:211-231

[32] Drury SS., Brett ZH., Henry C, Scheeringa M. The Association of a Novel Haplotype in the Dopamine Transporter with Preschool Age Posttraumatic Stress DisorderJournal of Child and Adolescent Psychopharmacology 2013. Vol. 23, No. 4https://doi.org/10.1089/cap.2012.0072